FIRST AID

Q&A
for the
NBDE
PART I

DEREK M. STEINBACHER, MD, DMD

University of Pennsylvania School of Dental Medicine
Class of 2001

Harvard Medical School
Class of 2004

Fellow, Plastic and Reconstructive Surgery
Johns Hopkins Hospital
Baltimore, Maryland

STEVEN R. SIERAKOWSKI, DMD, MDSc

University of Pennsylvania School of Dental Medicine
Class of 2001

Diplomate, American Board of Periodontology
Private Practice
Philadelphia, Pennsylvania

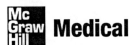 **Medical**

New York / Chicago / San Francisco / Lisbon / London / Madrid / Mexico City

Milan / New Delhi / San Juan / Seoul / Singapore / Sydney / Toronto

First Aid™ Q&A for the NBDE Part I

1 2 3 4 5 6 7 8 9 0   QPD/QPD   12 11 10 9 8

ISBN 978-0-07-150866-7
MHID 0-07-150866-X
ISSN 1932-5207

This book was set in Electra LH by International Typesetting and Composition.
The editors were Catherine A. Johnson and Peter J. Boyle.
The production supervisor was Sherri Souffrance.
Project management was provided by Gita Raman, International Typesetting and Composition.
Quebecor Dubuque was printer and binder.

This book is printed on acid-free paper.

To the contributors who dedicated their time, energy, and insight into the creation of this book,

and

To our families and loved ones who supported us through this endeavor.

Derek M. Steinbacher, MD, DMD
Steven R. Sierakowski, DMD, MDSc

CONTENTS

CONTRIBUTORS

Karl C. Bruckman, DDS
Class of 2008
College of Dental Medicine
Columbia University
New York, New York

Resident
Department of Oral and Maxillofacial Surgery
Jefferson Medical College
Thomas Jefferson University
Philadelphia, Pennsylvania

Derek J. Conover, DMD
Class of 2008
University of Pennsylvania
School of Dental Medicine
Philadelphia, Pennsylvania

Blaine A. Keister, DMD
Class of 2008
University of Pennsylvania
School of Dental Medicine
Philadelphia, Pennsylvania

First Aid Q&A for the NBDE Part I serves as the ideal companion manual for the *First Aid for the NBDE Part I,* Second Edition. Included are 800 questions simulating actual NBDE examination items. These are divided equally among the four sections included on the test: Anatomic Sciences, Biochemistry and Physiology, Microbiology and Pathology, and Dental Anatomy and Occlusion. Following each block of questions are concise answer explanations. Best of luck as you venture through the first standardized exam in dental school.

ACKNOWLEDGMENTS

We appreciate all authors and medical and dental students who have contributed to this work in both practice and concept. Special thanks to Karl Bruckman, DDS for exhibiting incredible diligence, reliability, and productivity.

Thanks to our publisher, McGraw-Hill, for recognizing the need for this book and for the assistance of their staff. Thanks to Catherine Johnson, our editor, for her continued support and guidance.

HOW TO CONTRIBUTE

We welcome your comments, suggestions, ideas, corrections, or other submissions to help with this and future editions of *First Aid Q&A for the NBDE Part I*. What information can you contribute?

- Critiques related to the content or questions contained herein
- Additional example questions
- Test-taking tips and study strategies for the exam
- Suggestions for mnemonics, diagrams, figures, and tables

If you wish to contribute, e-mail your entries or suggestions to the following address:

nbde_firstaid@yahoo.com

Please include your name, address, e-mail address, and school affiliation.

NOTE TO CONTRIBUTORS

All contributions become property of the authors and are subject to editorial manipulation. In the event that similar or duplicate entries are received, only the first entry received will be used. Please include a reference to a standard textbook to verify the factual data.

Anatomic Sciences

Questions 1-3 pertain to the following clinical vignette:

A 23-year-old female presents to the emergency department following a head-first collision with a teammate during a lacrosse match. The patient was stabilized, and vital signs were assessed. EMT on site mentioned that the contact caused lateral overextension of the neck as well as trauma to the shoulder area.

1. Damage to the lateral and medial cords of the brachial plexus would result in altered motor movements to each of the following muscles EXCEPT

   A. interosseus muscles.
   B. thenar muscles.
   C. extensor carpi ulnaris.
   D. flexor carpi ulnaris.
   E. flexor carpi radialis.

2. Traumatic dislocation of the clavicle at the sternoclavicular joint, in a posterior direction, can cause compromise to all of the following structures EXCEPT

   A. subclavian artery.
   B. brachial plexus.
   C. trachea.
   D. subclavian vein.
   E. all of the above.

3. The cervical plexus can also be damaged with injury to the cervical spine. Motor innervation to each of the following muscles would be affected by damage to the cervical plexus EXCEPT

   A. sternohyoid.
   B. stylohyoid.
   C. omohyoid.
   D. sternothyroid.
   E. none of the above.

Questions 4-8 pertain to the following clinical vignette:

A 42-year-old male presents to your office complaining of weakness on one side of his face, as well as intense headaches that have persisted. The patient is worked up, and sent for imaging, which reveals a lesion located in the petrous temporal bone.

4. Suppose a lesion compromises the lower motor neuron of CN VII, occurring proximal to the greater petrosal nerve and chorda tympani. All of the following clinical signs will be shown EXCEPT

   A. ipsilateral weakness to musculature of facial expression.
   B. diminished taste sensation to the posterior 1/3 of the tongue.
   C. ipsilateral dryness of eye due to lost function of lacrimal gland.
   D. compromised function of sublingual and submandibular glands.
   E. hyperacusis in ipsilateral ear.

5. A lesion to the upper motor neuron of CN VII would cause which of the following?

   A. Partial facial muscle paralysis on the ipsilateral side of the lesion to the lower face only
   B. Total facial muscle paralysis on the ipsilateral side of the lesion to the upper and lower face
   C. Partial facial muscle paralysis on the contralateral side of the lesion to the lower face only
   D. Total facial muscle paralysis of the contralateral side of the lesion to the upper and lower face

6. Which branchial arch has its derivatives innervated by CN VII?

   A. I
   B. II
   C. III
   D. IV

7. The common facial vein receives drainage from each of the following veins EXCEPT

   A. maxillary vein.
   B. anterior retromandibular vein.

C. retromandibular vein.

D. anterior facial vein.

E. internal jugular vein.

8. All of the following statements regarding blood and associated vasculature is true EXCEPT

A. approximately 45% of the blood is composed of formed elements/cellular material.

B. blood plasma lacking fibrinogen and clotting factors is considered serum.

C. the tunica adventitia of blood vessel walls is the most internal layer, endothelial in nature, and is composed of simple squamous epithelium.

D. sinusoids are fenestrated capillaries which allow the passage of phagocytic cells.

E. individuals with type O blood contain erythrocytes which lack A and B antigens, and are, thus, considered universal donors.

Questions 9-12 pertain to the following clinical vignette:

A 29-year-old female presents to the ED status post blunt trauma to the back of the head. The patient complains of severe head pain, and is sent for imaging. MRI shows bleeding within the cranium, and CT shows fractures of the skull.

9. Which of the following vessels is involved in an epidural hematoma?

A. Anterior communicating artery

B. Posterior cerebral artery

C. Anterior cerebral artery

D. Posterior communicating artery

E. Middle meningeal artery

10. All of the following structures are located within the posterior cranial fossa EXCEPT

A. occipital lobes.

B. jugular foramen.

C. cerebellum.

D. hypoglossal canal.

E. optic foramen.

11. Which of the following cranial nuclei of the thalamus are involved with mediating facial sensation and pain?

A. Ventral posterior medial nuclei (VPM)

B. Ventral anterior nucleus

C. Lateral geniculate nucleus

D. Ventral posterior lateral nuclei (VPL)

E. Ventral lateral nucleus

12. All of the following are brainstem nuclei involved with cranial nerve function EXCEPT

A. superior salivatory nucleus.

B. nucleus ambiguus.

C. nucleus of the solitary tract.

D. ventromedial nucleus.

E. inferior salivatory nucleus.

Questions 13 and 14 pertain to the following clinical vignette:

A 65-year-old male under your care is experiencing crushing chest pain. He is mentioning that the pain is radiating outward to his left shoulder, and that shortness of breath is also affecting him. After proper care is administered, it was later determined that the patient had experienced a myocardial infarct.

13. The tricuspid valve can be auscultated at which of the following anatomic locations?

A. Level of the 5th intercostal space, at the midclavicular line

B. Level of the 2nd intercostal space, at the right sternal border

C. Level of the 2nd intercostal space, at the left sternal border

D. Level of the 5th intercostal space, left of the sternal border

E. None of the above

14. Occlusion of which of the following arteries would most directly cause ischemia in the lateral wall of the left ventricle?

A. Left circumflex

B. Right coronary

C. Left anterior descending

D. Acute marginal

E. Posterior descending

15. Which of the following areas of the mediastinum contains the vagus nerve?

    A. Superior
    B. Posterior
    C. Anterior
    D. Middle
    E. None of the above

16. Regarding the fetal circulation, oxygenated blood bypasses the pulmonary circulation by way of which communication?

    A. Left atrium to left ventricle
    B. Left atrium to right atrium
    C. Right atrium to right ventricle
    D. Right atrium to left atrium
    E. Left atrium to left ventricle

17. Which of the following structures of the adult heart is a remnant of the foramen ovale in the fetal heart?

    A. Crista terminalis
    B. Fossa ovalis
    C. Sulcus terminalis
    D. Right auricle
    E. Atrial appendage

18. Regarding the fetal circulation, which of the following vasculature serves as a conduit between the aorta and pulmonary artery?

    A. Ductus venosus
    B. Umbilical arteries
    C. Ductus arteriosus
    D. Portal vein
    E. Umbilical vein

19. Which of the following germ layer derivatives comprise the epithelial lining of the cardiovascular system?

    A. Mesoderm
    B. Endoderm
    C. Ectoderm
    D. All of the above
    E. None of the above

20. Which TWO of the following embryonic structures combine to form the superior vena cava?

    1. Bulbus cordis
    2. Right common cardinal vein
    3. Truncus arteriosus
    4. Right anterior cardinal vein
    5. Right horn of sinus venosus

    A. 1 and 2
    B. 2 and 3
    C. 4 and 5
    D. 2 and 4
    E. None of the above

21. Which TWO of the following embryonic structures cause an atrial septal defect if they fail to completely fuse?

    1. Ostium secundum
    2. Ostium primum
    3. Septum primum
    4. Septum secundum
    5. Septum spurium

    A. 1 and 2
    B. 2 and 3
    C. 2 and 4
    D. 3 and 4
    E. 3 and 5

22. Which of the following is a derivative of the 4th aortic arch?

    A. Hyoid artery
    B. Stapedial artery
    C. Right subclavian artery
    D. Common carotid artery
    E. Pulmonary arteries

23. All of the following structures form the boundary known as the femoral triangle EXCEPT

    A. sartorius muscle.
    B. inguinal ligament.
    C. adductor longus muscle.
    D. cremaster muscle.
    E. pectineus muscle.

24. Which of the following statements regarding musculature of the abdomen is FALSE?

A. The external oblique muscle contracts to increase abdominal pressure.
B. The internal oblique muscle is innervated by the lower intercostal, iliohypogastric, and ilioinguinal nerves.
C. The external oblique muscle is innervated only by the lower intercostal nerves.
D. The transverse muscle contracts to flex the vertebral column.
E. The rectus abdominis muscle originates at the pubic symphysis and inserts into the xiphoid process, as well as costal cartilages 5-7.

25. Regarding connective tissue attachments, which of the following statements is TRUE?

A. Tendons form attachments between bone and bone.
B. Aponeuroses are merely sheetlike layers of tendon.
C. Nearly all connective tissue is of neural crest origin, with head and neck regions of connective tissue being of mesodermal origin.
D. Ligaments form attachments between muscle and bone.
E. None of the above are correct.

26. Which of the following statements regarding the thoracic region is FALSE?

A. The neurovascular bundles of the intercostal spaces run along the costal groove at the superior surface of each rib.
B. Musculature of respiration includes the intercostal muscles, diaphragm, and accessory muscles.
C. The costal groove of each rib protects the nerve (of the neurovascular bundle) the least when injury occurs.
D. The rib cage contains 12 ribs: ribs I-VI are true, VII-X are false, and XI-XII are floating.
E. Fracture of the left 10th and 11th ribs can cause injury to the spleen.

27. All of the following questions pertaining to the diaphragm are correct EXCEPT

A. blood supply to the diaphragm is via the musculophrenic artery.
B. the aorta passes through two crura when passing through the aortic opening.
C. the caval opening allows passage of the superior vena cava.
D. during the act of inspiration, the diaphragm contracts, thus, flattening out and creating a negative intrathoracic pressure.
E. innervation to the diaphragm is via the phrenic nerve (C3, C4, C5).

28. Relative to the thymus, which of the following statements is FALSE?

A. Growth continues and peaks at puberty, and then atrophies and is replaced by adipose tissue.
B. Lymphatic circulation returns via afferent vessels so that lymph may be filtered.
C. It is the site of T-cell maturation.
D. Thymic corpuscles/epithelioreticular cells are contained within the inner medulla.
E. The outer cortex holds the largest concentration of lymphocytes.

29. Which of the following statements is TRUE regarding vision and optic nerve fibers?

A. Left medial/nasal fibers decussate and cross over at the optic chiasm en route to the right primary visual cortex of the occipital lobe.
B. Left medial/nasal fibers decussate and stay ipsilateral at the optic chiasma en route to the left primary visual cortex of the occipital lobe.
C. Left lateral/temporal fibers decussate and cross over at the optic chiasma en route to the right primary visual cortex of the temporal lobe.
D. Right lateral/temporal fibers decussate and stay ipsilateral at the optic chiasma en route to the right primary visual cortex of the temporal lobe.

30. Which of the following extraocular muscles is innervated by abducens nerve?

    A. Superior oblique muscle
    B. Medial rectus muscle
    C. Inferior rectus muscle
    D. Lateral rectus muscle
    E. Superior rectus muscle

31. Regarding the pupillary light reflex, which of the following is TRUE?

    A. When shining light onto the left eye, the direct response elicits ipsilateral afferent firing via CN III and subsequent ipsilateral efferent firing via CN III to left eye.
    B. When shining light onto the left eye, the consensual response elicits ipsilateral afferent firing via CN II and subsequent contralateral efferent firing via CN III to right eye.
    C. When shining light onto the left eye, the consensual response elicits ipsilateral afferent firing via CN III and subsequent contralateral efferent firing via CN III to right eye.
    D. When shining light onto the right eye, the direct response elicits contralateral afferent firing via CN II and subsequent contralateral efferent firing via CN III to left eye.

32. In order to test for patency of the trochlear nerve, one would shine a light source directed at the pupil, and have patient follow it in what direction?

    A. Superiorly
    B. Superiorly and medially
    C. Inferiorly
    D. Laterally
    E. Inferiorly and laterally

33. Which of the following lesions involving vision occurring in patients with syphilis and diabetes allows the eye to accommodate but causes a loss of miosis function?

    A. Internuclear ophthalmoplegia
    B. Ophthalmoplegia

    C. Marcus-Gunn/relative afferent pupil
    D. Argyll Robertson/pupillary light-near dissociation pupil
    E. Horner syndrome

34. All of the following blood vessels comprise the circle of Willis EXCEPT

    A. middle cerebral artery.
    B. posterior cerebral artery.
    C. internal carotid artery.
    D. posterior communicating artery.
    E. anterior communicating artery.

35. Which of the following small, thin-walled vessels can rupture and, thus, are commonly involved in stroke?

    A. Left anterior cerebral
    B. Right posterior cerebral
    C. Lenticulostriate
    D. Left vertebral
    E. Left internal carotid

36. If damaged, all of the following bony structures would directly alter movement of the tongue EXCEPT

    A. genial tubercles.
    B. hamulus.
    C. hyoid bone.
    D. styloid process.
    E. none of the above.

37. Which of the following portions of the lung contain the lingula?

    A. Middle lobe of right lung
    B. Superior lobe of right lung
    C. Superior lobe of left lung
    D. Inferior lobe of left lung
    E. Inferior lobe of right lung

38. Which of the following wraps around the ligamentum arteriosum?

    A. Right recurrent laryngeal nerve
    B. Left brachiocephalic vein
    C. Right subclavian vein
    D. Superior laryngeal nerve
    E. Left recurrent laryngeal nerve

39. Each of the following statements concerning the foramen magnum are true EXCEPT

    A. it is located in the occipital bone.
    B. it allows passage of the medulla oblongata/spinal cord.
    C. it allows passage of the spinal accessory nerve.
    D. it is located in the parietal bone.
    E. it allows passage of the vertebral arteries.

40. The articulating surface of the mandibular condyle is covered with

    A. dense fibrocartilage.
    B. loose connective tissue.
    C. elastic cartilage.
    D. hyaline cartilage.
    E. none of the above.

41. The articulating disc of the temporomandibular joint attaches to the condyle via

    A. stylomandibular ligament.
    B. collateral ligaments.
    C. temporomandibular ligament.
    D. sphenomandibular ligament.
    E. none of the above.

42. Which of the following directions does the articulating disc of the temporomandibular joint most often displace?

    A. Anteromedially
    B. Laterally
    C. Inferiorly
    D. Superiorly
    E. Posteromedially

43. The pituitary gland is seated superiorly on which sinus?

    A. Frontal
    B. Maxillary
    C. Anterior ethmoid
    D. Posterior ethmoid
    E. Sphenoid

Questions 44-46 pertain to the following clinical vignette:

A 22-year-old male presents to your office for routine extraction of a malposed tooth No. 17. The dentist decides to attempt extraction of the tooth with a mandibular cowhorn forceps. The tooth is extracted without immediate complication.

44. If the patient is complaining of altered taste sensation to the anterior 2/3 of the tongue, as well as generalized paresthesia to the left lateral tongue, which of the following structures may have been compromised by the extraction?

    A. Buccal nerve
    B. Lingual nerve
    C. Middle superior alveolar nerve
    D. Hypoglossal nerve
    E. Inferior alveolar nerve

45. Prior to the extraction, if an infection had formed at the root apices of tooth No. 17, which fascial plane would the infection most likely travel within?

    A. Sublingual
    B. Parapharyngeal
    C. Masticator
    D. Submandibular
    E. Parotid

46. Emergency management of a patient with airway obstruction/compromise may involve a cricothyrotomy. During this procedure, an airway is established by incising between the

    A. hyoid bone and thyroid cartilage.
    B. cartilaginous rings of trachea.
    C. thyroid cartilage and cricoid cartilage.
    D. thyroid gland.
    E. left 3rd and 4th intercostal muscles, laterally.

47. When performing an inferior alveolar nerve block, the needle is accidentally directed too far posteriorly. Which of the following structures will be penetrated?

    A. Buccinator
    B. Lateral pterygoid
    C. Medial pterygoid
    D. Mylohyoid
    E. Parotid gland

48. Which of the following structures converge to form the pterygomandibular raphe?

    A. Superior pharyngeal constrictor and mylohyoid
    B. Medial pterygoid and mylohyoid
    C. Buccinator and superior pharyngeal constrictor
    D. Buccinator and mylohyoid
    E. Medial pterygoid and superior pharyngeal constrictor

Questions 49-53 pertain to the following clinical vignette:

A 55-year-old female presents to your office for deep scaling and root planing as part of treatment for periodontitis.

49. Due to large pocket depths surrounding the mandibular right molars, anesthesia of this quadrant is necessary to adequately scale and plane the roots. In order to locate area where anesthesia is distributed for inferior alveolar nerve block, you palpate which structure?

    A. Lingula
    B. Coronoid notch
    C. Antilingula
    D. Angle of the mandible
    E. External oblique ridge of the mandible

50. As is the case with periodontal disease, periodontal attachment loss is evident. Which of the following principal collagen fibers of the PDL course at right angles from the cementum to adjacent alveolar bone?

    A. Horizontal
    B. Apical
    C. Interradicular
    D. Transseptal
    E. Oblique

51. Principal collagen fibers of the PDL are comprised of which of the following type(s) of collagen?

    A. Type I only
    B. Type II only
    C. Type III only
    D. Type I and III
    E. Type II and III

52. Which of the following is the most abundant cell of a healthy periodontal ligament?

    A. Lymphocytes
    B. Neutrophils
    C. Osteoblasts
    D. Cementoblasts
    E. Fibroblasts

53. All of the following vessels contribute to Kisselbach plexus EXCEPT

    A. lesser palatine artery.
    B. sphenopalatine artery.
    C. lateral nasal branches of facial artery.
    D. superior labial artery.
    E. anterior ethmoid arteries of internal carotid artery.

Questions 54-58 pertain to the following clinical vignette:

A 26-year-old male presents to the emergency department following a bar fight. He mentions that he was punched in the area of his right eye, and is complaining of a headache. You note periorbital edema of his right eye, as well as complaints of pain when palpating right midfacial region inferolateral to his right eye (which also seems slightly depressed).

54. Each of the following bones are part of the orbit EXCEPT

    A. frontal.
    B. zygoma.
    C. ethmoid.
    D. lacrimal.
    E. temporal.

55. Which of the following arteries is the MAJOR blood supply to the orbit and eye?

    A. Facial
    B. Ophthalmic
    C. Maxillary
    D. Transverse facial
    E. Infraorbital

56. Which of the following muscles has its origin on the zygomatic process of maxilla (superficially) and zygomatic arch (deep)?

A. Lateral pterygoid
B. Temporalis
C. Buccinator
D. Masseter
E. Medial pterygoid

57. The superior orbital fissure is located between which of the following bones?

   A. Lesser wing of sphenoid and frontal.
   B. Ethmoid and maxilla.
   C. Greater wing of sphenoid and maxilla.
   D. Greater wing of sphenoid and lesser wing of sphenoid.
   E. Lesser wing of sphenoid and ethmoid.

58. All of the following are TRUE regarding the nasolacrimal apparatus EXCEPT

   A. the nasolacrimal duct empties into the superior meatus.
   B. relative to the orbit, the nasolacrimal apparatus is located superolaterally.
   C. tears wash across the globe in a superolateral → inferomedial direction.
   D. the lacrimal puncta collects tears and then drains directly into the lacrimal canals.
   E. the lacrimal sac drains directly into the nasolacrimal duct.

59. Each of the following is TRUE regarding the lacrimal gland EXCEPT

   A. it receives postganglionic parasympathetic fibers via the lacrimal nerve.
   B. preganglionic fibers synapse at the pterygopalatine ganglion.
   C. preganglionic fibers to the lacrimal gland are carried via greater petrosal nerve.
   D. the lacrimal gland is mucous secreting.
   E. the superior salivatory nucleus sends preganglionic fibers to the lacrimal gland.

60. The platysma is innervated by which of the following nerves?

   A. Trigeminal
   B. Facial
   C. Glossopharyngeal
   D. Spinal accessory
   E. Vagus

61. Which layer of fascia contains lymphatic vessels within the neck?

   A. Pretracheal
   B. Prevertebral
   C. Subcutaneous
   D. Investing
   E. None of the above

62. Which of the following ligaments connects the liver to the anterior abdominal wall?

   A. Falciform
   B. Gastrocolic
   C. Hepatoduodenal
   D. Gastroduodenal
   E. Gastrohepatic

63. Which of the following describes the teniae coli of the digestive tract?

   A. Fatty globules on the serosal surface of the colon
   B. Lymphoid tissue of the cecum
   C. Formed pouches within the colon
   D. Villous-like projections involved with absorption
   E. Smooth muscle bands of the colon

64. Coordination of muscle movement, as well as maintenance of equilibrium and posture, are controlled by which structure of the brain?

   A. Medulla
   B. Pons
   C. Cerebrum
   D. Thalamus
   E. Cerebellum

65. Which of the following types of cartilage has the ability to calcify?

   A. Fibrocartilage
   B. Hyaline
   C. Elastic
   D. Elastic and hyaline
   E. Hyaline and fibrocartilage

66. The one-cell thick layer of osteoprogenitor cells on the inner surface of bone is

    A. endosteum.
    B. haversian canal.
    C. Volkmann canal.
    D. lacuna.
    E. periosteum.

67. Which of the following is a type of syndesmosis?

    A. Tooth in socket.
    B. Cranial sutures.
    C. Temporomandibular joint.
    D. Epiphyseal plate of long bones.
    E. Connection between radius and ulna.

68. All of the following statements regarding the blood are true EXCEPT

    A. the majority of blood is plasma, which makes up 55% of the total.
    B. albumin regulates the vascular oncotic pressure.
    C. hematocrit measures the portion of proteins in a blood sample.
    D. blood comprises 8% of the total body weight.
    E. plasma is made up of 80% water.

69. Which of the following is a granulocyte?

    A. T cell.
    B. Macrophage.
    C. Platelet.
    D. Neutrophil.
    E. B cell.

70. Each of the following zones of the adrenal gland is of mesodermal origin EXCEPT

    A. zona fasciculate.
    B. chromaffin cells.
    C. zona glomerulosa.
    D. zona reticularis.
    E. none of the above.

71. Which of the following pharyngeal muscles shortens the velum?

    A. Muscularis uvula
    B. Palatopharyngeus
    C. Palatoglossal

D. Levator veli palatini
E. Tensor veli palatine

72. Which of the following nuclei is the primary controller of swallowing?

    A. Superior salivatory
    B. Nucleus ambiguus
    C. Inferior salivatory
    D. Facial nucleus
    E. Nucleus of the solitary tract

73. The pharyngeal plexus is comprised of which of the following combination of nerves?

    A. CN V, IX, X
    B. CN IX, X, XII
    C. CN IX, X, XI
    D. CN V, VII, IX
    E. CN V, IX, X

74. Which of the following nerves innervates the stapedius muscle of the middle ear?

    A. CN V-1
    B. CN V-2
    C. CN VII
    D. CN V-3
    E. CN VIII

75. Relative to the oral cavity, which of the layers of mucosa interdigitates with rete pegs?

    A. Stratum granulosum
    B. Papillary layer of lamina propria
    C. Stratum corneum
    D. Reticular layer of lamina propria
    E. Stratum spinosum

76. The formative cells of the enamel structure of teeth arise from the

    A. inner enamel epithelium.
    B. dental follicle.
    C. dental papilla.
    D. dental follicle and papilla.
    E. inner enamel epithelium and dental papilla.

77. When do ameloblasts begin to secrete enamel matrix?

A. During the cap stage
B. After the odontoblasts form dentin
C. Before the odontoblasts form dentin
D. After root formation begins
E. Before cap stage

78. In the growing fetus, which specific structure separates the external lips and cheeks from the internal jaw structures?

A. Tuberculum impar
B. Buccopharyngeal membrane
C. Vestibular lamina
D. Hypobranchial eminence
E. Lateral lingual swellings

79. The cribriform plate is located within which bone?

A. Sphenoid
B. Ethmoid
C. Frontal
D. Maxilla
E. Vomer

80. Suppose one would necessitate anesthesia of the anterior palatal mucosa. Which of the following nerves innervates this area?

A. Nasopalatine
B. Middle superior alveolar
C. Posterior superior alveolar
D. Maxillary
E. Lesser palatine

81. Which of the following articulations of the cervical vertebrae do NOT contain an intervertebral disk?

A. C4 and C5
B. C5 and C6
C. C2 and C3
D. C1 and C2
E. None of the above

82. The spinal accessory nerve is composed of motor rootlets from which of the following nerves?

A. C1-C5
B. C3-C5
C. C6
D. C1-C3 only
E. C1 and C2 only

83. Each of the following arteries is a branch of the subclavian artery EXCEPT

A. right carotid.
B. thyrocervical.
C. suprascapular.
D. transverse cervical.
E. vertebral.

84. The external jugular vein is formed by which two veins?

A. Anterior retromandibular and anterior facial
B. Maxillary vein and anterior facial
C. Posterior retromandibular and anterior retromandibular
D. Posterior auricular and posterior retromandibular
E. Common facial and posterior retromandibular

85. The stylomandibular ligament has its origin at which of the following bones?

A. Temporal
B. Sphenoid
C. Occipital
D. Maxilla
E. Parietal

86. Each of the following bones is unpaired EXCEPT

A. occipital.
B. sphenoid.
C. ethmoid.
D. frontal.
E. none of the above.

87. Which of the following is TRUE regarding the attachment of the mylohyoid muscle?

    A. It attaches superiorly at the lateral border of the mandible and inferiorly at the body of the hyoid.
    B. It attaches superiorly at the medial border of the mandible and inferiorly at the lesser horn of the hyoid.
    C. It attaches superiorly at the medial border of the mandible and inferiorly at the greater horn of the hyoid.
    D. It attaches superiorly at the medial border of the mandible and inferiorly at the body of the hyoid.
    E. It attaches superiorly at the lateral border of the mandible and inferiorly at the body of the hyoid.

88. Which of the following nerves innervates the anterior belly of the digastric muscle?

    A. Inferior alveolar nerve
    B. Mental nerve
    C. Mylohyoid nerve
    D. Auriculotemporal nerve
    E. Facial nerve

89. The infrahyoid musculature of the neck receives motor innervation from

    A. C4-C6.
    B. ansa cervicalis.
    C. lesser occipital nerve.
    D. greater occipital nerve.
    E. C6-C8.

90. All of the following are branches of the external carotid artery EXCEPT

    A. ophthalmic artery.
    B. ascending pharyngeal artery.
    C. superior thyroid artery.
    D. posterior auricular artery.
    E. occipital artery.

91. The crista galli is a superior extension of which of the following bones?

    A. Sphenoid
    B. Ethmoid
    C. Vomer
    D. Frontal
    E. Maxilla

92. Hypothetically speaking, when preparing a cavity preparation on the crown of a fully formed permanent tooth, as you initially cut through enamel and into dentin, which structure is first being penetrated?

    A. Circumpulpal dentin
    B. Mantle dentin
    C. Odontoblasts
    D. Radicular dentin
    E. Circumpulpal and radicular dentin

93. Raschkow plexus is located

    A. within the cementum of a tooth.
    B. within the cell rich zone of tooth pulp.
    C. within the dentin of a tooth.
    D. within the cell free zone (of Weil) of tooth pulp.
    E. within the core of the dental pulp.

94. Which of the following structures of sperm development is analogous to the stratum basale of the skin?

    A. Spermatid
    B. Spermatogonium
    C. Primary spermatocyte
    D. Secondary spermatocyte
    E. Junctional complex

95. The macula densa is located in which portion of the kidney?

    A. Distal convoluted tubule
    B. Bowman capsule
    C. Loop of Henle
    D. Proximal convoluted tubule
    E. Collecting duct

96. When extracting a tooth, one of the roots fractures off and remains within the alveolus. Which of the following would have the highest likelihood of becoming dislodged in the maxillary sinus?

A. Buccal root of the maxillary 1st premolar
B. Root of the maxillary canine
C. Root of the maxillary lateral incisor
D. Lingual root of the maxillary 1st molar
E. Lingual root of the maxillary 1st premolar

97. All of the following bones articulate with the zygoma EXCEPT

A. temporal.
B. maxilla.
C. frontal.
D. sphenoid.
E. parietal.

98. An 18-year-old female presents to the emergency department with a chief complaint of not being able to manipulate her lower jaw. You determine that luxation of her mandible has occurred. In which of the following directions would the mandibular condyles most likely be positioned from normal?

A. Posterior and superior
B. Posterior and inferior
C. Lateral and inferior
D. Anteriorly
E. Medially

99. The inferior alveolar artery is a DIRECT branch from which of the following arteries?

A. Middle meningeal
B. Facial
C. External carotid
D. Maxillary
E. Buccal

100. Bile is produced by which of the following?

A. Head of the pancreas
B. Gall bladder
C. Liver
D. Tail of the pancreas
E. Duodenum

101. Damage to the medulla would impair function of which cranial nerve nuclei?

A. V, VII, IX
B. III, IV, VI

C. IX, X, XII
D. X, XI, XII
E. V, VII, X

102. If one had a malfunction of pancreatic delta cells, which of the following would be impaired?

A. Insulin production
B. Trypsinogen production
C. Glucagon production
D. Somatostatin production
E. Exocrine function

103. Each of the following is an apocrine function of sweat glands EXCEPT

A. involved intimately with regulation of body temperature.
B. produces pheromones.
C. secretion is via myoepithelial and duct cells.
D. strictly serous fluid secretion.
E. cells receive sympathetic adrenergic innervation.

104. Which of the following portions of the female reproductive tract is the site of fertilization?

A. Uterus
B. Endometrium
C. Ovary
D. Cervix
E. Ampulla

105. Which of the following provides localized attachment of epithelium to connective tissue?

A. Hemidesmosome
B. Zonula adherens
C. Zonula occludens
D. Desmosome
E. Gap junction

106. A-gamma fibers function in

A. touch sensation.
B. muscle spindle apparatus.
C. pressure sensation.
D. temperature sensation.
E. sharp pain sensation.

107. The most inferior portion of the trachea, the carina, divides into

    A. bronchioles.
    B. segmental bronchi.
    C. main stem bronchi.
    D. alveoli.
    E. lobar bronchi.

108. Hilar lymph nodes are located

    A. in the lateral thoracic cavity.
    B. superior to the clavicle and surrounding the carotid sheath.
    C. along the sternocleidomastoid muscle.
    D. at the root of the lungs.
    E. at the posterior base of the skull.

109. The submaxillary ganglion receives presynaptic efferent innervation from which nerve?

    A. Inferior alveolar
    B. Facial
    C. Buccinator
    D. Maxillary
    E. Lingual

110. Rivian ducts allow drainage from which of the following glands?

    A. Parotid
    B. Sebaceous
    C. Lacrimal
    D. Sublingual
    E. Mammary

111. Each of the following is true regarding the embryological growth of the kidney EXCEPT

    A. the ureteric bud contributes to the adult kidney.
    B. the mesonephros gives rise to the ureteric bud and mesonephric duct.
    C. the pronephros ultimately forms the epididymis and ductus deferens.
    D. the mesonephros forms before the metanephros.
    E. the kidney initially forms in the pelvis.

112. Of the following structures, the Wolffian duct ultimately aids in development of the

    A. epididymis.
    B. ureter.
    C. collecting tubules.
    D. ovaries.
    E. uterus.

113. Neuroepithelial cells (of the fetal neural tube) give rise to each of the following EXCEPT

    A. ependymal cells.
    B. leptomeninges.
    C. astrocytes.
    D. neuroblasts.
    E. oligodendrocytes.

114. Which of the following is the correct sequence of zygotic cell cleavage?

    A. zygote, morula, blastula, blastomere
    B. morula, zygote, blastula, blastomere
    C. blastula, blastomere, morula, zygote
    D. zygote, blastomere, morula, blastula
    E. blastula, morula, blastomere, zygote

115. After what stage of zygote development does the zona pellucida disintegrate?

    A. First cleavage division
    B. Two-cell stage
    C. Blastula
    D. Late morula
    E. Early morula

116. Which of the following locations would NOT be considered a location of ectopic pregnancy?

    A. uterus
    B. ovary
    C. fallopian tube
    D. cervix
    E. abdomen

117. Meiosis II of sperm development MOST LIKELY occurs

    A. in the uterine tube.
    B. in the epididymis.
    C. in the ejaculatory duct.
    D. in the testes.
    E. in the vagina.

118. Each of the following muscles receives motor innervation from the facial nerve EXCEPT

A. risorius.
B. masseter.
C. orbicularis oris.
D. mentalis.
E. buccinator.

119. The jaw-jerk reflex involves efferent signals from which of the following cranial nerves?

A. V-1
B. V-3
C. VII
D. V-2
E. IX

120. Each of the following is TRUE with regard to the carotid sheath EXCEPT

A. the sternocleidomastoid muscle lies medial to it in the cervical region.
B. it lies anterior to the scalene musculature in the cervical region.
C. it lies anterior to the thyroid gland.
D. it contains the vagus nerve, jugular vein, and common carotid artery.
E. it is associated with the carotid sinus nerve, sympathetic nerves, and lymph nodes.

121. Suppose you are told that a patient has received damage to structures, which are contained in the submandibular triangle. Which of the following would you NOT consider to be affected?

A. CN XII
B. Nerve to mylohyoid
C. Lingual artery
D. CN X
E. Submandibular gland

122. If a patient is suffering from referred pain to the T4 dermatome, it will be felt at the

A. xiphoid.
B. umbilicus.
C. nipple.
D. inguinal ligament.
E. neck.

123. If a patient is unable to close his eyes (among other symptoms), one must consider damage to which of the following cranial nerve nuclei?

A. Main motor nucleus of VII
B. Nucleus of the solitary tract (of VII)
C. Spinal trigeminal nucleus of V
D. Mesencephalic nucleus of V
E. Motor nucleus of V

124. Each of the following is TRUE of nystagmus EXCEPT

A. irritation to the cerebellum and cerebral cortex can cause it.
B. it is defined as a rapid, involuntary movement of the eyes.
C. the caloric test using warm water will initiate nystagmus to the contralateral side.
D. the caloric test examines the vestibuloocular reflex.
E. it involves CN VIII lesions.

125. Movement of the head would be damaged in a patient with damage to which of the following spinal cord tracts?

A. Lateral spinothalamic
B. Tectospinal
C. Vestibulospinal
D. Reticulospinal
E. Anterior spinothalamic

126. Which of the following structures are involved in steroid synthesis and lipid/glycogen metabolism?

A. Smooth endoplasmic reticulum
B. Lysosomes
C. Peroxisomes
D. Rough endoplasmic reticulum
E. Mitochondria

127. Parafollicular cells are located within the

A. cortical bone.
B. kidney.
C. small intestine.
D. thyroid gland.
E. parathyroid gland.

128. The esophagus normally contains which type of epithelium?

    A. Nonkeratinized stratified squamous.
    B. Columnar.
    C. Keratinized stratified squamous.
    D. Cuboidal.
    E. Pseudostratified squamous.

129. Sperm is stored in the

    A. epididymis.
    B. urethra.
    C. testis.
    D. seminiferous tubules.
    E. prostate gland.

130. Each of the following is a function of skin EXCEPT

    A. sensation of touch, pain, and pressure.
    B. synthesis of vitamin E from ultraviolet light.
    C. excretion via sweat glands.
    D. homeostatic regulation of body temperature.
    E. protection against physical and chemical stresses.

131. The sphincter of Boyden is located at the

    A. ampulla of Vater.
    B. lower portion of the esophagus.
    C. common bile duct.
    D. rectum.
    E. opening of the duodenum.

132. The posterior 1/3 of the tongue drains directly into the

    A. deep cervical nodes.
    B. submental nodes.
    C. submandibular nodes.
    D. rectopharyngeal nodes.
    E. supraclavicular nodes.

133. Damage to the gastric cardiac glands would affect which type of exocrine gland?

    A. Coiled
    B. Tubular
    C. Tubuloacinar
    D. Acinar
    E. Apocrine

134. Which of the following is FALSE regarding bone marrow of the maxilla and mandible?

    A. It is contained within the medullary spaces of spongy bone.
    B. Red marrow contains fatty cells and is the predominant marrow type in the mandibular ramus and condyles.
    C. Red marrow contains hematopoietic cells.
    D. Yellow marrow contains fatty cells.
    E. Yellow marrow is the predominant marrow type in the maxilla and mandible.

135. Which of the following combinations of epithelium is contained in the nasal cavities?

    A. Stratified squamous, pseudostratified ciliated columnar, olfactory
    B. Simple squamous, olfactory, simple columnar
    C. Stratified squamous, olfactory, stratified columnar
    D. Simple cuboidal, simple squamous, simple columnar
    E. Stratified columnar, simple squamous, simple columnar

Questions 136 and 137 pertain to the following clinical vignette:

Suppose a patient presents to you after having been struck in the chin. Upon examination, you note a laceration of the anterior portion of their tongue accompanied with profuse bleeding.

136. Each of the following supply blood to the tongue EXCEPT

    A. facial artery.
    B. ascending pharyngeal artery.
    C. lingual artery.
    D. superior laryngeal artery.
    E. external carotid artery.

137. Each of the following muscles could possibly be damaged in this situation EXCEPT

    A. longitudinal.
    B. styloglossus.
    C. hyoglossus.
    D. transverse.
    E. palatoglossus.

138. Which of the following combinations of cranial nerves provide motor innervation to the tongue?

    A. VII, X
    B. X, XII
    C. VII, XII
    D. V, XII
    E. VII, IX

139. Which type of taste would most likely be altered if the entire tip of the tongue were damaged?

    A. Sweet
    B. Salt
    C. Bitter
    D. Sour
    E. None of the above

140. Relative to fetal development, sclerotome cells form

    A. vertebrae and ribs.
    B. skeletal muscle within body.
    C. connective tissue of skin.
    D. skeletal muscle within limbs.
    E. skeletal muscle of the body wall.

141. Formation of which of the following is NOT altered in complete bilateral palatal clefting?

    A. Lip
    B. Primary palate
    C. Alveolar process
    D. Inferior nasal turbinate/concha
    E. Secondary palate

142. Which of the following is a characteristic of the eruptive stage of a tooth?

    A. Elongation of cervical loop and formation of HERS
    B. Fusion of the REE and oral epithelium
    C. Disappearance of the enamel knot
    D. Formation of the enamel organ
    E. Merging of the OEE with the IEE

143. Which of the following is FALSE regarding cartilage?

    A. It is vascularized.
    B. It contains lacunae.

C. Chondrocytes comprise a large portion of it.
D. It is specialized in areas such as the bronchi, Eustachian tube, and knee menisci.
E. It can grow both appositionally and interstitially.

144. Suppose a patient presents with altered hemostasis. Malfunction of which of the following may be the cause?

    A. Monocytes
    B. B cells
    C. Megakaryocytes
    D. Erythroblasts
    E. Granulocytes

145. If a patient has high levels of bile pigment excreted by the liver, increased destruction of which of the following may be the causative factor?

    A. Neutrophils
    B. Eosinophils
    C. Erythrocytes
    D. Platelets
    E. Macrophages

146. Which of the following regarding gingival crevicular fluid is TRUE?

    A. It is comprised mostly of PMNs and leukocytes.
    B. It lacks plasma proteins and epithelial cells.
    C. It is contained mostly within the vestibule of the buccal mucosa.
    D. It lacks function in immune defense.
    E. It is not located within the gingival sulcus.

147. The most likely diagnosis for a young patient presenting with brownish pigmentation and mottling of his dentition would be

    A. congenital syphilis.
    B. nutritional deficiency.
    C. fluorosis.
    D. hypocalcification.
    E. hypomineralization.

148. Malfunction of which cranial nerve would affect the efferent output of the gag reflex?

    A. CN XII
    B. CN V
    C. CN IX
    D. CN VII
    E. CN X

149. Each of the following carries deoxygenated blood EXCEPT

    A. hepatic vein.
    B. superior vena cava.
    C. inferior vena cava.
    D. pulmonary vein.
    E. coronary sinus.

150. The gastroepiploic artery forms an anastomosis between which two arteries?

    A. Right gastric and hepatic proper
    B. Left gastric and right gastric
    C. Right gastric and short gastric
    D. Splenic and gastroduodenal
    E. Hepatic proper and splenic

151. The supraoptic nucleus is intricately involved in which of the following bodily functions?

    A. Aggression
    B. Satiety
    C. Hunger
    D. Water balance
    E. Circadian rhythm

152. Sensory innervation to the hypothenar region of the hand travels via the

    A. radial nerve.
    B. ulnar nerve.
    C. musculocutaneous nerve.
    D. median nerve.
    E. axillary nerve.

153. Which of the following muscles divides the maxillary artery into three distinct anatomical segments?

    A. Lateral pterygoid
    B. Masseter
    C. Posterior belly of digastric
    D. Stylohyoid
    E. Anterior belly of digastric

154. Each of the following structures receives blood from the external carotid EXCEPT

    A. thyroid.
    B. brain.
    C. salivary glands.
    D. teeth.
    E. jaw bones.

155. The vertebral artery enters the spine at which level?

    A. C6
    B. T2
    C. T1
    D. C5
    E. C7

156. The function of the salpingopharyngeus muscle is to

    A. open the auditory tube.
    B. raise the mandible.
    C. propel food down pharynx.
    D. retract the tongue.
    E. protrude the mandible.

157. Within which bone is the vestibulocochlear nerve most contained?

    A. Parietal
    B. Occipital
    C. Temporal
    D. Frontal
    E. Maxilla

158. Which of the following regarding the pectoralis major muscle is TRUE?

    A. It acts to protract and depress the glenoid of the scapula.
    B. It is an accessory muscle of respiration.
    C. It is innervated by the lateral and medial pectoral nerves.
    D. It inserts at the coracoid process.
    E. It is located superiorly to the pectoralis minor.

159. Which of the following arteries supplies the maxillary canines and incisors?

   A. Pterygoid
   B. Sphenopalatine
   C. Descending palatine
   D. Infraorbital
   E. Pharyngeal

160. The cisterna chyli drains lymph from each of the following EXCEPT

   A. thoracic duct.
   B. abdomen.
   C. pelvis.
   D. inguinal region.
   E. lower extremities.

161. As the dentin ages, which of the following is typically seen?

   A. Increased dentinal tubule diameter
   B. Decreased reparative dentin
   C. Decreased dead tracts
   D. Decreased sclerotic dentin
   E. Increased deposition of peritubular dentin

162. A 17-year-old patient presents at your office asking why there is a brownish-gray band across each of her teeth. You suspect that she was previously prescribed a regimen of tetracycline most likely at which of the following ages?

   A. 10
   B. 11
   C. 5
   D. 14
   E. 17

163. Which of the following vitamin deficiencies is LEAST likely to directly affect enamel structure?

   A. A
   B. B
   C. C
   D. K
   E. Calcium

164. Which type of epithelium is most commonly found lining closed body cavities?

   A. Simple columnar
   B. Simple squamous
   C. Transitional
   D. Stratified squamous
   E. Pseudostratified columnar

165. Which of the following is TRUE of the basement membrane?

   A. Lamina lucida is electron dense.
   B. Lamina densa is a product of the connective tissue.
   C. Type IV collagen is typically found in the basal lamina.
   D. Reticular lamina contains anchoring fibrils.
   E. It does not have a filtering function.

166. Which of the following oral epithelial types is keratinized?

   A. Sulcular epithelium
   B. Alveolar mucosa
   C. Junctional epithelium
   D. Attached gingiva
   E. Gingival col

167. Which of the following has the LOWEST organic composition?

   A. Cementum
   B. Dentin
   C. Pulp
   D. Enamel
   E. Alveolar bone

168. With increased age of the pulp, each of the following occurs EXCEPT

   A. decreased collagen content.
   B. decreased size of apical foramen.
   C. decreased sensitivity.
   D. decreased cellularity.
   E. increased calcification.

169. Which of the following portions of the tooth or its associated structures allows for orthodontic movement?

    A. Enamel
    B. Cementum
    C. Dentin
    D. Epithelial attachment
    E. Alveolar bone

170. What type of nerve ending is most common in the periodontal ligament?

    A. Coiled
    B. Spindle
    C. Free
    D. Meissner
    E. Ruffini

171. Which of the following is the depression of the interdental gingiva that connects the lingual and facial papillae?

    A. Gingival col.
    B. Alveolar mucosa.
    C. Attached gingiva.
    D. Mucogingival junction.
    E. Interdental papilla.

172. Which of the following is FALSE regarding the primary palate?

    A. It can be involved in facial clefting.
    B. It contains the incisive foramen.
    C. It usually contains no teeth.
    D. It is mesenchymal in origin.
    E. It is formed by fusion of two median nasal processes.

173. Which of the following best describes circumpulpal dentin?

    A. Most is produced in the form of intertubular dentin.
    B. It is the initial 150 μm of dentin laid down.
    C. It lacks hydroxyapatite.
    D. It forms before mantle dentin.
    E. It lacks dead tracts.

174. During amelogenesis, enamel is laid down each day at a rate of

    A. 0.04 μm.
    B. 1 mm.
    C. 0.1 mm.
    D. 4 μm.
    E. 4 mm.

175. Formation of which of the following brain structures normally occurs LAST in the fetus?

    A. Cerebellum
    B. Ventricles
    C. Neural tube
    D. Hemispheres
    E. Temporal lobe

176. During odontogenesis, which of the following cells determine the type of tooth to be formed?

    A. Mesoderm
    B. Mesenchyme
    C. Ectomesenchyme
    D. Endoderm
    E. Ectoderm

177. The area of skin covering the parotid gland receives sensory innervation from which nerve?

    A. Transverse cervical
    B. Superficial temporal
    C. Long buccal
    D. Lesser occipital
    E. Great auricular

178. Each of the following is TRUE regarding the sacral plexus EXCEPT

    A. one of its main branches is the obturator nerve.
    B. it is located in the posterior pelvic wall.
    C. it provides motor innervation to parts of the leg.
    D. it supplies sensory innervation to the lower back.
    E. it is comprised of L4-L5 and S1-S4.

179. Which of the following cranial nerves does NOT have an efferent involuntary parasympathetic function?

A. VII
B. V
C. X
D. III
E. IX

180. Which is TRUE regarding general visceral afferent function of the vagus nerve?

A. It is involved with chemo- and baroreception from the carotid body and sinus.
B. It travels through the jugular foramen.
C. Its origin of cell bodies is the nucleus ambiguus.
D. It transmits sensation from the posterior meninges.
E. It is involved with taste sensation.

181. Which of the following is FALSE regarding the adrenal gland?

A. Zona fasciculata secretes glucocorticoids.
B. Outer cortex contains chromaffin cells.
C. Aldosterone is a mineralocorticoid produced here.
D. Sex steroids are secreted from the innermost layer of the outer cortex.
E. Inner medulla secretes catecholamines.

182. If a patient is suffering from lack of peristalsis in the large intestine, which of the following may be affected?

A. Microvilli
B. Myenteric plexus
C. Plicae circulares
D. Teniae coli
E. Crypts of Lieberkühn

183. Bile contains each of the following EXCEPT

A. lipoproteins.
B. plasmin.
C. albumin.
D. prothrombin.
E. alpha and beta globulins.

184. The temporal bone articulates with each of the following bones EXCEPT

A. parietal.
B. occipital.

C. zygoma.
D. ethmoid.
E. sphenoid.

185. Terminal differentiation occurs during which stage of the cell cycle?

A. G1
B. S
C. G0
D. G2
E. Mitosis

186. Which of the following glands has paracrine function?

A. Gastroenteropancreatic glands.
B. Adrenal glands.
C. Gonads.
D. Salivary glands.
E. Pituitary glands.

187. The embryological stomodeum is lined by

A. endoderm.
B. mesoderm.
C. neural crest.
D. ectoderm.
E. ectomesenchyme.

188. Which of the following structures has its embryological origin located further cranial in a 4- to 5-week-old fetus?

A. Stapes
B. Internal carotid artery
C. Vagus nerve
D. Glossopharyngeal nerve
E. Stylopharyngeus muscle

189. Which of the following best describes the decidual reaction of embryogenesis?

A. Breakdown of the zona pellucida
B. The first zygotic cleavage
C. Invasion of the syncytiotrophoblast into the uterine endometrium
D. Release of an ovum from the ovary
E. Enlargement of the endometrium with lipid and glycogen accumulation

190. Which of the following is the number of chromosomes present after fusion of sperm and egg?

    A. $\frac{1}{2}N$
    B. N
    C. 2N
    D. 3N
    E. 4N

191. Each of the following contains sinusoids EXCEPT

    A. epidermis.
    B. liver.
    C. lymphatic tissue.
    D. endocrine glands.
    E. spleen.

192. Peroxisomes contain which of the following enzymes?

    A. Elastase
    B. Collagenase
    C. Trypsin
    D. Chymotrypsin
    E. Catalase

193. Production of vitamin D occurs at which of the following sites?

    A. Large intestine
    B. Kidney
    C. Spleen
    D. Liver
    E. Epidermis

194. Which of the following directly controls lens accommodation in the eye?

    A. Ciliary body
    B. Neural retina
    C. Choroids body
    D. Pupil
    E. Iris

195. Serum includes each of the following EXCEPT

    A. electrolytes.
    B. fibrinogen.
    C. immunoglobulins.
    D. water.
    E. albumin.

196. Which of the following is TRUE of the heart?

    A. The pericardium contains cardiac muscle.
    B. The endocardium has a layer of simple squamous endothelium.
    C. The innermost layer of the heart is pericardium.
    D. Normally the thickest portion of the heart is the endocardium.
    E. A layer of columnar epithelium surrounds the pericardium.

197. Which of the following is FALSE regarding heart conduction?

    A. The bundle of His conducts electric current to the Purkinje fibers.
    B. The SA node regulates the rate of electrical conductance.
    C. The autonomic nervous system regulates the rhythm of cardiac contraction.
    D. Cardiac muscle maintains an intrinsic rhythmicity.
    E. The pacemaker of the heart is the SA node.

198. Which of the following is TRUE of platelets?

    A. They range 200,000-400,000 per mm^3 blood.
    B. They are involved in immunoregulation.
    C. The average lifespan is upward of 120 days.
    D. They are nucleated.
    E. They function in blood gas transport.

199. Which of the following is the site of B-cell maturation?

    A. Lymph nodes
    B. Blood
    C. Thymus
    D. Bone marrow
    E. Target tissue

200. Thyroxine is secreted from

    A. follicular cells.
    B. outer cortex of adrenals.
    C. pars distalis.
    D. pars intermedia.
    E. parafollicular cells.

1. **The correct answer is C.** The extensor carpi ulnaris is innervated by the radial nerve (C6-C8), which is part of the posterior cord. The radial nerve innervates the extensor muscles of the arm/forearm.

   Answer A is incorrect. The interosseus muscles of the hand are innervated by the ulnar nerve (C8-T1).

   Answer B is incorrect. The thenar muscles of the hand are innervated by the median nerve (C5-T1).

   Answer D is incorrect. The flexor carpi ulnaris is innervated by the ulnar nerve (C8-T1).

   Answer E is incorrect. The flexor carpi radialis is innervated by the median nerve (C5-T1).

   Note that the median nerve includes the lateral and medial cords. It innervates muscles involved in forearm flexion. The ulnar nerve includes the medial cord. It provides innervation to flexor muscles of the wrist and fingers.

2. **The correct answer is E.** All of the structures listed run in close proximity and could be injured in the event of a clavicular fracture.

   Answer A is incorrect. The subclavian artery and vein run along the posterior border of the clavicle. Vasculature arising from the arch of the aorta first branches off as the brachiocephalic artery, which then gives rise to the right common carotid artery before continuing as the right subclavian artery. The arch of the aorta then gives rise directly to the left common carotid artery and, subsequently, the left subclavian artery. Venous drainage from the head and neck region eventually drain into the internal and external jugular veins, which combine to form the subclavian vein.

   Answer B is incorrect. The brachial plexus tracts posterior to the clavicle (along with the subclavian vessels), en route to innervating the shoulder girdle and upper limb.

   Answer C is incorrect. The trachea is an inferior continuation of the pharynx (after branching off into the esophagus) which runs posterior to the sternum. It extends from the C5-C6 level inferiorly to the sternal angle/T4-T5 level, before branching at the Carina into the left and right mainstem bronchi.

   Answer D is incorrect. The subclavian vein then forms the brachiocephalic vein, which empties into the superior vena cava and then right atrium of the heart.

3. **The correct answer is B.** The stylohyoid muscle is innervated by CN VII, and is considered a suprahyoid muscle. Motor innervation from the cervical plexus includes the genioglossus muscle (C1 by way of CN XII) and infrahyoid muscles.

   Answer A is incorrect. The sternohyoid is an infrahyoid muscle. It is innervated by the ansa cervicalis (C1-C3).

   Answer C is incorrect. The omohyoid is an infrahyoid muscle. It is innervated by the ansa cervicalis (C1-C3).

   Answer D is incorrect. The sternothyroid is an infrahyoid muscle. It is innervated by the ansa cervicalis (C1-C3).

   Note that the thyrohyoid muscle is also an infrahyoid muscle. It is innervated by C1.

4. **The correct answer is B.** Taste sensation to the posterior 1/3 of the tongue is mediated by CN IX (taste to the base of the tongue is by way of CN X). With this lesion, one would expect decreased taste sensation to the anterior 2/3 of the tongue. Taste fibers leave the tongue via the chorda tympani, which travels with the lingual nerve through the petrotympanic fissure and into the infratemporal fossa, and synapses with the geniculate ganglion. Fibers then follow the solitary tract and synapse at the (gustatory) nucleus of the solitary tract, en route to the VPM of the thalamus and then gustatory cortex.

   Answer A is incorrect. Ipsilateral weakness to musculature of facial expression will occur. Motor fibers of CN VII leave the main motor nucleus (of the pons), enter the internal acoustic meatus and through the facial canal, before exiting the skull base via the stylomastoid foramen. The nerve then courses through the parotid gland, and gives off five branches, including motor innervation to the muscles of facial expression (as well as the posterior belly of the digastric, stapedius, and stylohyoid).

Answer C is incorrect. Ipsilateral dryness of eye due to lost function of lacrimal gland will occur. The greater petrosal nerve gives fibers to the lacrimal, submandibular, and sublingual glands. Parasympathetic preganglionic fibers first leave the superior salivatory nucleus, synapsing at the geniculate ganglion (as well as giving off sympathetics), joins the deep petrosal nerve, and leaves the cranium via the foramen lacerum. Fibers then either travel with the chorda tympani to synapse at the submandibular ganglion (thus, parasympathetic innervation to the submandibular and sublingual glands).

Answer D is incorrect. Compromised function of sublingual and submandibular glands will occur. An alternate path of the deep petrosal nerve may enter the pterygoid canal (instead of the chorda tympani), which gives preganglionics to the pterygopalatine ganglion, and subsequent postganglionic fibers to supply parasympathetic innervation to the lacrimal gland.

Answer E is incorrect. Hyperacusis in ipsilateral ear will occur. This is due to motor innervation from the cranial nerve to the stapedius muscle.

5. **The correct answer is C.** A lesion affecting the upper motor neuron of CN VII would cause impairment to the facial musculature of expression (on the contralateral side) of the lower face only.

Answer A is incorrect. The ipsilateral side of the lower face is left unaffected by an upper motor lesion.

Answer B is incorrect. The ipsilateral side of the lower face is left unaffected by an upper motor lesion.

Answer D is incorrect. The ipsilateral side of the lower face is left unaffected by an upper motor lesion.

Note that this is because the musculature of facial expression of the upper face receives bilateral innervation from CN VII. The facial musculature of the lower face which is innervated by CN VII receives only unilateral innervation. The crossover occurs after the fibers leave the motor area of the cortex (thus traveling via the corticobulbar tract) and before they synapse at the pons.

6. **The correct answer is B.** The embryonic branchial arches are mesodermal ridges, formed from neural crest cells. Each arch contains a nerve, artery, cartilaginous bar, and musculature. The four main branchial arches develop at week 4 of life. Arch II consists of the hyoid and stapedial artery, CN VII, musculature of facial expression (also stapedius, stylohyoid, posterior belly of digastric), and stapes, styloid process, stylohyoid ligament, lesser cornu (of hyoid), and part of hyoid bone.

Answer A is incorrect. Arch I (gives rise to mandible and most of maxilla) is comprised of the maxillary artery, CN V, muscles of mastication (also tensor tympani, mylohyoid, tensor veli palatine, anterior belly of digastric), and malleus, incus, sphenomandibular ligament, and Meckel cartilage.

Answer C is incorrect. Arch III is comprised of the internal carotid artery, CN IX, stylopharyngeus muscle, greater cornu (of hyoid), hypobranchial eminence, and part of hyoid bone.

Answer D is incorrect. Arch IV consists of the right subclavian artery and aorta, CN X, pharyngeal and laryngeal musculature, and laryngeal cartilages. The tongue is formed from contributions made by each arch.

Note that branchial grooves and pouches also exist, which give rise to adult structures. Groove 1 gives rise to the external ear and external auditory meatus, while grooves 2-4 contribute to form the cervical sinus. Pouch 1 gives rise to the middle ear/auditory tube, pouch 2 contributes to the supratonsillar fossa, pouch 3 forms the thymus and inferior parathyroid gland, and pouch 4 contributes to the superior parathyroid gland, as well as postbranchial body.

7. **The correct answer is E.** The common facial vein eventually drains into the internal jugular vein. Venous drainage from the head and neck (superior to inferior) starts at the superficial temporal vein, which then merges with the maxillary vein. The internal jugular vein joins the subclavian vein. This merging of the internal jugular vein with the subclavian vein creates the large brachiocephalic vein. The left and right brachiocephalic veins merge and form the superior vena cava.

Answer A is incorrect. The maxillary vein receives drainage from the pterygoid plexus of veins. It combines with the superficial temporal vein. This union forms the retromandibular vein, which then divides at the angle of the mandible into anterior and posterior segments. The posterior segment of the retromandibular vein joins with the posterior auricular vein which then forms the external jugular vein, which eventually empties into the subclavian vein.

Answer B is incorrect. The anterior segment of the anterior retromandibular vein anastomoses with the anterior facial vein and creates the common facial vein.

Answer C is incorrect. The retromandibular vein has two segments: anterior and posterior. It is formed by the maxillary vein and superficial temporal vein.

Answer D is incorrect. The anterior facial vein is formed from the angular vein (which is a union of the supraorbital and supratrochlear veins) and it drains into the internal jugular vein.

8. **The correct answer is C.** This statement describes the tunica intima. The tunica adventitia is the outermost, connective tissue, layer of the blood vessel wall, and contains collagen, elastic fibers, and (if applicable) vasa vasora. Moving inward toward the lumen, next is the tunica media, which contains smooth muscle and elastic fibers. The innermost layer is the tunica intima.

Answer A is incorrect. Blood is composed of plasma (55%) (which is the liquid portion containing water, protein, and electrolytes/gases, etc), and formed elements/cellular portion (45%) (which is composed of erythrocytes, leukocytes, and platelets).

Answer B is incorrect. Serum is defined as blood plasma lacking fibrinogen and clotting factors.

Answer D is incorrect. Sinusoids are defined as fenestrated capillaries which allow the passage of phagocytic cells.

Answer E is incorrect. ABO blood typing is with regard to the antigen present on an individual's erythrocytes. For example, a person with blood type A has erythrocytes contains the A antigen, and, thus, plasma lacking anti-A and containing anti-B antibodies.

9. **The correct answer is E.** The middle meningeal artery is ruptured in the case of an epidural hematoma, as it lies within the epidural space between the periosteum of the inner surface of the skull and dura mater. A subdural hematoma involves a bridging vein being ruptured within the subdural space between the dura mater and arachnoid.

Answer A is incorrect. A subarachnoid hemorrhage involves a ruptured aneurysm, for example, involving the anterior communicating artery.

Answer B is incorrect. The posterior cerebral artery is not directly involved in an epidural hematoma.

Answer C is incorrect. The anterior cerebral artery is not directly involved in an epidural hematoma.

Answer D is incorrect. The posterior communicating artery is not directly involved in an epidural hematoma.

Note that the meningeal layer, from outermost to innermost, surrounding the brain and spinal cord is: periosteum of inner skull surface, epidural space, dura mater, subdural space, arachnoid, subarachnoid space, pia mater, and then the brain/spinal cord. The subarachnoid space holds cerebrospinal fluid, and is a prime location for a spinal tap.

10. **The correct answer is E.** The optic foramen is located within the middle cranial fossa. Also contained within the middle cranial fossa (temporal, parietal, and sphenoid bones) are temporal lobes, pituitary gland, superior orbital fissure, carotid canal, trigeminal ganglion, foramen rotundum, ovale, and spinosum.

    Answer A is incorrect. The occipital lobes are located within the posterior cranial fossa.

    Answer B is incorrect. The jugular foramen is located within the posterior cranial fossa.

    Answer C is incorrect. The cerebellum is located within the posterior cranial fossa.

    Answer D is incorrect. The hypoglossal canal is located within the posterior cranial fossa.

    Note that the anterior cranial fossa (frontal and ethmoid bones) contains frontal lobes, cribriform plate, foramen cecum, and crista galli. The posterior cranial fossa (occipital and temporal bones) contains the above mentioned and brainstem, internal acoustic meatus, and foramen magnum.

11. **The correct answer is A.** The VPM of the thalamus is involved with facial sensation and pain. Thalamus is a sensory relay station, en route to higher cortical areas. Lateral auditory sensation is mediated by the medial geniculate nucleus.

    Answer B is incorrect. The ventral anterior nucleus each mediates motor function.

    Answer C is incorrect. The lateral geniculate nucleus is involved with visual sensation.

    Answer D is incorrect. VPL is involved with proprioception, pressure, touch, and vibration.

    Answer E is incorrect. The ventral lateral nucleus mediates motor function.

12. **The correct answer is D.** The ventromedial nucleus is located within the hypothalamus, and functions as the satiety center involved with body homeostasis.

    Answer A is incorrect. The superior salivatory nucleus functions with CN VII, and gives off parasympathetic efferent fibers (from the cortex) which control salivation (of submandibular and sublingual glands), as well as glandular secretion.

    Answer B is incorrect. Also giving off parasympathetic efferents is the nucleus ambiguous of CN IX and X, which controls swallowing.

    Answer C is incorrect. Sensory afferents to the brainstem (eventually relayed to the thalamus and cortex) nucleus of the solitary tract, involved with CN VII, IX, and X, mediate taste sensation.

    Answer E is incorrect. The inferior salivatory nucleus gives off parasympathetic efferent fibers by way of CN IX to cause salivation by way of the parotid gland.

    Note that all cranial nerves (except CN I and II) originate in the brainstem.

13. **The correct answer is D.** The tricuspid valve, which has three cusps and separates the right atrium from the right ventricle, can be auscultated left of the sternal border in the 5th intercostal space.

    Answer A is incorrect. As for the mitral valve, which also contains three cusps and divides the left atrium from left ventricle, it can be heard at the midclavicular line at the level of the 5th intercostal space.

    Answer B is incorrect. The aortic valve is auscultated at the level of the 2nd intercostal space, just lateral to the sternal border in the right, 2nd intercostal space. This valve is considered semilunar (thus, containing two cusps), and divides the left ventricle from the ascending aorta.

    Answer C is incorrect. At the level of the 2nd intercostal space, left and lateral to the sternal border, the pulmonic valve can be heard.

It is also semilunar, and separates the right ventricle from the pulmonary arteries.

14. **The correct answer is A.** Blood supply to the lateral wall of the left ventricle is via the left circumflex artery. The coronary arteries are the first branches of the aorta, and fill during the diastole stage of the heart cycle.

Answer B is incorrect. The right coronary artery branches off as the acute marginal and posterior descending arteries.

Answer C is incorrect. The left anterior descending artery provides blood supply to the anterior wall of left ventricle and interventricular septum.

Answers D and E are incorrect. Such vasculature supplies blood to the posterior and inferior walls of the left ventricle, as well as the entire right ventricle and atrioventricular node.

Note that the left coronary artery to branch from the aorta is the left main coronary artery, which subsequently gives off the circumflex (blood supplied to the lateral wall of the left ventricle) and left descending arteries.

15. **The correct answer is B.** The vagus nerve travels through the posterior portion of the inferior mediastinum. It contains the thoracic duct, descending aorta, azygous vein, hemiazygous vein, esophagus, vagus nerves, splanchnic nerves, and lymph nodes. Within the thorax, between and medial to the lungs, lies an area termed the mediastinum, which is divided into a superior and inferior portion.

Answer A is incorrect. The superior mediastinum contains the following: thoracic duct, ascending and descending aorta, aortic arch (and branches), superior vena cava, brachiocephalic veins, thymus (childhood), trachea, esophagus, cardiac nerve, and left recurrent laryngeal nerve.

Answer C is incorrect. The anterior mediastinum (subdivision of the inferior mediastinum) contains the thymus, connective tissue, lymph nodes, and branches of internal thoracic artery.

Answer D is incorrect. The middle mediastinum (subdivision of the inferior mediastinum) contains the pericardium, heart, roots of great vessels, and phrenic nerve.

16. **The correct answer is D.** Oxygenated blood bypasses the pulmonary circulation by a communication in the fetal heart called the foramen ovale. This opening connects the right atrium to the left atrium. Blood, therefore, is oxygenated by the mother and enters the fetal heart by way of the inferior vena cava. The blood is then shunted from the right to left atrium, where it proceeds to flow through the left ventricle, and subsequently out through the aorta to supply the fetal head. Prostaglandins, as well as inspiration, help to close the foramen ovale upon birth.

Answers A, B, C, and E are incorrect. Oxygenated blood does not bypass the pulmonary circulation via these routes.

17. **The correct answer is B.** The fossa ovalis, which lies on the atrial septum (separating the right and left atria) is the adult remnant of the fetal foramen ovale. Its upper margin is the anulus ovalis.

Answer A is incorrect. The crista terminalis lies between the vena cavae openings, and is a vertical ridge which represents the sinus venosus and fetal heart.

Answer C is incorrect. The sulcus terminalis, a vertical groove lying externally on the right atrium, represents the internal location of the crista terminalis.

Answer D is incorrect. The right auricle is an appendage of the right atrium.

Answer E is incorrect. The atrial appendage serves as a connection (in concert with the crista terminalis) of the pectinate musculature of the right atrium.

18. **The correct answer is C.** The ductus arteriosus connects the pulmonary artery to the aorta, thus assisting in the pumping of blood throughout the fetal vasculature.

Answer A is incorrect. The ductus venosus is a continuation of the umbilical vein, and carries blood back to the inferior vena cava.

Answer B is incorrect. The umbilical arteries return deoxygenated blood from the fetus to the mother/placenta.

Answer D is incorrect. The poral vein returns blood back to the heart by pumping through the liver, then the ductus venosus and inferior vena cava.

Answer E is incorrect. The umbilical veins deliver oxygenated blood from the mother/placenta en route to the fetal heart.

19. **The correct answer is A.** Mesoderm makes up the epithelial lining of the cardiovascular system, as well as most of the urogenital system. It also comprises all muscle types (cardiac, smooth, skeletal), and all connective tissue (including cartilage, bone, and red/white blood cells).

    Answer B is incorrect. The endodermal layer leads to growth of epithelial lining for the gastrointestinal tract, as well as for organs budding from the endodermal tube: pharyngeal gland derivatives (thymus, palatine tonsils, parathyroids, thyroid), the respiratory system, digestive organs (liver, pancreas), and terminal urogenital system.

    Answer C is incorrect. As for ectoderm, it makes up superficial epithelium/epidermis, and all nervous tissue (CNS tissue is from neuroectoderm, brain and spinal cord from neural tube, and PNS tissue from neural crest).

20. **The correct answer is D.** The right common cardinal vein and right anterior cardinal vein combine to form the superior vena cava. Of the arterial structures comprising the heart, the truncus arteriosus eventually forms the ascending aorta and pulmonic trunk.

    Answer A is incorrect. The bulbus cordis eventually becomes the smooth part of the right and left ventricles. The right common cardinal vein becomes part of the superior vena cava.

Answer B is incorrect. The truncus arteriosus forms the ascending aorta and pulmonic trunk.

Answer C is incorrect. The right anterior cardinal vein combines with the right common cardinal vein to form the superior vena cava.

Note that the primitive ventricle comprises the trabeculated portions of the right and left ventricles. The primitive atrium develops into the trabeculated areas of the right and left atria. As for the venous portions, the left horn of the sinus venosus becomes the coronary sinus, while the right horn of the sinus venosus develops into the smooth portion of the right atrium.

21. **The correct answer is D.** The septum primum grows downward toward the atrial cushion in the developing heart, eventually meeting with the septum secundum, which grows next to it.

    Answer A is incorrect. The ostium secundum grows next to the septum primum, and undergoes apoptotic changes to form a hole.

    Answer B is incorrect. The septum primum grows just a bit further inferiorly to the septum secundum, thus, formation of the atrial septum.

    Answer C is incorrect. The ostium primum is the opening left by the downgrowth of the septum primum.

    Answer E is incorrect. The septum spurium is a fold which demarcates the uniting of right and left venous valves.

    Note that incomplete fusion of the ostium secundum and septum primum results in formation of an atrial septal defect (which is typically symptomatic until middle age is encountered).

22. **The correct answer is C.** The derivative of the 4th aortic arch is the right subclavian artery and aortic trunk.

    Answer A is incorrect. The hyoid arteries are derivatives of the 2nd aortic arch.

Answer B is incorrect. The stapedial arteries are a derivative of the 2nd aortic arch.

Answer D is incorrect. The common carotid artery is a derivative of the 3rd aortic arch.

Answer E is incorrect. The pulmonary arteries are a derivative of the 6th aortic arch.

Note that the aortic arch gives rise to arteries of the cardiac system at approximately week 4 of development. This structure arises from the distal truncus arteriosus/aortic sac. It fuses with the paired dorsal aortae in week 5 to form the descending thoracic and abdominal aortae. The 1st aortic arch also develops into the maxillary artery, the 3rd into the interior carotid arteries, 5th involutes, and 6th develops into the ductus arteriosus.

23. **The correct answer is D.** The cremaster muscle, a continuation of the internal oblique musculature in the lower abdominal region, is not a part of the femoral triangle.

Answer A is incorrect. The sartorius muscle forms part of the boundary known as the femoral triangle. It forms the lateral border.

Answer B is incorrect. The inguinal ligament forms part of the boundary known as the femoral triangle. It forms the superior border.

Answer C is incorrect. The adductor longus muscle forms part of the boundary known as the femoral triangle. It forms the medial border.

Answer E is incorrect. The pectineus muscle forms part of the boundary known as the femoral triangle. It forms the floor of the triangle.

Note that (running laterally → medially the triangle contains the femoral nerve, artery, and vein (in that order).

24. **The correct answer is D.** The transversus abdominis muscle contracts to increase abdominal pressure. The rectus abdominis contracts to flex the vertebral column, as well as increase abdominal pressure.

Answer A is incorrect. The external oblique muscle contracts to increase abdominal pressure.

Answer B is incorrect. The internal oblique muscle is innervated by the lower intercostal, iliohypogastric, and ilioinguinal nerves.

Answer C is incorrect. The external oblique muscle is innervated only by the lower intercostal nerves.

Answer E is incorrect. The rectus abdominis muscle originates at the pubic symphysis and inserts into the xiphoid process, as well as costal cartilages 5-7.

25. **The correct answer is B.** Aponeuroses are simply sheetlike layers of tendon.

Answer A is incorrect. Tendons are connective tissue attachments between muscle and bone.

Answer C is incorrect. Connective tissue of the head and neck region originates from neural crest, but most other connective tissue of the body is mesodermally derived.

Answer D is incorrect. Ligaments connect two separate bones.

26. **The correct answer is A.** The neurovascular bundle of the intercostal space runs within the costal groove on the inferior surface of each rib. Each of the other statements is correct pertaining to the thoracic cavity.

Answer B is incorrect. Musculature of respiration includes the intercostal muscles, diaphragm, and accessory muscles.

Answer C is incorrect. The costal groove of each rib protects the nerve (of the neurovascular bundle) the least when injury occurs.

Answer D is incorrect. The rib cage contains 12 ribs: ribs I-VI are true, VII-X are false, and XI-XII are floating.

Answer E is incorrect. Fracture of the left 10th and 11th ribs can cause injury to the spleen.

27. **The correct answer is C.** The caval opening of the diaphragm allows passage of the inferior vena cava. Other openings of the diaphragm include the esophageal (passage of the esophagus) and aortic (passage of the aorta, thoracic

duct, azygous and hemiazygous veins). Other structures that pass through the diaphragm include the posterior and anterior vagal trunks, splanchnic nerves, sympathetic trunk, and superior epigastric artery. When expiration occurs, the diaphragm relaxes, thus, moves upward and forms a dome, which creates a positive intrathoracic pressure. Forceful expiration involves contraction of the abdominal musculature.

Answer A is incorrect. Blood supply to the diaphragm is via the musculophrenic artery.

Answer B is incorrect. The aorta passes through two crura when passing through the aortic opening.

Answer D is incorrect. During the act of inspiration, the diaphragm contracts, thus, flattening out and creating a negative intrathoracic pressure.

Answer E is incorrect. Innervation to the diaphragm is via the phrenic nerve (C3, C4, C5).

28. **The correct answer is B.** The thymus communicates via efferent lymph vessels only to the systemic circulation; there are no afferent vessels, and the lymph is not filtered here.

Answer A is incorrect. Growth continues and peaks at puberty, and then atrophies and is replaced by adipose tissue.

Answer C is incorrect. The thymus is the site of T-cell maturation.

Answer D is incorrect. Thymic corpuscles/epithelioreticular cells are contained within the inner medulla.

Answer E is incorrect. The outer cortex holds the largest concentration of lymphocytes.

29. **The correct answer is A.** Objects are received by the retina by lateral/temporal and medial/nasal fibers.

Answer B is incorrect. The left medial/nasal fibers decussate and cross over at the optic chiasma en route to the right primary visual cortex of the occipital lobe.

Answer C is incorrect. The left lateral/temporal fibers decussate and stay ipsilateral

at the optic chiasma en route to the left primary visual cortex in the occipital lobe.

Answer D is incorrect. The right lateral/temporal fibers decussate and stay ipsilateral at the optic chiasma en route to the right primary visual cortex in the occipital lobe.

Note that left and right lateral/temporal fibers of the optic nerve decussate ipsilaterally to the left and right primary visual cortex of the occipital lobe, respectively, where images are developed. Left and right medial/nasal fibers of the optic nerve decussate and cross over at the optic chiasma, whereby left medial/nasal fibers are received by the right primary visual cortex of the occipital lobe (and right fibers received by the left primary visual cortex) where images are developed.

30. **The correct answer is D.** The abducens nerve (CN VI) innervates the lateral rectus muscle.

Answer A is incorrect. The superior oblique muscle is innervated by the trochlear nerve (CN IV).

Answer B is incorrect. The medial rectus muscle is innervated by the oculomotor nerve (CN III).

Answer C is incorrect. The inferior rectus muscle is innervated by the oculomotor nerve (CN III).

Answer E is incorrect. The superior rectus muscle is innervated by the oculomotor nerve (CN III).

Note that all other extraocular muscles (superior, inferior, and medial rectus, inferior oblique) are innervated by the oculomotor nerve (CN III).

31. **The correct answer is B.** The papillary light reflex involves stimulus to the eye (eg, right eye), which then causes afferent firing via the optic nerve (CN II), synapsing at the Edinger-Westphal nucleus and then ciliary ganglia. From here, postganglionic fibers, by way of the short ciliary nerve/oculomotor nerve/CN III, then stimulate the constrictor pupillae muscle.

Answer A is incorrect. When shining light onto the left eye, the direct response elicits ipsilateral afferent firing via CN II and subsequent ipsilateral efferent firing via CN III to left eye.

Answer C is incorrect. When shining light onto the left eye, the consensual response elicits ipsilateral afferent firing via CN II and subsequent contralateral efferent firing via CN III to right eye.

Answer D is incorrect. When shining light onto the right eye, the direct response elicits ipsilateral afferent firing via CN II and subsequent ipsilateral efferent firing via CN III to left eye.

Note that there are two distinct responses: direct and consensual. The direct response is when light is shined, for example, on the left eye. Ipsilateral afferents are sent via CN II followed by subsequent efferents via CN III to the ipsilateral (left) eye. The consensual response is when light is shined, again, on the left eye, thus, eliciting ipsilateral afferents via CN II followed by subsequent contralateral efferents via CN III to the right eye.

32. **The correct answer is E.** The trochlear nerve (CN IV) innervates the superior oblique muscle. The main action of the superior oblique muscle is to move the eyeball in an inferior and lateral direction. It is important to note that clinical testing of the extraocular eye muscles does not follow the same anatomical movements.

Answer A is incorrect. Superior movement of the eye is the main movement of the superior rectus muscle.

Answer B is incorrect. Superior and medial movement of the eye is the main movement of the inferior oblique muscle.

Answer C is incorrect. Downward movement of the eye is the main movement of the inferior rectus muscle.

Answer D is incorrect. Lateral movement of the eye is the main movement of the lateral rectus muscle.

33. **The correct answer is D.** Argyll-Robertson/papillary light-near dissociation pupil affects patients with syphilis and diabetes, and causes accommodation with no reaction of the pupil. Therefore, the pupil does not constrict with near stimulus (accommodation-convergence); that is, there is no miosis with either direct or consensual light.

Answer A is incorrect. Internuclear ophthalmoplegia involves a lesion of the medial longitudinal fasciculus, thus, lost connection of CNs III, IV, and VI. For example, if the lesion is on the right side, when looking laterally to the right, both eyes will follow; when looking laterally to the left, only the left eye follows, and the right eye stares straight. This is due to lost function of the medial rectus muscle, although, it still functions in accommodation.

Answer B is incorrect. Ophthalmoplegia involves either internal or external lesions: internal lesions spare the extraocular muscles but cause lost function of autonomics to the papillary sphincter and ciliary muscles, and external lesions cause lost function of all except for the superior oblique, superior rectus, papillary sphincter, and ciliary muscles. The external lesion is seen in diabetes mellitus neuropathy.

Answer C is incorrect. Marcus-Gunn/relative afferent pupil is a lesion of the optic nerve seen with multiple sclerosis optic neuritis. Therefore, by use of the swinging flashlight test, by shining a light source into the good eye, both pupils will constrict; quickly shining light source into the damaged eye will cause immediate pupillary dilation of both eyes, due to lost afferent function of the optic nerve.

Answer E is incorrect. Horner syndrome is due to lost oculosympathetic function. Thus, sympathetic fibers from the superior cervical ganglion are damaged, causing apparent enophthalmos, miosis, ptosis, and hemianhidrosis.

34. **The correct answer is A.** The middle cerebral, although the largest branch of the internal carotid artery, is not considered part of the circle of Willis.

Answer B is incorrect. The posterior cerebral artery is part of the circle of Willis.

Answer C is incorrect. The internal carotid artery is part of the circle of Willis.

Answer D is incorrect. The posterior communicating artery is part of the circle of Willis.

Answer E is incorrect. The anterior communicating artery is part of the circle of Willis.

Note that these arterial anastomoses function to prevent blockage of blood flow by offering collateral circulation, which is critical to prevent ischemia to brain tissue. Along with the internal carotid, the vertebral and basilar arteries indirectly feed blood to the circle of Willis.

35. **The correct answer is C.** The lenticulostriate arteries, sometimes known as the "arteries of stroke," are a branch of the middle cerebral artery (which, in turn, branches from the internal carotid). Blockage of the middle cerebral artery can cause severe ischemic injury, as well.

    Answer A is incorrect. The left anterior cerebral artery is not commonly involved in stroke.

    Answer B is incorrect. The right posterior cerebral artery is not commonly involved in stroke. It is part of the circle of Willis.

    Answer D is incorrect. Left vertebral artery is not commonly involved in stroke. It gives blood to the basilar artery.

    Answer E is incorrect. The left internal carotid artery is not commonly involved in stroke. It is part of the circle of Willis.

36. **The correct answer is B.** The hamulus is not directly involved in attachment and movement of the tongue. It attaches the tensor veli palatini muscle.

    Answer A is incorrect. The genial tubercles directly affect movement of the tongue. They attach the genioglossus muscle.

    Answer C is incorrect. The hyoid bone directly affects movement of the tongue. It attaches the hyoglossus muscle.

    Answer D is incorrect. The styloid process directly affects movement of the tongue. It attaches the styloglossus muscle.

Note that each of these muscles receives innervation via the motor division of CN XII.

37. **The correct answer is C.** The lingual is a tongue-shaped depression that is present on the superior lobe of the left lung. This structure corresponds with the middle lobe of the right lung.

    Answer A is incorrect. The middle lobe of the right lung does not contain the lingula.

    Answer B is incorrect. The superior lobe of the right lung does not contain the lingula.

    Answer D is incorrect. The inferior lobe of the left lung does not contain the lingula.

    Answer E is incorrect. The inferior lobe of the right lung does not contain the lingula.

38. **The correct answer is E.** The left recurrent laryngeal nerve, a branch of the vagus nerve (CN X), wraps around the arch of the aorta, also known as the ligamentum arteriosum, as it ascends in the mediastinum.

    Answer A is incorrect. The right recurrent laryngeal nerve does not wrap around the ligamentum arteriosum. It wraps around the right subclavian artery.

    Answer B is incorrect. The left brachiocephalic vein does not wrap around the ligamentum arteriosum.

    Answer C is incorrect. The right subclavian vein does not wrap around the ligamentum arteriosum.

    Answer D is incorrect. The superior laryngeal nerve does not wrap around the ligamentum arteriosum.

39. **The correct answer is D.** The foramen magnum is located within the inferior aspect of the occipital bone, and acts as a passageway for the exit of the spinal cord from the cranium.

    Answer A is incorrect. The foramen magnum is located within the occipital bone.

    Answer B is incorrect. The foramen magnum allows passage of the medulla oblongata/spinal cord.

Answer C is incorrect. The foramen magnum allows passage of the spinal accessory nerve.

Answer E is incorrect. The foramen magnum allows passage of the vertebral arteries.

40. **The correct answer is A.** The articulating surface of the mandibular condyle is covered with dense fibrocartilage, which is dense connective tissue. Although, most articulating surfaces of diarthrodial joints are covered with hyaline cartilage.

    Answer B is incorrect. The condyle is not covered by loose connective tissue. This is typically found associated with the epithelium.

    Answer C is incorrect. The condyle is not covered by elastic cartilage. This is typically found associated with the outer ear and larynx.

    Answer D is incorrect. The condyle is not covered by hyaline cartilage. This is typically found covering the ends of articulating joints.

41. **The correct answer is B.** The collateral ligaments of the TMJ connect the meniscus to the medial and lateral poles of the condyle. These ligaments function to limit movement of the condyle in lateral excursion. Tearing of these ligaments will allow the lateral pterygoid muscle to displace the meniscus.

    Answer A is incorrect. The stylomandibular ligament connects to the styloid process and the angle of the mandible.

    Answer C is incorrect. The temporomandibular ligament connects the temporal bone to the mandibular condyle.

    Answer D is incorrect. The sphenomandibular ligament connects the mandible to the sphenoid bone. It joins from the lingula of the mandible to the spine of the sphenoid.

42. **The correct answer is A.** When the collateral ligaments which attach the meniscus to the mandibular condyle tear, attachment will be lost. Thus, the lateral pterygoid muscle will cause anteromedial displacement of the articulating disc, upon contraction.

    Answers B, C, D, and E are incorrect. See above.

43. **The correct answer is E.** The pituitary gland is seated in the middle cranial fossa on the sphenoid bone, just superior to the sphenoid sinus.

    Answer A is incorrect. The frontal sinus is anterosuperior to the pituitary. It is normally empty.

    Answer B is incorrect. The maxillary sinuses are each located anterolateral to the pituitary. It is normally empty, but can often be filled with secretions and infectious material.

    Answer C is incorrect. The anterior ethmoid sinus is located anterior to the pituitary. It is normally empty.

    Answer D is incorrect. The posterior ethmoid sinus is located anterior to the pituitary. It is normally empty.

44. **The correct answer is B.** The lingual nerve runs just medial to the lingual cortical plate of the posterior mandible. This nerve contains sensory fibers, which function in taste recognition in the anterior 2/3 of the tongue (CN VII), as well as general sensation to the ipsilateral side of the tongue (CN V). Thus, iatrogenic impingement of such nerve near mandibular third molars may cause the aforementioned symptoms.

    Answer A is incorrect. The buccal nerve would not be compromised by this type of extraction. It is located lateral to the buccal shelf and within the cheek. It is a branch of CN V3.

    Answer C is incorrect. The middle superior alveolar nerve would not be compromised by this type of extraction. It is located within the maxilla, superior to the dentition. It is a branch of CN V2.

    Answer D is incorrect. The hypoglossal nerve (CN XII) would not be compromised by this type of extraction. It enters the tongue from the region of the posterior digastric muscle.

45. **The correct answer is D.** Odontogenic infection involving the root apices of a mandibular molar would most likely travel within the submandibular fascial plane via piercing of the mylohyoid muscle. This type of infection, if not

treated appropriately, can eventually course posteriorly and, thus, cause airway compromise.

Answer A is incorrect. The sublingual fascial plane is bound by the genioglossus, geniohyoid, and mylohyoid muscles.

Answer B is incorrect. The parapharyngeal fascial plane runs from the base of the skull to the hyoid bone, and it is bound laterally by the masticator and retropharyngeal space and medially by the oropharynx.

Answer C is incorrect. The masticator fascial plane is formed by the temporal, pterygoids, and masseter muscle.

Answer E is incorrect. The parotid fascial plane encompasses the parotid gland.

46. **The correct answer is C.** In an emergency situation where an airway must be obtained, an incision is made by palpating the membrane inferior to the thyroid cartilage and superior to the cricoid cartilage, thus, the cricothyroid membrane. This location will bypass any superior airway obstruction or laryngospasm, and allow air into the trachea to maintain oxygen distribution to the lungs.

Answer A is incorrect. An incision here would not directly place you into an airway.

Answer B is incorrect. An incision into the trachea would be considered a tracheotomy.

Answer D is incorrect. An incision into the thyroid gland would not directly place you into an airway.

Answer E is incorrect. An incision between the left 3rd and 4th intercostal muscles, laterally, would access an airspace, but also cause a pneumothorax.

47. **The correct answer is E.** When attempting an inferior alveolar nerve block, the parotid gland may be infiltrated if the needle is advanced too far posteriorly. Thus, CN VII can be damaged, which would cause an ipsilateral facial paralysis.

Answer A is incorrect. In order to pierce the buccinator muscle, one must direct the needle in a posterolateral direction.

Answer B is incorrect. In order to pierce the lateral pterygoid muscle, one must direct the needle in superior direction.

Answer C is incorrect. In order to pierce the medial pterygoid muscle, one must direct the needle in an inferolateral direction.

Answer D is incorrect. In order to pierce the mylohyoid muscle, one must direct the needle in an inferomedial direction.

48. **The correct answer is C.** The pterygomandibular raphe is formed by the convergence of the buccinator and the superior pharyngeal constrictor. These two muscles meet on the anterior border to the mandibular ramus.

Answer A is incorrect. The superior pharyngeal constrictor and mylohyoid muscles do not meet to form the pterygomandibular raphe.

Answer B is incorrect. The medial pterygoid and mylohyoid do not meet to form the pterygomandibular raphe.

Answer D is incorrect. The buccinator and mylohyoid muscles do not meet to form the pterygomandibular raphe.

Answer E is incorrect. The medial pterygoid and superior pharyngeal constrictor do not meet to form the pterygomandibular raphe.

49. **The correct answer is B.** In order to achieve an inferior alveolar nerve block in a particular mandibular quadrant, one must first locate the area where the inferior alveolar nerve enters the mandibular body. After exiting the cranial base via the foramen ovale, CN V3 courses inferiorly along the anteromedial border of the ramus and gives off numerous branches. It is within the coronoid notch, a depression on the anteromedial border of the ramus, that inferior alveolar branch is exposed and most vulnerable to anesthetic deposition. The inferior alveolar nerve then enters the body of the mandible via the mandibular foramen, provides sensory to the mandibular posterior teeth, and exits anteriorly via the mental foramen.

Answer A is incorrect. The lingula is located on the medial border of the ramus and connects the sphenomandibular ligament.

Answer C is incorrect. The antilingula is located on the lateral border of the ramus and marks the position of the lingula (on the medial border).

Answer D is incorrect. Palpating the angle of the mandible would not assist in locating the inferior alveolar nerve. It is located too far inferior.

Answer E is incorrect. The external oblique ridge of the mandible would not assist in locating the inferior alveolar nerve. It is located too far anterior.

50. **The correct answer is A.** The horizontal fibers of the PDL run from the cementum, at right angles, to the alveolar bone.

    Answer B is incorrect. The apical fibers extend from the apical region of cementum to alveolar bone.

    Answer C is incorrect. The interradicular fibers run from radicular cementum to interradicular alveolar bone (ONLY in multirooted teeth)

    Answer D is incorrect. The transseptal fibers run from cementum to cementum of two adjacent teeth.

    Answer E is incorrect. The oblique fibers run from cementum to alveolar bone in an oblique fashion.

51. **The correct answer is D.** The principal collagen fibers of the periodontal ligament are composed mostly of Type I collagen, as well as some Type III.

    Answer A is incorrect. Type I collagen fibers comprise tendons and parts of bone.

    Answer B is incorrect. Type II collagen fibers comprise hyaline and articular cartilage.

    Answer C is incorrect. Type III collagen fibers comprise bone, tendon, and cartilage, amongst other connective tissue.

    Answer E is incorrect. Principal collagen fibers of the PDL are not made of Type III collagen.

52. **The correct answer is E.** Fibroblasts are the most abundant cells of the PDL. They are

necessary to produce the extensive extracellular matrix of the PDL, namely the ground substance (which is made of water (~ 70%)) and proteoglygans, glycosaminoglycans, glycoproteins.

Answer A is incorrect. Lymphocytes are located within the PDL, but are not the most abundant cells.

Answer B is incorrect. Neutrophils are located within the PDL, but are not the most abundant cells.

Answer C is incorrect. Osteoblasts are located within the PDL, but are not the most abundant cells.

Answer D is incorrect. Cementoclasts are located within the PDL, but are not the most abundant cells.

53. **The correct answer is A.** The lesser palatine artery is not part of Kiesselbach plexus. This plexus of five arterial anastomoses includes the above arteries, as well as the greater palatine artery. Any of these vessels are typically involved in cases of epitasis owing to trauma to the nasal mucosa.

    Answer B is incorrect. The sphenopalatine artery is considered a part of Kiesselbach plexus.

    Answer C is incorrect. The lateral nasal branches of the facial artery are considered a part of Kiesselbach plexus.

    Answer D is incorrect. The superior labial artery is considered a part of Kiesselbach plexus.

    Answer E is incorrect. The anterior ethmoid arteries of internal carotid artery are considered a part of Kiesselbach plexus.

54. **The correct answer is E.** The temporal bone is not part of the orbit. The orbit of the eye is composed of seven separate bones: frontal, zygoma, sphenoid, lacrimal, maxilla, palatine, and ethmoid.

    Answer A is incorrect. The frontal bone contributes to part of the orbital cavity.

    Answer B is incorrect. The zygoma bone contributes to part of the orbital cavity.

Answer C is incorrect. The ethmoid bone contributes to part of the orbital cavity.

Answer D is incorrect. The lacrimal bone contributes to part of the orbital cavity.

55. **The correct answer is B.** The ophthalmic artery serves as the major blood supply of the eye and orbit. It is a branch of the internal carotid and, after branching, enters the orbit via the optic canal (along with CN II).

Answer A is incorrect. The facial artery supplies blood to the superficial facial tissues.

Answer C is incorrect. The maxillary artery supplies blood to the internal maxillary area.

Answer D is incorrect. The transverse facial artery supplies blood to the masseter muscle and parotid gland.

Answer E is incorrect. The infraorbital artery supplies blood to the anterior maxillary teeth and some extraocular muscles.

56. **The correct answer is D.** The masseter muscle has both a deep (zygomatic arch) and superficial (zygomatic process of maxilla) as its origin, and a superficial (angle of mandible) and deep (lateral ramus) insertion. This muscle of mastication serves as an elevator of the mandible, as well as assisting in retrusion and lateral excursions (ipsilaterally) of the mandible.

Answer A is incorrect. The lateral pterygoid muscle attaches to the articular disk (of the TMJ) and originates from the lateral pterygoid plate of the sphenoid bone.

Answer B is incorrect. The temporalis muscle originates on the temporal bone and inserts into the coronoid process.

Answer C is incorrect. The buccinator muscle attaches to the pterygomandibular raphe and originates from the alveolar processes of the maxilla and mandible.

Answer E is incorrect. The medial pterygoid muscle at the medial border of the mandible and originates from the lateral pterygoid plate of the sphenoid bone.

57. **The correct answer is D.** The superior orbital fissure is located between the greater and lesser wings of the sphenoid bone, in the posterior portion of the orbit. This foramina transmits CN III, IV, V1, VI, and superior ophthalmic vein. These nerves then provide motor function to the musculature associated with eye movement (III, IV, VI), glandular function (lacrimal of V1), and sensation (frontal and nasociliary of V1).

Answer A is incorrect. The superior orbital fissure is not located between the lesser wing of the sphenoid and frontal bones.

Answer B is incorrect. The superior orbital fissure is not located between the ethmoid and maxilla bones.

Answer C is incorrect. The superior orbital fissure is not located between the greater wing of the sphenoid and maxilla bones.

Answer E is incorrect. The superior orbital fissure is not located between the lesser wing of the sphenoid and ethmoid bones.

58. **The correct answer is A.** The nasolacrimal duct drains into the inferior meatus of the nasal cavity.

Answer B is incorrect. The lacrimal gland, which is located in the superolateral portion of the orbit, produces tears which are collected into the lacrimal puncta.

Answer C is incorrect. Tears wash across the globe in a superolateral → inferomedial direction.

Answer D is incorrect. The puncta then drains into inferior and superior lacrimal canals and joins the lacrimal sac before draining into the nasolacrimal duct.

Answer E is incorrect. The lacrimal sac drains directly into the nasolacrimal duct.

59. **The correct answer is D.** The lacrimal glands are serous secreting.

Answer A is incorrect. The lacrimal gland receives postganglionic parasympathetic fibers via the lacrimal nerve.

Answer B is incorrect. Preganglionic fibers to the lacrimal gland synapse at the pterygopalatine ganglion.

Answer C is incorrect. Preganglionic fibers to the lacrimal gland are carried via greater petrosal nerve.

Answer E is incorrect. The superior salivatory nucleus sends preganglionic fibers to the lacrimal gland.
Note: The paired lacrimal glands receive parasympathetic innervation via the following pathway: superior salivatory nucleus (of brainstem) → greater petrosal nerve/VII (preganglionics) → pterygopalatine ganglion → lacrimal nerve/V1 (postganglionics) → lacrimal gland and serous fluid production.

60. **The correct answer is B.** The platysma, considered a muscle of facial expression, is innervated by the facial nerve (CN VII).

Answer A is incorrect. The trigeminal nerve innervates the muscles of mastication.

Answer C is incorrect. The glossopharyngeal nerve innervates the stylopharyngeal muscle.

Answer D is incorrect. The spinal accessory muscle innervates the trapezius and sternocleidomastoid muscles.

Answer E is incorrect. The vagus nerve innervates multiple involuntary muscles.

61. **The correct answer is C.** The subcutaneous layer of neck fascia contains lymphatic vessels. This layer of fascia is also known as the superficial cervical fascia, and also contains blood vessels, (cutaneous) nerves, fat, and the anterolateral portion of the platysma. Tissue layers of the neck proceed as follows (superficial → deep): skin → superficial/subcutaneous fascia → deep/muscular fascia (investing → pretracheal → prevertebral). The deep fascial layer supports the thyroid gland, musculature, and deep lymph nodes.

Answer A is incorrect. The pretracheal layer contains the pharynx, trachea, thyroid, esophagus, and larynx.

Answer B is incorrect. The prevertebral layer contains the subclavian vein and brachial nerves.

Answer D is incorrect. The investing layer contains the trapezius muscle.

62. **The correct answer is A.** The falciform ligament helps suspend the liver by connecting it to the anterior abdominal wall. It also contains the ligamentum teres.

Answer B is incorrect. The gastrocolic ligament connects the greater curvature of the stomach to the transverse colon.

Answer C is incorrect. The hepatoduodenal ligament connects liver to first part of duodenum.

Answer D is incorrect. The gastroduodenal ligament connects lesser curvature of stomach to duodenum.

Answer E is incorrect. The gastrohepatic ligament connects liver to the lesser curvature of the stomach.

63. **The correct answer is E.** Teniae coli are three smooth muscle bands which are located within the colon.

Answer A is incorrect. Epiploic appendages are fatty globules on the serosal surface of the colon.

Answer B is incorrect. Lymphoid tissue of the cecum would be considered GALT (gut-associated lymphoid tissue).

Answer C is incorrect. Formed pouches within the colon wall are called haustra.

Answer D is incorrect. Fingerlike projections involved with absorption in the intestine are called villi.

64. **The correct answer is E.** The cerebellum is involved with coordinating skeletal muscle movements of the body, including maintenance of posture and equilibrium. Proprioceptive/positional inputs are received via the dorsal columns.

Answer A is incorrect. The medulla controls autonomic functions of the body.

Answer B is incorrect. The pons serves as a relay center between the cerebrum and cerebellum.

Answer C is incorrect. The cerebrum is the part of the brain which functions in memory, olfaction, communication, and motor skills.

Answer D is incorrect. The thalamus is involved with sleep and is intimately involved with numerous other functions from different regions of the brain.

65. **The correct answer is B.** Hyaline is the only type of cartilage which has the ability to calcify. This is seen in formation of the condyle. Also, hyaline cartilage is found within long bones (articulating surfaces), nose, trachea, bronchi, and costal cartilages of ribs.

    Answer A is incorrect. Fibrocartilage does not have the ability to calcify.

    Answer C is incorrect. Elastic cartilage does not have the ability to calcify.

    Answer D is incorrect. Hyaline cartilage does have the ability to calcify, but elastic does not.

    Answer E is incorrect. Hyaline cartilage does have the ability to calcify, but fibrocartilage does not.

66. **The correct answer is A.** The endosteum of bone is one-cell thick, and is located on the inner surface of bone (whereas, periosteum surrounds the outer surface of bone). This layer is mostly osteoprogenitor cells, and also contains bone marrow.

    Answer B is incorrect. The haversian canals are formed by lamellae within compact bone. They offer a means of communication between osteocytes.

    Answer C is incorrect. The Volkmann canals offer connection between the periosteum and osteons. They are perpendicular to haversian canals.

    Answer D is incorrect. Lacuna is the area which surrounds an osteocyte.

    Answer E is incorrect. The periosteal layer is a fibrous connective tissue capsule which also holds osteoprogenitor cells, as well as fibroblasts and collagen.

67. **The correct answer is E.** An example of a syndesmosis involves the radius and ulna bones.

    Answer A is incorrect. A gomphosis is a joint such as a tooth in socket.

    Answer B is incorrect. The cranial bones are held together by cranial/sutural joints.

    Answer C is incorrect. The TMJ is a synovial joint.

    Answer D is incorrect. The epiphyseal plates of long bones are synchondroses.

68. **The correct answer is C.** The amount of hematocrit found in blood is actually a measure of the erythrocyte percentage. Normally, in males the value is 45%; in females it is 40%.

    Answer A is incorrect. Blood, as a whole, is 55% plasma and 45% formed elements/cellular material.

    Answer B is incorrect. Albumin regulates the vascular oncotic pressure.

    Answer D is incorrect. Another portion of plasma is comprised of 8% protein (55% albumin, 38% globulins, 7% clotting factors/ fibrinogen), and the remainder (2%) is electrolytes, blood gases, hormones, enzymes, and metabolic products. The formed elements include erythrocytes, leukocytes, and platelets.

    Answer E is incorrect. Plasma is broken down as 80% water.

69. **The correct answer is D.** Granulocytes include neutrophils, basophils, and eosinophils.

    Answer A is incorrect. T cells are formed from lymphoid stem cells. They are lymphocytes.

    Answer B is incorrect. Macrophages are formed from myeloid stem cells. They are considered myelogenous cells.

    Answer C is incorrect. Platelets are formed from the breakdown of megakaryocytes.

Answer E is incorrect. B cells are formed from lymphoid cells. They are lymphocytes.

Note: The process of hematopoiesis begins with pluripotent stem cells, which are then capable of forming lymphoid (T and B cells) or myeloid (granulocyte, monocyte, erythroblast, megakaryocyte) stem cells. Hematopoiesis is regulated by colony stimulating factors and erythropoietin, mostly, and occurs primarily in the bone marrow. Lymphocytes then mature in the lymphatic tissue.

70. **The correct answer is B.** The chromaffin cells of the adrenal glands are located within the inner/medullary portion of the gland, and are of neural crest origin.

Answer A is incorrect. The cells of the zona fasciculata are of mesodermal origin.

Answer C is incorrect. The cells of the zona glomerulosa are of mesodermal origin.

Answer D is incorrect. The cells of the zona reticularis are of mesodermal origin.

71. **The correct answer is A.** The muscularis uvula (CN XI) constricts to shorten the velum.

Answer B is incorrect. The palatopharyngeus (CN X) depresses the velum, as well as raises and constricts the pharynx.

Answer C is incorrect. The palatoglossal muscle (CN X) works to raise the velum.

Answer D is incorrect. The levator veli palatini (CN X) works to raise the velum.

Answer E is incorrect. The tensor veli palatini (CN V) tenses the velum.
Note: Failure of these muscles to function leads to velopharyngeal incompetence.

72. **The correct answer is B.** The nucleus ambiguus (CN X) is located within the medulla oblongata, and receives sensory afferents from the pharynx. It sends special visceral efferents to the pharyngeal constrictors, palatopharyngeus, levator veli palatine, palatoglossus, and laryngeal musculature.

Answer A is incorrect. The superior salivatory nucleus functions with the facial nerve to control motor stimulation to various glands.

Answer C is incorrect. The inferior salivatory nucleus functions with the glossopharyngeal nerve to control motor stimulation to the parotid gland.

Answer D is incorrect. The facial nucleus is a lower motor neuron which controls the muscles of facial movement.

Answer E is incorrect. The nucleus of the solitary tract receives afferents from cranial nerve VII, IX, X, and XI. It functions with special sensation (taste).

73. **The correct answer is C.** The pharyngeal plexus is innervated by CNs IX, X, and XI. Thus, motor innervation is sent to the pharyngeal constrictors (IX and X), palatoglossus (X), palatopharyngeus (XI), and cricopharyngeus (X).

Answers A, B, D, and E are incorrect. See above.

74. **The correct answer is C.** The stapedius muscle receives motor stimulus from a branch of the facial nerve (CN VII). It is important to distinguish this from innervation to the tensor tympani (CN V3).

Answer A is incorrect. Cranial nerve V1 does not provide motor stimulation to any muscles of the ear.

Answer B is incorrect. Cranial nerve V2 does not provide motor stimulation to any muscles of the ear.

Answer D is incorrect. Cranial nerve V3 provides motor innervation to the tensor tympani (a muscle of the middle ear).

Answer E is incorrect. Cranial nerve VIII does not provide motor innervations to any muscles of the ear. It is purely sensory.

75. **The correct answer is B.** The papillary layer of the lamina propria contains fingerlike projections that interdigitate with the epithelial rete pegs. This wavy, ridgelike interface can

be appreciated histologically to differentiate between the epithelium and connective tissue.

Answer A is incorrect. The stratum granulosum is the layer which contains live cells, such as squamous cells.

Answer C is incorrect. The stratum corneum is the outermost layer of cells (nonliving) which protect the skin.

Answer D is incorrect. The reticular layer of the lamina propria is the innermost layer. It is synthesized by connective tissue.

Answer E is incorrect. The stratum spinosum helps to provide structural support by synthesizing intermediate filaments to join adjacent cell layers.

76. **The correct answer is A.** The inner enamel epithelium provides the formative cells of the enamel structure of teeth. These cells, along with the outer enamel epithelium, are considered the enamel organ, and form during the cap stage of tooth development. The enamel organ is altogether a downgrowth of the dental lamina.

    Answer B is incorrect. The dental follicle gives rise to cementoblasts, osteoblasts, and fibroblasts.

    Answer C is incorrect. The dental papilla contains the odontoblasts. It forms the pulp and dentin.

    Answer D is incorrect. Both the dental follicle and papilla are not the formative cells of the tooth.

    Answer E is incorrect. The IEE contains the formative cells of enamel, but not the dental papilla.
    Note: The tooth germ is comprised of the enamel organ, dental papilla, and dental follicle.

77. **The correct answer is B.** Ameloblasts begin secreting the enamel matrix after the odontoblasts first form dentin. Preameloblasts are first formed when the inner enamel epithelium elongates and becomes columnar. Once

this occurs, the dental papilla nearby follows suit, and differentiates into odontoblasts. Odontoblasts then begin to secrete the dentin matrix. Enamel matrix deposition then follows via ameloblasts.

Answer A is incorrect. During the cap stage, the cells of the tooth begin to arrange. The dental papilla, dental follicle, and enamel organ are all present.

Answer C is incorrect. Ameloblasts do not begin to secrete enamel matrix prior to odontoblast formation of dentin.

Answer D is incorrect. Ameloblasts begin to secrete dentin prior to root formation.

Answer E is incorrect. Ameloblasts begin to secrete dentin prior to the cap stage.

78. **The correct answer is C.** The vestibular lamina separates the lips and cheeks (externally) from the jaw structures (internally) in the developing fetus.

    Answer A is incorrect. The tuberculum impar forms the central part of the tongue.

    Answer B is incorrect. The buccopharyngeal membrane separates the primitive stomodeum from the pharynx.

    Answer D is incorrect. Hypobranchial eminence forms the root of the tongue.

    Answer E is incorrect. The lateral lingual swellings form the lateral aspects of the tongue.

79. **The correct answer is B.** The ethmoid bone contains the cribriform plate. This structure is located in the superiormost portion of the nasal cavity, and transmits sensory afferents by way of CN I from the olfactory epithelium. The olfactory nerve projects to the primary olfactory/pyriform cortex.

    Answer A is incorrect. The sphenoid bone does not contain the cribriform plate.

    Answer C is incorrect. The frontal bone does not contain the cribriform plate.

    Answer D is incorrect. The maxilla does not contain the cribriform plate.

Answer E is incorrect. The vomer does not contain the cribriform plate.

80. **The correct answer is A.** The nasopalatine nerve supplies sensory innervation to the mucosa of the anterior hard palate. This nerve is a branch of CN V3.

    Answer B is incorrect. The middle superior alveolar nerve supplies sensation to the adult premolars and buccal gingival. It is a branch of CN V2.

    Answer C is incorrect. The posterior superior alveolar nerve supplies sensation to the adult molars and buccal gingival. It is a branch of CN V2.

    Answer D is incorrect. The greater palatine nerve supplies sensation to the hard palate mucosa and anterior portion of the soft palate.

    Answer E is incorrect. The lesser palatine nerve supplies sensation to the soft palate.

81. **The correct answer is D.** The joint created between cervical vertebrae 1 (axis) and 2 (atlas) contains no intervertebral disk. This allows for an increased range of motion for the axis (and, thus, the head), on the atlas.

    Answer A is incorrect. There is an intervertebral disk in the joint between C4 and C5.

    Answer B is incorrect. There is an intervertebral disk in the joint between C5 and C6.

    Answer C is incorrect. There is an intervertebral disk in the joint between C2 and C3.

82. **The correct answer is A.** The spinal accessory nerve is a combination of motor rootlets from C1 to C5. Once these nerves unite, they pass back through the foramen magnum, then exit the cranium via the jugular foramen as CN XI.

    Answer B is incorrect. C3 is part of the ansa cervicalis. C4 is a part of the cervical plexus, and C5 part of the brachial plexus, as well as the cervical plexus. C3-C5 also form the phrenic nerve.

    Answer C is incorrect. C6 is part of the brachial plexus.

Answer D is incorrect. C1-C3 forms the ansa cervicalis.

Answer E is incorrect. C1 and C2 are part of the ansa cervicalis.

83. **The correct answer is A.** The right carotid artery is a branch of the brachiocephalic trunk. Once giving off the carotid, the brachiocephalic trunk then continues as the subclavian artery. This then branches off as the thyrocervical, vertebral, and suprascapular arteries. The transverse cervical is a branch of the thyrocervical artery.

    Answer B is incorrect. The thyrocervical artery is a branch of the subclavian.

    Answer C is incorrect. The suprascapular artery is a branch of the subclavian.

    Answer D is incorrect. The transverse cervical artery is a branch of the subclavian.

    Answer E is incorrect. The vertebral artery is a branch of the subclavian.

84. **The correct answer is D.** The external jugular vein is formed by a communication between the posterior auricular and posterior retromandibular veins. This structure drains the skin, parotid gland, and musculature of the face and neck before emptying into the subclavian vein.

    Answer A is incorrect. The retromandibular vein unites and continues on with the facial vein.

    Answer B is incorrect. The maxillary and anterior facial veins do not meet and form any structures.

    Answer C is incorrect. The anterior and posterior retromandibular veins do not meet and form any structures.

    Answer E is incorrect. The retromandibular vein unites and continues on with the facial vein.

85. **The correct answer is A.** The stylomandibular ligament has its origin at the styloid process, which projects from the temporal bone. The ligament then inserts into the angle of the

mandible. It is also considered an accessory ligament to the temporomandibular joint.

Answer B is incorrect. The sphenomandibular ligament has its origin at the sphenoid bone.

Answer C is incorrect. The stylomandibular ligament does not have its origin at the occipital bone.

Answer D is incorrect. The stylomandibular ligament does not have its origin at the maxillary bone.

Answer E is incorrect. Stylomandibular ligament does not have its origin at the parietal bone.

86. **The correct answer is D.** The frontal bone forms as two separate entities, which later fuse together to appear as one bone. Occipital, sphenoid, and ethmoid bones each are unpaired, singular bones of the cranium.

    Answers A, B, and C are incorrect. See above.

87. **The correct answer is D.** The mylohyoid muscle attaches superiorly at the mylohyoid line, which is located on the medial portion of the mandible. The muscle then tracks inferiorly and eventually attaches to the body of the hyoid bone.

    Answers A, B, C, and E are incorrect. See above.

88. **The correct answer is C.** The mylohyoid nerve (branch of CN V3) innervates the anterior belly of the digastric muscle, which is considered part of the suprahyoid musculature of the neck. This nerve also innervates the mylohyoid muscle.

    Answer A is incorrect. The inferior alveolar nerve (branch of CN V3) innervates the dentition of the mandible. It continues on anteriorly as the mental nerve.

    Answer B is incorrect. The mental nerve (branch of CN V3), a continuation of the inferior alveolar nerve, innervates the lower lip and buccal mucosa of anterior mandible.

Answer D is incorrect. The auriculotemporal nerve (branch of CN V3) provides sensory innervations to the auricle, tympanic membrane, and external auditory meatus. It also innervates skin of the temporal region of the head.

Answer E is incorrect. The facial nerve (CN VII) innervates the muscles of facial expression.

89. **The correct answer is B.** The ansa cervicalis is comprised of cervical nerves 1-3, and provides motor innervation to the infrahyoid muscles of the neck (omohyoid, sternohyoid, thyrohyoid, sternothyroid). As a generality, these muscles work together to depress the hyoid and larynx.

    Answer A is incorrect. Nerves C4-C6 are not part of the ansa cervicalis. C4 provides innervations to the cervical plexus and phrenic nerve. C5 provides innervation to the brachial plexus, cervical plexus, and phrenic nerve. C6 is part of the brachial plexus.

    Answer C is incorrect. The lesser occipital nerve is a branch of C2 and innervates the scalp and lateral head.

    Answer D is incorrect. The greater occipital nerve is a branch of C2. It innervates the scalp and areas of skin covering the parotid gland.

    Answer E is incorrect. C6-C8 are part of the brachial plexus.

90. **The correct answer is A.** The ophthalmic artery is a branch of the internal carotid artery. The other arteries listed in the question are branches of the external carotid artery, as well as the facial, maxillary, lingual, and temporal arteries.

    Answer B is incorrect. The ascending pharyngeal artery is a branch of the external carotid artery.

    Answer C is incorrect. The superior thyroid artery is a branch of the external carotid artery.

    Answer D is incorrect. The posterior auricular artery is a branch of the external carotid artery.

Answer E is incorrect. The occipital artery is a branch of the external carotid artery.

91. **The correct answer is B.** The crista galli is a superior projection of the ethmoid bone. It is located in the midline of the cranium.

    Answers A, C, D and E are incorrect. See above.

92. **The correct answer is B.** As one is preparing a cavity preparation on the crown of a permanent tooth, once the bur penetrates through the enamel and meets the dentinoenamel junction, from the list given in the question, the first structure penetrated would be the mantle dentin, which is classified as the initial 150-μm dentin laid down in a tooth. The odontoblast then secretes dentin matrix as it retreats toward the pulp.

    Answer A is incorrect. The circumpulpal dentin, as well as odontoblasts, would be located nearer the pulp.

    Answer C is incorrect. Odontoblasts are located most closely to the pulp.

    Answer D is incorrect. Radicular dentin is within the root, thus, would not first be encountered in preparing the crown of a tooth.

    Answer E is incorrect. Circumpulpal dentin is the layer just occlusal to that of the odontoblasts.

93. **The correct answer is D.** Raschkow (parietal) plexus is located within the cell free zone of Weil, a portion of the pulp which is lacking cellular material in the mature tooth. Also located here is vasculature of the tooth.

    Answer A is incorrect. The cementum layer of the tooth contains attachments of the periodontal ligament fibers.

    Answer B is incorrect. The cell rich zone of the pulp contains undifferentiated mesenchymal cells. It also contains fibroblasts.

    Answer C is incorrect. The dentin layer of the tooth contains odontoblastic processes and other proteins.

    Answer E is incorrect. The core of the dental pulp contains the tooth's vasculature and nerve supply.

94. **The correct answer is B.** The stratum basale of the skin and the spermatogonium (of the Sertoli cell) are similar relative to the fact they are both the least differentiated, most immature cellular layer in the development of their respective structures.

    Answer A is incorrect. The spermatid is a form of male gamete. It is $1^{1}/_{2}$N.

    Answer C is incorrect. The primary spermatocyte is a form of male gamete. It is 2N (diploid).

    Answer D is incorrect. The secondary spermatocyte is a form of male gamete. It is N (haploid).

    Answer E is incorrect. The junctional complex consists of tight junction, intermediate junction, and desmosome.

95. **The correct answer is A.** The macula densa is a structure which is located on the distal convoluted tubule. It is a specialized collection of cells that function as part of the juxtaglomerular apparatus (along with the juxtaglomerular cells) to monitor body fluid concentration, and, thus, systemically release renin when appropriate.

    Answer B is incorrect. The Bowman capsule is a part of the nephron. It initially filters the solute through which will enter the nephron.

    Answer C is incorrect. The loop of Henle is a part of the nephron. Its primary function is reabsorption of water and solutes via a countercurrent multiplier.

    Answer D is incorrect. The proximal convoluted tubule is a part of the nephron. Its primary function is the reabsorption of sodium.

    Answer E is incorrect. The collecting duct is a part of the nephron. Its primary function is the reuptake of water.

96. **The correct answer is D.** Of the following options, the lingual root of the maxillary 1st

molar would have the highest probability of becoming dislodged into the maxillary sinus upon excessive force of a hand instrument in an apical direction. The maxillary sinus typically dips down inferiorly as it encounters the region of the maxillary 1st molar. Thus, as the other options are placed anterior to this location, they would have a lower probability of sinus penetration than the lingual root of the maxillary 1st molar.

Answer A is incorrect. The buccal root of the maxillary 1st premolar would not typically fracture and become dislodged in the maxillary sinus. In most cases, it is placed too far anteriorly.

Answer B is incorrect. The root of the maxillary canine would not typically fracture and become dislodged in the maxillary sinus. In most cases, it is placed too far anteriorly.

Answer C is incorrect. The root of the maxillary lateral incisor would not typically fracture and become dislodged in the maxillary sinus. In most cases, it is placed too far anteriorly.

Answer E is incorrect. The lingual root of the maxillary 1st premolar would not typically fracture and become dislodged in the maxillary sinus. In most cases, it is placed too far anteriorly.

97. **The correct answer is E.** The parietal bone does not articulate with the zygoma.

    Answer A is incorrect. The zygoma articulates with the temporal bone posteriorly.

    Answer B is incorrect. The zygoma articulates with the maxilla anteriorly.

    Answer C is incorrect. The zygoma articulates with the frontal bone superiorly.

    Answer D is incorrect. The zygoma articulates with the sphenoid bone (specifically the greater wing) medially.

98. **The correct answer is D.** Luxation of the mandible occurs when the lower jaw becomes overextended in a manner that causes the condyles to sufficiently translate over the articular eminence. Thus, the condyles will

most likely be displaced in an anterior direction, necessitating hand manipulation of the mandible to reseat the condylar heads in the glenoid fossa. In the case of subluxation, the joint will autoreduce.

Answer A is incorrect. The mandibular condyles most likely would not luxate in a posterior and superior direction. This is because the articular eminence does not interrupt its path back into the joint.

Answer B is incorrect. The mandibular condyles most likely would not luxate in a posterior and inferior direction. This is because the articular eminence does not interrupt its path back into the joint.

Answer C is incorrect. The mandibular condyles most likely would not luxate in a lateral and inferior direction. This is because the articular eminence does not interrupt its path back into the joint.

Answer E is incorrect. The mandibular condyles most likely would not luxate in a medial direction. This is because the articular eminence does not interrupt its path back into the joint.

99. **The correct answer is D.** The inferior alveolar artery directly branches from the maxillary artery, which in turn is a branch of the external carotid artery.

    Answer A is incorrect. The inferior alveolar artery does not branch from the middle meningeal artery. The middle meningeal artery is a branch of the internal carotid and enters the skull through foramen spinosum. The middle meningeal artery is medial to the TMJ and can be injured during TMJ procedures.

    Answer B is incorrect. The inferior alveolar artery does not branch directly from the facial artery. The facial artery first branches off into the maxillary artery before it gives off the inferior alveolar.

    Answer C is incorrect. The inferior alveolar artery does not branch directly from the external carotid artery. The external carotid first branches off as the facial and then maxillary artery prior to the inferior alveolar.

Answer E is incorrect. The inferior alveolar artery does not branch from the buccal artery. This artery is a branch of the maxillary artery.

100. **The correct answer is C.** Bile is formed by hepatocytes within the liver. From here, bile is transported and stored within the gall bladder until it receives stimuli from enzymes which are secreted by the stomach and duodenum. From here, bile travels through a network of ducts from the gall bladder and eventually is deposited into the duodenum by way of the ampulla of Vater.

    Answer A is incorrect. The head of the pancreas produces insulin and glucagon, amongst other digestive enzymes.

    Answer B is incorrect. The gall bladder stores the bile which is produced by the liver.

    Answer D is incorrect. The tail of the pancreas produces insulin and glucagon, amongst other digestive enzymes.

    Answer E is incorrect. The duodenum produces the digestive enzymes cholecystokinin and secretin.

101. **The correct answer is C.** The medulla houses the nuclei of cranial nerves IX, X, and XII, thus, impairment of certain functions involving the glossopharyngeal, vagus, and hypoglossal nerves.

    Answer A is incorrect. CN V and VII nuclei are located in the pons.

    Answer B is incorrect. CN III and IV nuclei are located in the midbrain. CN VI is in the pons.

    Answer D is incorrect. CN XI nucleus is located in the medulla.

    Answer E is incorrect. CN V nucleus is located in the pons.

102. **The correct answer is D.** Somatostatin is produced by delta cells of the endocrine pancreas (ie, pancreatic islet cells). Somatostatin functions to inhibit glucagon and insulin.

Answer A is incorrect. Insulin is produced in the pancreatic beta cells of the islet of Langerhans.

Answer B is incorrect. Trypsinogen is a proenzyme produced by the exocrine pancreas.

Answer C is incorrect. Glucagon is produced in the pancreatic alpha cells of the islet of Langerhans.

Answer E is incorrect. The exocrine function of the pancreas would not be disturbed in this situation.

103. **The correct answer is A.** Eccrine, not apocrine, glands are involved with regulating body temperature. Eccrine glands, also known as sweat glands, also have myoepithelial and duct cells, as well as clear and dark, and are located throughout the body (except on lips and portions of the external genitalia). Eccrine cells receive sympathetic cholinergic innervation.

    Answer B is incorrect. Apocrine glands produce pheromones.

    Answer C is incorrect. Secretion of apocrine glands is via myoepithelial cells.

    Answer D is incorrect. Apocrine gland secretion is strictly serous fluid.

    Answer E is incorrect. Apocrine sweat gland cells receive sympathetic adrenergic innervation.

104. **The correct answer is E.** Fertilization occurs in the ampulla, which is the longest extension of the oviduct (a part of the fallopian tubes).

    Answer A is incorrect. The uterus is the site of embryonic and fetal development.

    Answer B is incorrect. The endometrium is the layer of the uterus which the zygote implants into (or is shed during menstruation).

    Answer C is incorrect. The ovary is the site of ovum development.

    Answer D is incorrect. The cervix produces fluid which bathes the vaginal cavity.

105. **The correct answer is A.** Hemidesmosomes provide attachment of the epithelial layer of the cell to the connective tissue layer.

   Answer B is incorrect. Zonula adherens (intermediate junction) is a beltlike junction around a cell while leaving an intercellular space.

   Answer C is incorrect. Zonula occludens (tight junction) is a beltlike junction around a cell which closes-off intercellular spaces between cells.

   Answer D is incorrect. Desmosomes (macula adherens) provide localized adhesion between adjacent cells.

   Answer E is incorrect. Gap junctions allow cell-to-cell communication.

106. **The correct answer is B.** The muscle spindle apparatus, which senses proprioception within a muscle, communicates with the CNS via A-gamma fibers.

   Answer A is incorrect. Touch sensation is mediated by A-beta fibers.

   Answer C is incorrect. Pressure sensation is mediated by A-beta fibers.

   Answer D is incorrect. Temperature sensation is mediated by C fibers.

   Answer E is incorrect. Sharp pain sensation is mediated by A-delta fibers.
   Note: A-alpha fibers function with proprioception and motor nerves, A-beta with sensory, touch, and pressure, and A-delta with sharp pain, temperature, and touch. B fibers are involved with preganglionic autonomic nerves, and C fibers with dull pain, temperature, and postganglionic autonomic nerves.

107. **The correct answer is C.** The trachea extends inferiorly in the superior mediastinum and bifurcates (marked by the carina) into right and left main stem bronchi. Main stem bronchi then divide (as they course inferiorly in each lung) into lobar bronchi, segmental bronchi, bronchioles, and then alveoli.

   Answer A is incorrect. Bronchioles are a continuation of the segmental bronchi, and lead into the alveoli.

   Answer B is incorrect. Segmental bronchi are a continuation of the lobar bronchi, and lead into the bronchioles.

   Answer D is incorrect. Alveoli are the terminal end of the bronchioles.

   Answer E is incorrect. Lobar bronchi are branches of the main stem bronchi, and lead into the segmental bronchi.

108. **The correct answer is D.** Hilar lymph nodes are located at the root of the lungs, and thus are involved in lymphatic drainage of the lungs.

   Answer B is incorrect. The supraclavicular nodes drain the head and neck, and are located laterally at the base of the neck, superior to the clavicle.

   Answer C is incorrect. Superficial cervical nodes are located along the sternocleidomastoid muscle and drain the head and neck.

   Answer E is incorrect. The occipital nodes are located at the posterior base of the skull and drain the scalp.

109. **The correct answer is E.** The lingual nerve provides presynaptic efferents to the submaxillary ganglion.

   Answer A is incorrect. The inferior alveolar nerve gives postsynaptic sensory innervation to the teeth of the mandible.

   Answer B is incorrect. The facial nerve mainly provides motor innervation to the muscles of facial expression.

   Answer C is incorrect. The buccinator nerve innervates the buccinator muscle.

   Answer D is incorrect. The maxillary nerve provides mainly sensory innervation to structures of the midface/maxillary region.

110. **The correct answer is D.** The sublingual gland drains into the oral cavity via the rivian ducts.

   Answer A is incorrect. The parotid gland drains by Stensen duct into the oral cavity.

Answer C is incorrect. The lacrimal glands drain via numerous interlobular ducts onto the globe.

Answer B is incorrect. The sebaceous glands empty into sweat pores.

Answer E is incorrect. The mammary glands drain by way of lactiferous ducts.

111. **The correct answer is C.** The pronephros does not give rise to any structures of the adult kidney. Rather, it regresses shortly after formation in the 4th week of fetal development. The pronephros forms first, followed by the mesonephros (gives rise to mesonephric duct and ureteric bud) and then metanephros (the adult kidney, formed by ureteric bud and metanephric mass). The early adult kidney forms in the pelvis before ascending into the abdominal region.

Answer A is incorrect. The ureteric bud contributes to the adult kidney.

Answer B is incorrect. The mesonephros gives rise to the ureteric bud and mesonephric duct.

Answer D is incorrect. The mesonephros forms before the metanephros.

Answer E is incorrect. The kidney initially forms in the pelvic region.

112. **The correct answer is A.** The Wolffian duct is synonymous with the mesonephric duct. Thus, it develops (in the male) into the ductus deferens, epididymis, ejaculatory duct, and seminal vesicles. It is obliterated in females.

Answers B, C, D and E are incorrect. The ureter, the collecting tubules, the ovaries and the uterus are NOT formed from the Wolffian duct.

113. **The correct answer is B.** Leptomeninges are formed from neural crest cells. The neural crest gives rise to sensory ganglia, dorsal root ganglia, Schwann cells, enterochromaffin cells, melanocytes, odontoblasts, parasympathetic/sympathetic ganglia, and parafollicular cells.

Mesenchymal cells of the neural tube give rise to microglia.

Answer A is incorrect. The ependymal cells are formed from neuroepithelial cells. They form the epithelial lining of the ventricles of the brain.

Answer C is incorrect. The astrocytes are formed from neuroepithelial cells. They are glial cells of the brain which work with endothelial cells.

Answer D is incorrect. The neuroblasts are formed from neuroepithelial cells. They give rise to neurons and glia.

Answer E is incorrect. The oligodendrocytes are formed from neuroepithelial cells. They offer insulation to axons.

114. **The correct answer is D.** Once fertilization occurs, the zygote undergoes cell division and cleavage. The first cell division leads to the blastomere (×2), then after multiple cleavage divisions, the morula forms, followed by the blastula.

Answer A is incorrect. The blastomere forms before the morula.

Answer B is incorrect. The zygote forms before the morula, and the blastomere prior to formation of the morula.

Answer C is incorrect. The zygote forms first, followed by the blastomere, morula, and blastula.

Answer E is incorrect. This order is reversed from the correct one.

115. **The correct answer is C.** The zona pellucida protects the zygote from the initial fertilization up until the multiple cleavages have occurred through the blastula stage. Once the blastula forms, the zona pellucida breaks down, and implantation into endometrial tissue of the uterus occurs.

Answer A is incorrect. The zona pellucida has already disintegrated by this point.

Answer B is incorrect. The zona pellucida has already disintegrated by this point.

Answer D is incorrect. The zona pellucida has already disintegrated by this point.

Answer E is incorrect. The zona pellucida has already disintegrated by this point.

116. **The correct answer is A.** Normal pregnancy involves implantation of the cleaved zygote into the uterine endometrial walls. Thus, if implantation does not occur here, it is considered ectopic.

    Answers B, C, D, and E are incorrect. The ovaries, the fallopian tubes, the cervix and the abdomen are potential locations of ectopic pregnancy.

117. **The correct answer is A.** Regarding sperm development, the 2nd meiotic cell division does not occur until postfertilization of the ovum. Thus, the most likely place for this to occur is within the uterine tube (where the sperm typically fertilizes the ovum).

    Answers B, C, D and E are incorrect. Meiosis II has not yet occurred at these points in development.

118. **The correct answer is B.** The masseter receives innervation from the 3rd branch of the trigeminal nerve.

    Answer A is incorrect. The risorius is innervated by CN VII. This muscle is involved with movement of the angle of the mouth.

    Answer C is incorrect. The orbicularis oris is innervated by CN VII. This muscle is involved with puckering of the lips.

    Answer D is incorrect. The mentalis is innervated by CN VII. This muscle elevates the skin on the chin.

    Answer E is incorrect. The buccinator is innervated by CN VII. This muscle compresses the buccal mucosa up against the dentition.
    Note: Also innervated from CN VII is the platysma, orbicularis oculi, frontalis, stapedius, and occipitalis muscles.

119. **The correct answer is B.** The mandibular branch of the trigeminal nerve is responsible for the efferent signaling of the jaw-jerk reflex.

This motion begins with tapping of the chin (mouth open in a physiologic rest position), thus, activating proprioceptive afferents of V3. Upon processing, efferents are sent by way of V3 which causes closure of the mouth.

Answer A is incorrect. CN V1 is responsible for sensation on the forehead and part of the upper face.

Answer C is incorrect. CN VII is responsible for movement of the muscles of facial expression.

Answer D is incorrect. CN V2 is responsible for sensation in the midface.

Answer E is incorrect. CN IX is responsible for motor innervations to the stylopharyngeus muscle and special sensation to the tongue.

120. **The correct answer is C.** The carotid sheath lies posterior to the thyroid gland. It contains the common carotid artery, jugular vein, and vagus nerve, as well as sympathetic nerves, lymph nodes, and carotid sinus nerve. The sheath begins at the root of the neck, extending medial to the sternocleidomastoid muscle and anterior to the scalene musculature, bilaterally, up to the base of the cranium.

    Answer A is incorrect. The sternocleidomastoid muscle lies lateral to the carotid sheath in the cervical region.

    Answer B is incorrect. The carotid sheath lies anterior to the scalene musculature in the cervical region.

    Answer D is incorrect. The carotid sheath contains the vagus nerve, jugular vein, and common carotid artery.

    Answer E is incorrect. The carotid sheath is associated with the carotid sinus nerve, sympathetic nerves, and lymph nodes.

121. **The correct answer is D.** The vagus nerve is contained within the anterior triangle of the neck.

    Answer A is incorrect. CN XII passes through the submandibular triangle prior to inserting into and innervating the tongue musculature.

Answer B is incorrect. The nerve to the mylohyoid passes through the submandibular triangle prior to innervating the mylohyoid muscle.

Answer C is incorrect. The lingual artery passes through the submandibular triangle after branching from the inferior alveolar artery and prior to inserting into the tongue.

Answer E is incorrect. The submandibular gland rests within the submandibular triangle.

Note: The submandibular triangle is bounded inferiorly by the bellies of the digastrics and superiorly by the inferior border of the mandible, the "roof" being the skin, superficial fascia, platysma, and deep fascia, and the "floor" being the mylohyoid and hyoglossus muscles. This formed area contains the submandibular gland and lymph nodes, hypoglossal and mylohyoid nerves, and lingual and facial arteries/veins.

122. **The correct answer is C.** The T4 dermatome refers pain to the area of the nipples.

Answer A is incorrect. As for the xiphoid process, it is relative to the T7 dermatome.

Answer B is incorrect. The umbilicus refers to the T10 dermatome.

Answer D is incorrect. The inguinal ligament refers to the L1 dermatome.

Answer E is incorrect. The neck refers to the C3 dermatome.

123. **The correct answer is A.** The main motor nucleus of the facial nerve is involved with motor movements of the facial musculature involved with expression. Thus, as the orbicularis oculi muscle mediates closing of the eyelids and its motor innervation is received via CN VII, one must suspect damage to the main motor nucleus of VII. Also affected by damage to this nuclei includes other muscles of facial expression, posterior belly of the digastric, stylohyoid, and stapedius muscles. Musculature which is involved with the upper face would be affected bilaterally, and of the lower face unilaterally.

Answer B is incorrect. The nucleus of the solitary tract mediates taste sensation.

Answer C is incorrect. The spinal trigeminal nucleus mediates pain and temperature.

Answer D is incorrect. The mesencephalic nucleus mediates proprioception.

Answer E is incorrect. The motor nucleus of V mediates motor sensation to masticatory musculature.

124. **The correct answer is C.** The caloric test is one of which nystagmus is initiated by application of warm and then cool water to the external auditory meatus. For example, cool water stimulation applied to the right ear will cause nystagmus to the left side, and warm water stimulation to the right ear will cause nystagmus to the right side.

Answer A is incorrect. Nystagmus can occur when irritation occurs to any or all of the following: labyrinth, vestibular nerve/nuclei, cerebellum, visual system, and cerebral cortex.

Answer B is incorrect. Nystagmus itself is a fast, involuntary movement of the eyes.

Answer D is incorrect. This is a test of the vestibuloocular reflex, involving CN VIII.

Answer E is incorrect. Nystagmus involves CN VIII lesions.

125. **The correct answer is B.** Damage to the tectospinal tract of the spinal cord would affect movement of the head.

Answer A is incorrect. The lateral spinothalamic tract of the spinal cord transmits sensation of pain and temperature.

Answer C is incorrect. The vestibulospinal tract transmits equilibrium sense.

Answer D is incorrect. The reticulospinal tract carries sensation involved with muscle tone and sweat gland function.

Answer E is incorrect. The anterior spinothalamic tract transmits touch and pressure sensation.

126. **The correct answer is A.** Smooth endoplasmic reticulum is an intracellular organelle which has differing functions dependent on its cellular location. For example, within the

liver, the SER is involved in the metabolism of glycogen and lipids, whereas in the adrenal cortex and testis, it functions in steroid anabolism as well as calcium sequestrum in skeletal and cardiac muscle.

Answer B is incorrect. Lysosomes contain digestive enzymes which breakdown invading pathogens and dead cells.

Answer C is incorrect. Peroxisomes contain enzymes which breakdown toxic products in the cell.

Answer D is incorrect. Rough endoplasmic reticulum is an organelle which produces proteins within a cell.

Answer E is incorrect. Mitochondria are organelles which produce the majority of ATP in a cell.

127. **The correct answer is D.** Parafollicular cells are located within the thyroid gland. Their function is to secrete calcitonin, which acts on the intestines, kidneys, and osteoclasts, to ultimately decrease the level of blood calcium.

Answer A is incorrect. Cortical bone does not contain parafollicular cells.

Answer B is incorrect. The kidney does not contain parafollicular cells. They do, though, contain other cells which produce hormones involved with acid-base balance.

Answer C is incorrect. The small intestine does not contain parafollicular cells. They contain cells which produce digestive enzymes, though.

Answer E is incorrect. The parathyroid gland does not contain parafollicular cells. They contain parathyroid cells which produce parathyroid hormone.

128. **The correct answer is A.** The esophagus, in normal conditions, is lined with nonkeratinized stratified squamous epithelium. This type of epithelium is found in areas of the body which are continually kept moist, and is a protective layer which turns over rapidly. Thus, in states of esophageal pathology, metaplastic changes may occur in the epithelium

which changes the lining layer from squamous to columnar (especially in the lower esophagus → as with Barrett esophagus).

Answer B is incorrect. Columnar epithelium is found in the stomach and intestines, amongst other areas.

Answer C is incorrect. Keratinized stratified squamous epithelium is found comprising the outer covering of skin.

Answer D is incorrect. Cuboidal epithelium is found lining the kidney tubules.

Answer E is incorrect. Pseudostratified squamous epithelium is found lining the trachea.

129. **The correct answer is A.** Sperm travels to the epididymis, where it matures and is stored until ejaculation.

Answer B is incorrect. The urethra serves as a pathway for the exit of ejaculate and urine from the male body.

Answer C is incorrect. The testis produces male sex hormones.

Answer D is incorrect. Sperm is produced in the seminiferous tubules (of the testis).

Answer E is incorrect. The prostate gland provides the fluid which mixes with sperm prior to ejaculation.

130. **The correct answer is B.** The skin uses ultraviolet light to produce vitamin D. Vitamin E is an essential vitamin, which must be ingested by humans. The skin functions include protection, homeostasis, synthesis, sensation, and excretion.

Answer A is incorrect. The skin functions to achieve the sensation of touch, pain, and pressure.

Answer C is incorrect. The skin serves to excrete via sweat glands.

Answer D is incorrect. The skin functions include homeostatic regulation of body temperature.

Answer E is incorrect. The skin provides protection against physical and chemical stresses.

131. The correct answer is C. The sphincter of Boyden is located in the common bile duct.

Answer A is incorrect. The ampulla of Vater contains the sphincter of Oddi, which allows communication between pancreatic duct and common bile duct.

Answer B is incorrect. The lower esophageal sphincter seals the opening into the stomach.

Answer D is incorrect. The rectum contains an internal and external sphincter.

Answer E is incorrect. The pyloric sphincter separates the stomach from the duodenum.

132. The correct answer is A. The posterior 1/3 of the tongue drains directly into the deep cervical lymph nodes.

Answer B is incorrect. The submental nodes drain the tip of the tongue, anterior floor of mouth, and anterior buccal mucosa/lip region.

Answer C is incorrect. The submandibular nodes drain the anterior 2/3 of the tongue, submental nodes, upper lip, cheek, gingiva of hard palate, all teeth (except mandibular anteriors), and posterior floor of mouth.

Answer D is incorrect. The rectopharyngeal nodes drain the posterior nasal cavity, nasopharynx, soft palate, middle ear, and external auditory meatus.

Answer E is incorrect. The supraclavicular nodes receive lymphatic drainage from the entire body, and are common sites of metastasis.

133. The correct answer is D. The cardiac glands of the gastric mucosa are exocrine acinar glands. These types of glands are defined by their secretory portion which is a saclike dilation. The other exocrine glands listed in question 133 are not particularly involved with the gastric mucosa.

Answer A is incorrect. Coiled glands have a secretory portion shaped like a coiled tube, and an example is the eccrine sweat gland.

Answer B is incorrect. The tubular cells have a tube-shaped secretory portion, and are involved in intestinal glands.

Answer C is incorrect. The tubuloacinar cells are a combination of tubular and acinar cells, and comprise the major salivary glands.

Answer E is incorrect. Apocrine cells are defined by their secretory mechanism (as they are defined by their secretory unit), thus, having their secretory portion released into the cytoplasm. Examples of such are mammary and apocrine sweat glands.

134. The correct answer is B. The red marrow does NOT contain fatty cells, although, it is the predominant marrow type in the mandibular ramus and condyles.

Answer A is incorrect. Both types of marrow are located within the medullary spaces of spongy bone.

Answer C is incorrect. The red marrow does also contain hematopoietic cells.

Answer D is incorrect. Yellow marrow contains fatty cells, and is the predominant marrow type of the maxilla and mandible.

Answer E is incorrect. Yellow marrow is the predominant marrow type in the maxilla and mandible.

135. The correct answer is A. The nasal cavities are lined by stratified squamous epithelium to withstand stresses, pseudostratified ciliated columnar which aid in absorption, and specialized olfactory cells for smelling sense.

Answers B, C, D and E are incorrect. The nasal cavity is not lined by these types of epithelium.

136. The correct answer is D. The superior laryngeal artery does not supply blood to the tongue; it supplies the musculature of the larynx.

Answer A is incorrect. The facial artery (specifically its branches) supplies blood to the tongue. It is a branch of the external carotid artery.

Answer B is incorrect. The ascending pharyngeal artery supplies blood to the tongue. It is a branch of the external carotid artery.

Answer C is incorrect. The lingual artery supplies blood to the tongue. It is a branch of the external carotid artery.

Answer E is incorrect. The external carotid artery (specifically its branches) supplies blood to the tongue.

137. **The correct answer is E.** The palatoglossus inserts on the posterolateral portion of the tongue, and, thus, would not be damaged if the anterior portion of the tongue was lacerated.

    Answer A is incorrect. The longitudinal muscle (intrinsic muscle of the tongue) could possibly be affected in this situation.

    Answer B is incorrect. The styloglossus (extrinsic muscle of the tongue) inserts into the tongue near its anterior portion. Thus, it could possibly be damaged in this situation.

    Answer C is incorrect. The hyoglossus (extrinsic muscle of the tongue) inserts into the tongue near its anterior portion. Thus, it could possibly be damaged in this situation.

    Answer D is incorrect. The transverse (intrinsic muscle of the tongue) could possibly be affected in this situation.

138. **The correct answer is B.** The vagus and hypoglossal nerves provide motor innervation to the tongue. Cranial nerve X innervates the palatoglossus muscle, which elevates the tongue. The other extrinsic muscles are innervated by cranial nerve XII (genioglossus (protrusion), hyoglossus (depression), and styloglossus (retraction)). The intrinsic musculature of the tongue is also innervated by the hypoglossal muscle.

    Answer A is incorrect. CN VII does not provide motor innervation to the tongue. It innervates the muscles of facial expression.

    Answer C is incorrect. CN VII does not provide motor innervation to the tongue. It innervates the muscles of facial expression.

    Answer D is incorrect. CN V does not provide motor innervation to the tongue. It innervates the muscles of mastication.

Answer E is incorrect. CN IX does not provide motor innervation to the tongue. It innervates the stylopharyngeus muscle.

139. **The correct answer is A.** Receptors for sweet sensation are mostly congregated at the anterior tip of the tongue.

    Answer B is incorrect. As for salt receptors, they are bilaterally located, just a bit posterior to the sweet receptors.

    Answer C is incorrect. Bitter taste receptors are mostly found at the posterior portion of the tongue.

    Answer D is incorrect. Sour taste is sensed bilaterally in the middle portion of the tongue.

140. **The correct answer is A.** Somites are comprised of mesoderm and line the primitive neural tube. They eventually form dermatomes, myotomes, and sclerotomes. Sclerotome cells develop into vertebrae and ribs.

    Answer B is incorrect. Myotomes form skeletal muscle components of the body.

    Answer C is incorrect. Dermatomes eventually develop into connective tissue of the skin.

    Answer D is incorrect. Myotomes form skeletal muscle components of the body.

    Answer E is incorrect. Myotomes form skeletal muscle components of the body.

141. **The correct answer is D.** The formation of the inferior nasal turbinate/concha is not altered in a complete bilateral cleft palate. In this situation, there is incomplete fusion of the lip, primary (anterior) palate, secondary (posterior) palate, and alveolar process. Thus, surgical closure is necessary to restore normal anatomy.

    Answers A, B, C, and E are incorrect. Formation of these are compromised in complete bilateral palatal clefting.

142. **The correct answer is B.** Fusion of the reduced enamel epithelium with oral epithelium marks eruption of a tooth. This action forms the dentogingival junction/epithelial attachment.

Answer A is incorrect. Elongation of the cervical loop and formation of HERS is indicative of the root formation stage.

Answer C is incorrect. Disappearance of the enamel knot occurs in the bell stage.

Answer D is incorrect. The cap stage demonstrates formation of the enamel organ.

Answer E is incorrect. Merging of the OEE with IEE occurs during the appositional stage.

143. **The correct answer is A.** Cartilage is an avascular substance. This type of substance is formed by chondroblasts secreting an extensive extracellular matrix.

    Answer B is incorrect. Chondrocytes reside in lacunae once they have completed deposition of cartilaginous matrix.

    Answer C is incorrect. These chondroblasts then reside as chondrocytes within their individual lacunae.

    Answer D is incorrect. Cartilage can be specialized in different areas of the body (ie, hyaline, elastic, and fibrocartilage).

    Answer E is incorrect. Cartilage can grow by both interstitial and appositional stages.

144. **The correct answer is C.** The typical function of megakaryocytes is fragmentation into platelets. Platelets are the primary factor involved in the clotting of blood.

    Answer A is incorrect. Monocytes form macrophages.

    Answer B is incorrect. B cells are lymphocytes which are involved with the immune reaction.

    Answer D is incorrect. Erythroblasts form red blood cells.

    Answer E is incorrect. Granulocytes form white cells.

145. **The correct answer is C.** When the body breaks down erythrocytes, the by-products are excreted by the liver in the form of bile pigment. Thus, high levels of bile pigment would be indicative of increased breakdown of erythrocytes. The other cells would not cause such to occur.

    Answer A is incorrect. Increased breakdown of neutrophils would not cause high levels of bile excretion.

    Answer B is incorrect. Increased breakdown of eosinophils would not cause high levels of bile excretion.

    Answer D is incorrect. Increased breakdown of platelets would not cause high levels of bile excretion.

    Answer E is incorrect. Increased breakdown of macrophages would not cause high levels of bile excretion.

146. **The correct answer is A.** GCF is a fluid that is comprised of numerous cellular elements, such as PMNs and leukocytes.

    Answer B is incorrect. The GCF contains plasma proteins and epithelial cells.

    Answer C is incorrect. GCF is not contained within the vestibule of the buccal mucosa.

    Answer D is incorrect. It functions in the immune response, and some studies have shown that hyperactivity of such reaction may have implications regarding periodontal disease.

    Answer E is incorrect. Bacteria are also found in this fluid, which is contained mostly within the gingival sulcus.

147. **The correct answer is C.** When excessive fluoride uptake occurs in patients, they tend to suffer clinically from a brown pigmentation and mottling of their teeth. This process occurs prior to eruption of the teeth, where excessive fluoride is detrimental. Once the teeth erupt, fluoride treatment helps to improve the strength of the tooth by substituting with oxygen to form fluorapatite (rather than hydroxyapatite).

    Answer A is incorrect. Congenital syphilis presents with Hutchinson incisor and Mulberry molars.

    Answer B is incorrect. Nutritional deficiency would result in hypocalcification of the formed tooth.

Answer D is incorrect. Hypocalcification would present as a chalky white tooth which is soft.

Answer E is incorrect. Hypomineralization typically causes hypocalcification of the tooth.

148. **The correct answer is E.** The gag reflex is mediated via both the glossopharyngeal and vagus nerves. Stimuli which activates such activates afferents by way of CN IX. This occurs in a unilateral fashion. Efferents are then sent out via CN X bilaterally to cause constriction of the pharyngeal musculature.

Answer A is incorrect. CN XII would not be involved in this reflex. It provides motor innervation to the tongue.

Answer B is incorrect. CN V would not be involved in this reflex. It provides motor innervation to the muscles of mastication.

Answer C is incorrect. CN IX would not be affected in the efferent output of the gag reflex. It is responsible for the afferent aspect of it.

Answer D is incorrect. CN VII would not be involved in this reflex. It is responsible for innervation of the muscles of facial expression.

149. **The correct answer is D.** The pulmonary vein does not carry deoxygenated blood. This vein receives oxygenated blood from the lungs and returns it to the heart.

Answer A is incorrect. The hepatic vein carries deoxygenated blood from the liver to the inferior vena cava.

Answer B is incorrect. The superior vena cava carries deoxygenated blood from the upper extremities/head and neck region into the heart.

Answer C is incorrect. The inferior vena cava carries deoxygenated blood from the lower portions of the body into the heart.

Answer E is incorrect. The coronary sinus carries deoxygenated blood from the heart and returns it to the right atrium.

150. **The correct answer is D.** The gastroepiploic artery forms an anastomosis between the splenic and gastroduodenal arteries. Once it

branches from the celiac trunk, the gastroduodenal artery gives rise to the right gastric and right gastroepiploic arteries. The right gastroepiploic artery then courses along the stomach where it continues as the left gastroepiploic artery. The left gastroepiploic artery is attached to the splenic artery.

Answer A is incorrect. The right gastric and hepatic proper arteries do not anastomose into the gastroepiploic artery.

Answer B is incorrect. The left and right gastric arteries do not anastomose into the gastroepiploic artery.

Answer C is incorrect. The right gastric and short gastric arteries do not anastomose into the gastroepiploic artery.

Answer E is incorrect. The hepatic proper and splenic arteries do not anastomose into the gastroepiploic artery.

151. **The correct answer is D.** The supraoptic nucleus controls the body's balance of water. This nucleus is located within the hypothalamus. Production of such hormones as antidiuretic and oxytocin are produced here and released upon stimulation.

Answer A is incorrect. Aggression is controlled by the septal nucleus of the hypothalamus.

Answer B is incorrect. Satiety is controlled by the pineal gland of the epithalamus.

Answer C is incorrect. Hunger is controlled by the pineal gland of the epithalamus.

Answer E is incorrect. The circadian rhythm is controlled by the pineal gland of the epithalamus.

152. **The correct answer is B.** The ulnar nerve innervates the hypothenar region of the hand. This nerve provides sensory innervation for the medial $1/2$ digits (pinky finger), medial arm/forearm, and medial palm. As for motor function, the ulnar nerve flexes the wrist and fingers, ulnar two lumbricals, and interosseus musculature.

Answer A is incorrect. The radial nerve provides motor innervation to the triceps muscle as well as the extensors of the hand and wrist, and sensory innervation to the dorsal hand (excluding the pinky finger).

Answer C is incorrect. The musculocutaneous nerve provides motor innervation to the biceps, coracobrachialis, and portion of the brachialis muscles.

Answer D is incorrect. The median nerve provides motor innervation to multiple flexors of the forearm, 1st and 2nd lumbricals, thenar eminence, and sensory innervation on the palmar surface of the hand from the thumb to medial $1/2$ of the ring finger.

Answer E is incorrect. The axillary nerve provides motor innervation to the teres minor and deltoid muscles, and sensory innervation to the skin covering in the deltoid region as well as the shoulder joint.

153. **The correct answer is A.** The lateral pterygoid divides the maxillary artery into differing segments. The maxillary artery branches from the external carotid artery posterior to the ramus at the level of the mastoid process and continues on until it meets the lateral pterygoid muscle. It is here that the lateral pterygoid inserts into the meniscus of the temporomandibular joint. The maxillary artery is then divided in this region into the mandibular, pterygoid, and pterygopalatine arteries.

Answer B is incorrect. The masseter does not divide the maxillary artery.

Answer C is incorrect. The posterior belly of the digastric does not divide the maxillary artery.

Answer D is incorrect. The stylohyoid does not divide the maxillary artery.

Answer E is incorrect. The anterior belly of the digastric does not divide the maxillary artery.

154. **The correct answer is B.** The brain does not receive blood from the external carotid. Blood reaches the brain via the internal carotid artery as well as the vertebrobasilar system (see circle of Willis).

Answer A is incorrect. The thyroid gland receives blood supply via the superior thyroid artery.

Answer C is incorrect. The salivary glands receive blood supply via the facial artery.

Answer D is incorrect. The maxillary teeth receive blood supply via the posterior superior alveolar and infraorbital arteries. The mandibular teeth receive blood supply via the inferior alveolar artery.

Answer E is incorrect. The mandible receives blood supply via the inferior alveolar arteries and overlying periosteum (branches of the external carotid system). The maxilla receives its blood supply via the superior alveolar vessels, ascending pharyngeal, nasal vessels (primarily external carotid system).

155. **The correct answer is A.** The vertebral artery enters the spine at the 6th cervical vertebrae after branching off the subclavian artery. It then continues superiorly within the transverse processes/foramina of the spinal column until it reaches the skull base. Here it then combines with the contralateral vertebral artery to form the basilar artery.

Answers B, C, D and E are incorrect. See above.

156. **The correct answer is A.** The salpingopharyngeus is a muscle of the pharynx, and is actually part of the palatopharyngeus muscle. It is also considered a longitudinal pharyngeal muscle. It connects to cartilage of the auditory tube and, thus, upon contraction it opens it. It also elevates the nasopharynx. Motor innervation is supplied by CN XI (carried by CN X).

Answer B is incorrect. The action of raising the mandible is performed by the masseter and medial pterygoid muscles.

Answer C is incorrect. The action of propelling food down the pharynx is performed by the pharyngeal constrictors (superior, middle, inferior).

Answer D is incorrect. The action of retracting the tongue is performed by the styloglossus muscle.

Answer E is incorrect. The action of protruding the mandible is performed by the lateral pterygoid muscle.

157. **The correct answer is C.** The vestibulocochlear nerve (CN VIII) is mostly found within the confines of the temporal bone. It originates from the brainstem near the junction of the pons and medulla. Here is where the cochlear nucleus and the vestibular nuclear complex are located. This nerve functions in hearing and balance.

    Answer A is incorrect. The parietal bone does not house the majority of CN VIII.

    Answer B is incorrect. The occipital bone does not house the majority of CN VIII.

    Answer D is incorrect. The frontal bone does not house the majority of CN VIII.

    Answer E is incorrect. The maxilla does not house the majority of CN VIII.

158. **The correct answer is C.** The pectoralis major is innervated by the lateral and medial pectoral muscles.

    Answer A is incorrect. Its function is to medially rotate, flex, and adduct the humerus.

    Answer B is incorrect. The pectoralis major is not an accessory muscle of respiration.

    Answer D is incorrect. It originates on the medial half of the clavicle, as well as the costal cartilages and sternum and inserts at the greater tubercular crest.

    Answer E is incorrect. The pectoralis major is located inferiorly to the pectoralis minor.

159. **The correct answer is D.** The infraorbital artery supplies blood to the maxillary canines and incisors. It is a branch of the pterygopalatine artery, which in turn is a continuation of the maxillary artery. Blood supply to the maxillary molars and premolars is via the posterosuperior artery (also branched from the same source as the infraorbital artery).

Answer A is incorrect. The pterygoid artery supplies blood to the pterygoid muscles.

Answer B is incorrect. The sphenopalatine artery supplies blood to the anterior palate. It does this via anastomoses with the palatine arteries.

Answer C is incorrect. The descending palatine artery supplies blood to the mucosa of the soft palate.

Answer E is incorrect. The pharyngeal artery supplies blood to the pharynx.

160. **The correct answer is A.** The cisterna chyli is a central point of lymphatic drainage from the region inferior to the diaphragm. Thus, it drains lymph from the abdomen, pelvis, inguinal region, and lower extremities. From this point, the cisterna chyli continues superiorly and drains into the thoracic duct.

    Answer B is incorrect. The cisterna chyli receives lymphatic drainage from the abdomen.

    Answer C is incorrect. The cisterna chyli receives lymphatic drainage from the pelvis.

    Answer D is incorrect. The cisterna chyli receives lymphatic drainage from the inguinal region.

    Answer E is incorrect. The cisterna chyli receives lymphatic drainage from the lower extremities.

161. **The correct answer is E.** As the dentin increases in age, there is an increase in deposition of peritubular dentin.

    Answer A is incorrect. There is a decrease in dentinal tubule diameter.

    Answer B is incorrect. There is an increase in reparative dentin formation.

    Answer C is incorrect. There is an increase in dead tracts.

    Answer D is incorrect. There is an increase in sclerotic dentin formation.

162. **The correct answer is C.** This patient was probably taking tetracycline at the age of 5 years (of the given options). Tetracycline

causes this clinical phenomenon due to its ability to chelate divalent cations, thus incorporating into mineralizing tissue. Therefore, tetracycline should not be given to a patient under the age of 8, which marks the completion of calcification of the 2nd molars.

Answer A is incorrect. The age of 10 is too old. By this time, complete calcification of all teeth (except the permanent 3rd molars) should be complete.

Answer B is incorrect. The age of 11 is too old. By this time, complete calcification of all teeth (except the permanent 3rd molars) should be complete.

Answer D is incorrect. The age of 14 is too old. By this time, complete calcification of all teeth (except the permanent 3rd molars) should be complete.

Answer E is incorrect. The age of 17 is too old. By this time, complete calcification of all teeth (except the permanent 3rd molars) should be complete.

163. **The correct answer is D.** Vitamin K (of the options given) is least likely to directly affect enamel structure. This vitamin is most intimately involved in formation of blood clotting factors II, V, VII, and IX.

    Answer A is incorrect. Vitamin A can, in a deficient state, cause enamel pitting.

    Answer B is incorrect. Vitamin B can, in a deficient state, cause enamel pitting.

    Answer C is incorrect. Vitamin C can, in a deficient state, cause enamel pitting.

    Answer E is incorrect. Calcium can, in a deficient state, cause enamel pitting. This is due to the enamel matrix being less calcified than normal.

164. **The correct answer is B.** The internal lining of all closed body cavities is simple squamous epithelium. Another term used to classify this layer is mesothelium. This epithelial type has a barrier function.

    Answer A is incorrect. Simple columnar epithelium functions to transport, absorb, and secrete.

Answer C is incorrect. Transitional epithelium is a barrier which also allows for distension.

Answer D is incorrect. Stratified squamous epithelium is used as protection on the outer surface of skin.

Answer E is incorrect. Pseudostratified columnar epithelium functions to transport, absorb, and secrete.

165. **The correct answer is C.** The basal lamina contains type IV collagen. This layer is also known as the basement membrane.

    Answer A is incorrect. The lamina lucida is an electron-clear layer.

    Answer B is incorrect. The lamina densa is a product of the epithelium and contains proteoglycans, laminin, fibronectin, and type VII collagen (anchoring fibrils).

    Answer D is incorrect. The reticular layer (a product of the connective tissue) contains type III collagen, also known as reticular fibers.

    Answer E is incorrect. The basement membrane has a filtering function.

166. **The correct answer is D.** The attached gingiva, as is the case with all types of gingiva, is keratinized.

    Answer A is incorrect. The sulcular epithelium of the oral cavity is nonkeratinized.

    Answer B is incorrect. The alveolar mucosa of the oral cavity is nonkeratinized.

    Answer C is incorrect. The junctional epithelium of the oral cavity is nonkeratinized.

    Answer E is incorrect. The gingival col of the oral cavity is nonkeratinized.

167. **The correct answer is D.** The enamel layer has only approximately 4% organic composition.

    Answer A is incorrect. The cementum is comprised of 45% organic constituents.

    Answer B is incorrect. The dentin is comprised of 30% organic constituents.

Answer C is incorrect. The pulp is comprised of greater than 95% organic constituents.

Answer E is incorrect. The alveolar bone is comprised of nearly 50% organic constituents.

168. **The correct answer is A.** As one ages, the pulp becomes more collagenous.

    Answer B is incorrect. There is a decreased size of the apical foramen of the pulp as one ages.

    Answer C is incorrect. There is a decreased sensitivity of the pulp as one ages.

    Answer D is incorrect. There is a decreased cellularity of the pulp as one ages.

    Answer E is incorrect. There is an increased calcification of the pulp as one ages.
    Note that the overall size of the pulp chamber decreases due to continuous deposition of dentin.

169. **The correct answer is B.** Cementum affords the tooth resistance to resorption. This is due to continuous cementum deposition at the apex of the tooth's root. This resistance to resorption in cementum even surpasses that of alveolar bone.

    Answer A is incorrect. The enamel does not allow for orthodontic movement. It serves to protect the underlying structures of the tooth and assist in the tooth's normal functioning.

    Answer C is incorrect. The dentin does not allow for orthodontic movement. It serves to cushion the enamel during mastication.

    Answer D is incorrect. The epithelial attachment does not allow for orthodontic movement. It serves as an attachment for the gingival.

    Answer E is incorrect. The alveolar bone does not allow for orthodontic movement. It serves as a housing of the entire tooth apparatus.

170. **The correct answer is C.** Free nerve endings are the most abundant neuronal ending of the PDL. Generally speaking, they sense touch, temperature, and pain.

    Answer A is incorrect. The coiled nerve endings are found in the PDL and have a function with mechanoreception.

Answer B is incorrect. The spindle nerve endings are found in the PDL and have a function with mechanoreception.

Answer D is incorrect. Meissner nerve endings (touch) are not found in the PDL.

Answer E is incorrect. Ruffini corpuscles are also found in the PDL. They have a function with mechanoreception.
    Note that each of the PDL nerve endings is associated with the trigeminal nerve.

171. **The correct answer is A.** The gingival col is a depression located just apical to the contact of adjacent teeth. It is located in the interdental gingiva connecting the buccal and lingual papilla. It is nonkeratinized.

    Answer B is incorrect. The alveolar mucosa is not found in this location.

    Answer C is incorrect. The attached gingiva serves to line and protect the oral cavity.

    Answer D is incorrect. The mucogingival junction is the line formed between the gingival and alveolar mucosa.

    Answer E is incorrect. The interdental papilla is triangular in shape and located in the interproximal embrasure between two teeth.

172. **The correct answer is C.** The primary palate contains the central and lateral incisor.

    Answer A is incorrect. The primary palate can be involved in facial clefting.

    Answer B is incorrect. The primary palate is known as the premaxilla and also contains the incisive foramen.

    Answer D is incorrect. It is formed once mesenchyme differentiates lateral to the nasal placodes.

    Answer E is incorrect. The median nasal processes form from the primary palate and eventually fuse.

173. **The correct answer is A.** Circumpulpal dentin is most produced in the form of intertubular dentin.

Answer B is incorrect. It is secreted by odontoblasts and formed after mantle dentin (the initial 150 μm of dentin) is laid down.

Answer C is incorrect. It becomes mineralized and calcified over time by way of hydroxyapatite crystal fusion.

Answer D is incorrect. Circumpulpal dentin forms after mantle dentin formation.

Answer E is incorrect. This form of dentin contains dead tracts.

174. **The correct answer is D.** The enamel matrix is laid down at a rate of 4 μm per day. This is achieved by actively secreting ameloblasts. It is comprised mostly of amelogenins, among other proteins.

Answer A is incorrect. The rate of 0.04 μm/day is much too slow.

Answer B is incorrect. The rate of 1 mm/day is far too rapid a growth rate.

Answer C is incorrect. The rate of 0.1 mm/day is far too slow a growth rate.

Answer E is incorrect. The rate of 4 mm/day is far too rapid a growth rate.

175. **The correct answer is E.** This stage of development completes at around the 12th week of fetal development when the temporal lobe, sulci, and gyri begin to form.

Answer A is incorrect. The cerebellum forms at approximately the 5th week of development.

Answer B is incorrect. The ventricles form approximately the 5th week of development.

Answer C is incorrect. Development of the brain begins at the 3rd week of fetal life when the neural tube takes shape.

Answer D is incorrect. The hemispheres form approximately the 5th week of development.
  Note: This developmental stage continues on for the remainder of gestation.

176. **The correct answer is C.** As odontogenesis is initiated, the ectodermal layer of the oral cavity is induced to proliferate. This occurs via the underlying ectomesenchymal layer during approximately week 6 in utero. Thus, the site of a forming tooth is formed from this ectomesenchymal interaction with overlying ectoderm.

Answer A is incorrect. The mesodermal layer does not determine the shape of the tooth.

Answer B is incorrect. The mesenchyme layer does not determine the shape of the tooth.

Answer D is incorrect. The endoderm layer does not determine the shape of the tooth.

Answer E is incorrect. The ectoderm layer does have a part in determination of tooth shape, but the ectomesenchyme is the main mediator.

177. **The correct answer is E.** The great auricular nerve (C2/C3) offers sensory innervation to the area of skin covering the parotid gland, as well as posterior auricle and area of skin forming the area between the angle of the mandible and mastoid process.

Answer A is incorrect. The transverse cervical nerve (C2/C3) innervates the skin of the neck and scalp (posterosuperior to the auricle).

Answer B is incorrect. The superficial temporal nerve (CN V) innervates the skin in the temporal region.

Answer C is incorrect. The long buccal nerve (of CN V) innervates oral gingiva from the first mandibular molar posteriorly.

Answer D is incorrect. The lesser occipital nerve (C2) innervates skin of the anterior triangle of the neck.

178. **The correct answer is A.** The obturator nerve is a branch of the lumbar plexus (L1-L4).

Answer B is incorrect. This plexus is located in the posterior pelvic wall.

Answer C is incorrect. The sacral plexus provides motor innervation to parts of the lower limbs.

Answer D is incorrect. The sacral plexus provides sensory innervation to the pelvis and lower back.

Answer E is incorrect. The sacral plexus is made up of lumbar nerves 4 and 5, as well as sacral nerves 1-4.

Note: The sacral plexus branches off as the sciatic nerve, which is the largest nerve of the body, as well as the gluteal and greater splanchnic nerves.

179. **The correct answer is B.** The trigeminal nerve (CN V) does not have an efferent involuntary parasympathetic function. CN III distributes such efferents to the ciliary muscles, sphincter pupillae, dilator pupillae, and tarsal muscles.

Answer A is incorrect. CN VII distributes parasympathetic efferents to the lacrimal gland, and nasal and palatal glands.

Answer C is incorrect. CN X distributes efferent involuntary parasympathetics to numerous smooth muscles.

Answer D is incorrect. CN III distributes efferent involuntary parasympathetics to the ciliary muscle, sphincter pupillae, dilator pupillae, and tarsal muscles.

Answer E is incorrect. CN IX gives involuntary parasympathetic efferents to the parotid gland.

180. **The correct answer is B.** General visceral afferents of the vagus nerve travel through the cranial base via the jugular foramen.

Answer A is incorrect. CN IX is involved with afferent transmission from the carotid body and sinus.

Answer C is incorrect. This afferent function has cell bodies in the nodose ganglion and function to transmit sensation from viscera of the pharynx, larynx, thoracic, and abdominal regions (to the left colic flexure).

Answer D is incorrect. Sensation from the posterior meninges (and external ear) is a general somatic afferent function of CN X.

Answer E is incorrect. The nucleus ambiguus has cell bodies involved with special visceral efferents of CN X. Taste is a special visceral function of CN X.

181. **The correct answer is B.** Chromaffin cells are located within the inner medulla, and secrete catecholamines (epinephrine and norepinephrine).

Answer A is incorrect. The zona fasciculata secretes glucocorticoids. An example of this is cortisone.

Answer C is incorrect. The zona glomerulosa secretes mineralocorticoids. An example of this is aldosterone.

Answer D is incorrect. The inner layer, the zona reticularis, secretes gonadocorticoids. Examples of these are sex steroids.

Answer E is incorrect. The inner medulla secretes catecholamines.

182. **The correct answer is D.** Teniae coli are longitudinal bands of smooth muscle in the large intestine which function to regulate peristaltic movements within it.

Answer A is incorrect. Microvilli are located in the small intestine and are involved with reabsorption.

Answer B is incorrect. The myenteric (Auerbach) plexus maintains peristalsis in the small intestine.

Answer C is incorrect. The plicae circulares are involved in reabsorption.

Answer E is incorrect. The crypts of Lieberkühn are involved in reabsorption.

183. **The correct answer is B.** Plasmin is a protein involved in physiological regulation of blood clotting, and is not found in bile. Bile is composed of many proteins formed in the liver, as well as degradation products or red blood cells.

Answer A is incorrect. Lipoproteins are found comprising bile. They transport lipid.

Answer C is incorrect. Albumin is found comprising bile. It is a carrier protein.

Answer D is incorrect. Prothrombin is found comprising bile. It is involved in the clotting cascade.

Answer E is incorrect. Alpha and beta globulins are found comprising bile. Together they form hemoglobin molecules.

184. **The correct answer is D.** The ethmoid bone is located anteriorly within the internal aspect of the skull. Thus, it does not articulate with the temporal bone.

Answer A is incorrect. The parietal bone articulates with the temporal bone superiorly.

Answer B is incorrect. The occipital bone articulates with the temporal bone posteriorly.

Answer C is incorrect. The zygoma articulates with the temporal bone anteriorly.

Answer E is incorrect. The sphenoid bone articulates with the temporal bone anteriorly.

185. **The correct answer is C.** Terminal differentiation occurs in the G0 stage of the cell cycle. There is no cellular activity at this time. It is part of interphase.

Answer A is incorrect. The G1 phase is part of interphase. This is the 1st stage of cellular growth.

Answer B is incorrect. The S phase is part of interphase. Synthesis of DNA occurs here.

Answer D is incorrect. The G2 phase is part of interphase. This is the 2nd stage of cellular growth.

Answer E is incorrect. Mitosis consists of cell division.

186. **The correct answer is A.** Gastroenteropancreatic glands are an example of paracrine function. Paracrine-type glands affect cells within the same epithelium by way of secretion of products into the extracellular space. An example of this is the secretion of cholecystokinin by the pancreas into the small intestine.

Answer B is incorrect. The adrenal glands are endocrine in function. They secrete products into the blood stream.

Answer C is incorrect. The gonads are endocrine in function. They secrete products into the blood stream.

Answer D is incorrect. The salivary glands are exocrine in function. They secrete products nonspecifically via ducts.

187. **The correct answer is D.** The stomodeum, also known as the primitive mouth, is lined by ectoderm. This structure is separated from the pharynx by the buccopharyngeal membrane.

Answer A is incorrect. The endodermal layer lines the pharynx.

Answers B, C, and E are incorrect. These do not line the stomodeum.

188. **The correct answer is A.** The stapes is a derivative of the 2nd branchial arch, which is located further cranially than any of the corresponding branchial arches in the answers given above. At the 4th-5th week of embryonic development, the branchial arches are most evident and line up in a cranial-caudal fashion (arch 1 most cranial and arch 4 most caudal).

Answer B is incorrect. The internal carotid artery is a derivative of the 3rd branchial arch.

Answer C is incorrect. The vagus nerve is a derivative of the 4th branchial arch.

Answer D is incorrect. The glossopharyngeal nerve is a derivative of the 3rd branchial arch.

Answer E is incorrect. The stylopharyngeus muscle is a derivative of the 3rd branchial arch.

189. **The correct answer is E.** The decidual reaction occurs during week 2 of embryogenesis and involves endometrial enlargement via lipid and glycogen accumulating within this portion of the uterus.

Answer A is incorrect. The breakdown of the zona pellucida occurs once the blastula forms.

Answer B is incorrect. The first zygotic cleavage has no formal name.

Answer C is incorrect. Invasion of the syncytiotrophoblast into the endometrium of the uterus is part of implantation of the zygote.

Answer D is incorrect. The release of an ovum from the ovary occurs during the menstrual cycle.

190. **The correct answer is C.** The chromosomal number 2N represents the fusion of sperm and egg. This represents 46 chromosomes.

    Answer A is incorrect. The chromosomal number $1/2$ N does not occur in the normal physiological development of sperm and egg.

    Answer B is incorrect. Each male and female pronuclei has an N chromosome number (thus, 23 chromosomes).

    Answer D is incorrect. The chromosomal number 3N does not occur in the normal physiological development of sperm and egg.

    Answer E is incorrect. The chromosomal number 4N occurs prior to the first meiotic division in each of the sperm and egg.

191. **The correct answer is A.** The epidermis does not contain sinusoids. Sinusoids are modified capillaries that contain discontinuities within them referred to as fenestrae. These have a more complex structure than conventional capillaries and are also larger in overall size. This structure provides adaptation to reticuloendothelial cells infiltrating a particular region of tissue.

    Answer B is incorrect. The liver contains sinusoids. Drainage of blood from the portal circulation occurs here.

    Answer C is incorrect. The lymphatic tissue contains sinusoids. Here is where lymph is contained.

    Answer D is incorrect. Endocrine glands contain sinusoids. The function varies, but this is a place where one may find hormones.

    Answer E is incorrect. The spleen contains sinusoids. Here is where immune reactions occur.

192. **The correct answer is E.** Peroxisomes contain catalase. These organelles function to remove substances which may be toxic to the cell. For example, catalase is an enzyme which oxidizes hydrogen peroxide (which is cytotoxic) into water and other non toxic products. These organelles are typically found in the liver, and organ which has a detoxifying function for the body.

    Answer A is incorrect. Elastase is contained within the cell. Its function is the breakdown of elastin.

    Answer B is incorrect. Collagenase is contained within the cell. Its function is the breakdown of collagen.

    Answer C is incorrect. Trypsin is contained within the pancreas (as a proenzyme). It is a digestive enzyme.

    Answer D is incorrect. Chymotrypsin is contained in the pancreas. It is a digestive (proteolytic) enzyme.

193. **The correct answer is E.** The epidermis produces vitamin D. It must undergo other steps to become biologically active.

    Answer A is incorrect. Vitamin D is not produced at the large intestine. It has no function in vitamin D production.

    Answer B is incorrect. Vitamin D is not produced in the kidney. It does hydroxylate vitamin D, though, to a biologically active form.

    Answer C is incorrect. Vitamin D is not produced at the spleen. It has no function in vitamin D production.

    Answer D is incorrect. Vitamin D is not produced in the liver. It does hydroxylate vitamin D, though, to a biologically active form.

194. **The correct answer is A.** The ciliary body most directly controls accommodation. This portion of the eye contains smooth muscle and thus can receive neural input which alters lens shape.

    Answer B is incorrect. The neural retina contains rods and cones, so its function is photoreception.

    Answer C is incorrect. The choroid layer is involved with vascularity of the eye.

    Answer D is incorrect. The pupil is an aperture which allows light into the eyeball.

    Answer E is incorrect. The iris (which also contains smooth muscle) alters the shape of the eyeball's central aperture, the pupil.

195. **The correct answer is B.** Fibrinogen, as well as other clotting factors, is not found in serum. Serum is composed of all other elements found in the blood plasma.

Answer A is incorrect. Electrolytes are found within the blood serum.

Answer C is incorrect. Immunoglobulin is found within the blood serum.

Answer D is incorrect. Water is found within the blood serum.

Answer E is incorrect. Albumin is found within the blood serum.
   Note that blood gases, hormones, enzymes, and metabolic products are also found in the serum.

196. **The correct answer is B.** A layer of simple squamous endothelium can be found lining the lumen of the heart as part of the endocardium.

Answer A is incorrect. The pericardium is the outermost layer. It contains connective tissue and adipose tissue.

Answer C is incorrect. The endocardium is the innermost layer of the heart.

Answer D is incorrect. The thickest portion of the heart is the myocardium. It is in the center of the heart layers and contains cardiac musculature.

Answer E is incorrect. A layer of simple squamous epithelium surrounds the outermost layer, the pericardium.

197. **The correct answer is C.** The autonomic nervous system is involved with heart rate. This is accomplished by firing of neural signals onto the SA node, which then passes the current on to the AV node.

Answer A is incorrect. The bundle of His conducts electric current to the Purkinje fibers.

Answer B is incorrect. The SA node regulates the rate of electrical conductance.

Answer D is incorrect. The cardiac muscle maintains an intrinsic rhythmicity.

Answer E is incorrect. The pacemaker of the heart is the SA node.

198. **The correct answer is A.** Platelets range in number some 200,000-400,000 per mm^3 of blood.

Answer B is incorrect. Platelets are involved with hemostasis.

Answer C is incorrect. Platelets have a lifespan/turnover rate of 7-10 days.

Answer D is incorrect. Platelets are anucleate.

Answer E is incorrect. Platelets do not function in blood gas transport. They are involved in the blood clot.

199. **The correct answer is D.** Bone marrow is the site of B-cell maturation. Here is where pluripotent stem cells become phagocytes or lymphocytes.

Answer A is incorrect. The lymph nodes are the site for further lymphocyte differentiation as well as lymph filtering.

Answer B is incorrect. The blood is the site for further lymphocyte differentiation. Immunologic reactions also occur here.

Answer C is incorrect. The thymus is the site of T-cell maturation.

Answer E is incorrect. The target tissue is a site of further lymphocyte differentiation. Immunologic response also occurs here.

200. **The correct answer is A.** Thyroxine (T_4) is secreted from follicular cells of the thyroid gland, as is triiodothyronine (T_3). T_4 is produced from precursor thyroglobulin molecules.

Answer B is incorrect. The outer cortex of the adrenals produces steroids involved with sugar, salt, and sexual regulation.

Answer C is incorrect. The pars distalis is part of the anterior pituitary gland. It secretes prolactin and growth hormone.

Answer D is incorrect. The pars intermedia is part of the anterior pituitary gland. It secretes lipotropic hormone.

Answer E is incorrect. The parafollicular cells of the thyroid gland secrete calcitonin.

CHAPTER 2

Biochemistry and Physiology

1. The plateau in the cardiac action potential is caused by which of the following?

    A. Influx of Na^+
    B. Efflux of Na^+
    C. Influx of Ca^{2+}
    D. Efflux of Ca^{2+}
    E. Influx of K^+

2. The first law of thermodynamics states that the entropy of a closed system always increases. The second law of thermodynamics states that the total energy of a closed system is conserved.

    A. Both statements are true.
    B. Both statements are false.
    C. The first statement is true; the second statement is false.
    D. The first statement is false; the second statement is true.

3. Which of the following is not a peptide hormone?

    A. PTH
    B. Insulin
    C. GH
    D. Aldosterone
    E. ADH

4. Which of the following types of blood vessels is responsible for the greatest proportion of vascular resistance?

    A. Arteries
    B. Arterioles
    C. Capillaries
    D. Venules
    E. Veins

5. All of the following are true of carbonic anhydrase EXCEPT

    A. most isoforms contain a central zinc atom.
    B. interconverts carbon dioxide and bicarbonate.
    C. significantly increases the reaction rate.
    D. highly active in platelets.
    E. critical in osteoclastic activity.

6. All of the following are true of cardiac muscle EXCEPT

    A. contractile activity is mediated intrinsically.
    B. it contains T tubules.
    C. it does not contain troponin.
    D. each cell has one centrally located nucleus.
    E. it is striated.

7. What autosomal recessive disease is caused by a deficiency of muscle glycogen phosphorylase?

    A. Pompe disease
    B. McArdle syndrome
    C. Hunter syndrome
    D. Von Gierke disease
    E. Hurler syndrome

8. Extracellular fluid comprises what amount of total body water?

    A. 25%
    B. 33%
    C. 50%
    D. 66%
    E. 75%

9. Which of the following types of cartilage may calcify?

    A. Elastic
    B. Hyaline
    C. Fibrocartilage
    D. B and C
    E. All of the above

10. All of the following are key enzymes in DNA synthesis EXCEPT

    A. polymerase.
    B. exonuclease.
    C. aminotransferase.
    D. topoisomerase.
    E. helicase.

11. All of the following tissues are involved in a feedback axis with the hypothalamus EXCEPT

    A. thyroid.
    B. parathyroid.
    C. pituitary.
    D. adrenal.
    E. testicular.

12. Which of the following catalyze bond cleavage?

    A. Hydrolases and lyases
    B. Transferases and isomerases
    C. Ligases and oxidoreductases
    D. Transferases and lyases
    E. Hydrolases and isomerases

13. Which of the following decreases gastric motility?

    A. Gastrin
    B. Secretin
    C. GIP
    D. B and C
    E. All of the above

14. Which of the following respiratory volumes is incorrect?

    A. ERV = FRC – RV
    B. VC = TLV – RV
    C. TLV = IRV + TV + ERV + RV
    D. IC = IRV – TV
    E. VC = TV + IRV + ERV

15. Which of the following is TRUE of ΔG?

    A. Determines reaction rate
    B. Exergonic reactions will have a positive ΔG
    C. Determines reaction equilibrium
    D. Dependent on the path of the reaction
    E. Determines reaction direction

16. All of the following are true of the somatic nervous system EXCEPT

    A. it consists of 12 cranial nerves.
    B. it transmits temperature and pain.
    C. it innervates skeletal muscle.
    D. it has short preganglionic motor neurons.
    E. all are true of the somatic nervous system.

17. Which of the following is the most abundant glycosaminoglycan?

    A. Keratan sulfate
    B. Heparan sulfate
    C. Chondroitin sulfate
    D. Dermatan sulfate
    E. Hyaluronic acid

18. All of the following are true of the pulmonary circulation compared to the systemic circulation EXCEPT

    A. it has higher resistance.
    B. it has higher compliance.
    C. it has a lower blood pressure.
    D. it has a similar volume of blood flow.
    E. it conducts deoxygenated blood via the pulmonary artery.

19. Which of the following anterior pituitary hormones does not directly act on a specific target tissue?

    A. FSH
    B. GH
    C. ACTH
    D. Prolactin
    E. TSH

20. Which of the following is a type of frameshift mutation?

    A. Nonsense mutation
    B. Repeat mutation
    C. Transverse mutation
    D. Missense mutation
    E. None of the above

21. Aldosterone is secreted in a pathway in response to the release of which hormone?

    A. Renin
    B. ADH
    C. Vasopressin
    D. Erythropoietin
    E. ACTH

Biochemistry and Physiology

22. All of the following are true of plasma membranes EXCEPT

    A. Selectively permeable
    B. Function as barriers
    C. Symmetrical
    D. Contain cholesterol
    E. Have a hydrophobic inner layer

23. Most connective tissue (CT) originates from mesoderm. The majority of dense CT is regular in its cellular arrangement.

    A. Both statements are true.
    B. Both statements are false.
    C. The first statement is true, the second statement is false.
    D. The first statement is false, the second statement is true.

24. There are four basic tastes. Each taste cell can sense all of the basic tastes.

    A. Both statements are true.
    B. Both statements are false.
    C. The first statement is true, the second statement is false.
    D. The first statement is false, the second statement is true.

25. In general, reaction rate will increase as a result of all of the following EXCEPT

    A. an increase in temperature.
    B. an increase in enzyme concentration.
    C. an increase in activation energy.
    D. an increase in substrate concentration.
    E. a decrease in activation energy.

26. A sarcomere is defined as the area within a myofibril located between two

    A. A bands.
    B. H bands.
    C. I bands.
    D. M lines.
    E. Z lines.

27. All of the following are disaccharides EXCEPT

    A. sucrose.
    B. maltose.
    C. lactose.
    D. mannose.

28. The intrinsic coagulation pathway is initiated by which of the following clotting factors?

    A. I
    B. II
    C. VII
    D. VIII
    E. XII

29. What type of GI contraction is most common in the duodenum?

    A. Tonic contractions
    B. Peristalsis
    C. Segmentation
    D. None of the above

30. All of the following are zymogens EXCEPT

    A. clotting factor I.
    B. calmodulin.
    C. trypsinogen.
    D. clotting factor X.
    E. procollagen.

31. Hyperventilation results in all of the following EXCEPT

    A. increased P_{O_2}.
    B. hypocapnia.
    C. decreased cerebral blood flow.
    D. increased P_{CO_2}.
    E. respiratory alkalosis.

32. Which of the following is TRUE of protein synthesis?

    A. Aminoacyl-tRNA synthetase adds each amino acid to tRNA.
    B. mRNA carries the anticodon to each tRNA.
    C. Two ribosomal subunits of equal size bind to mRNA.
    D. Occurs only in cells that contain 80s ribosomes.
    E. Occurs in a 3′ to 5′ direction.

33. Local anesthetics function by

    A. activating Na^+ channels.
    B. blocking Na^+ channels.
    C. activating K^+ channels.
    D. blocking K^+ channels.
    E. none of the above.

34. Which of the following pressure changes will result in edema?

    A. Decreased capillary hydrostatic pressure
    B. Decreased interstitial oncotic pressure
    C. Decreased capillary oncotic pressure
    D. Increased interstitial hydrostatic pressure
    E. All of the above

35. A noncompetitive inhibitor increases K_m and decreases V_{max}.

    A. Both actions are true.
    B. Both actions are false.
    C. The first action is true; the second action is false.
    D. The first action is false; the second action is true.

36. Which of the following have been implicated in osteonecrosis of the jaws?

    A. Pamidronate
    B. Zolendronate
    C. Alendronate
    D. All of the above
    E. None of the above

37. All of the following are true of α-amylase EXCEPT

    A. it is secreted by the parotid gland.
    B. it cleaves α-1,6-glycosidic linkages.
    C. it catabolizes starch.
    D. it is a hydrolase.

38. Hyperparathyroidism will cause all of the following EXCEPT

    A. decreased renal phosphate reabsorption.
    B. increased renal calcium reabsorption.
    C. increased alveolar bone density.
    D. A and B.
    E. all are true of hyperparathyroidism.

39. All of the following are true of total peripheral resistance (TPR) EXCEPT

    A. it is influenced by sympathetic activation.
    B. it is directly proportional to cardiac output.
    C. it is directly proportional to mean arterial pressure.
    D. it is influenced by thermal changes.

40. Which of the following converts acetyl-CoA to malonyl-CoA?

    A. Vitamin E
    B. Vitamin B_1
    C. Vitamin B_6
    D. Vitamin B_{12}
    E. Biotin

41. Calmodulin functions by

    A. binding calcium.
    B. activating myosin light-chain kinase.
    C. hydrolyzing ATP.
    D. A and B.
    E. all of the above.

42. All of the following are true of allosteric regulation EXCEPT

    A. Follows simple Michaelis-Menten kinetics
    B. The allosteric and catalytic sites on the enzyme are spatially unique
    C. May involve feedback regulation
    D. Can raise K_m without an effect on V_{max}
    E. Can lower V_{max} without an effect on K_m

43. FSH is only functional in females. LH stimulates the production of testosterone in testicular Leydig cells.

    A. Both statements are true.
    B. Both statements are false.
    C. The first statement is true; the second statement is false.
    D. The first statement is false; the second statement is true.

44. What is the normal pH of blood?

    A. 5.8
    B. 6.6
    C. 7.0
    D. 7.4
    E. 8.2

45. Which of the following proteins functions in monitoring DNA integrity?

    A. p53
    B. p54
    C. p55
    D. p56
    E. p57

46. Insulin is released from which type of gland?

    A. Merocrine
    B. Acinar
    C. Tubular
    D. A and B
    E. None of the above

47. The total amount of oxygen carried in blood occurs via

    A. bicarbonate.
    B. dissolved O_2.
    C. bound to hemoglobin.
    D. B and C.
    E. all of the above.

48. Which of the following is not found in plasma membranes?

    A. Sphingomyelin
    B. Cholesterol
    C. G proteins
    D. Collagen
    E. Arachidonic acid

49. Which pathway transmits pain and temperature?

    A. Dorsal column pathway
    B. Anterior spinothalamic tract (of the anterolateral pathway)
    C. Lateral spinothalamic tract (of the anterolateral pathway)
    D. Corticospinal tract (of the pyramidal system)
    E. Medial lemniscal pathway

50. All of the following are true of glycolysis EXCEPT

    A. Converts glucose to two molecules of pyruvate
    B. Takes place in the cytosol
    C. Also called the Embden-Meyerhof pathway
    D. The rate-limiting step is the conversion of glucose-6-phosphate to fructose-6-phosphate
    E. Directly produces 4 ATP per glucose

51. The first heart sound (S1) indicates closure of the semilunar valves. It is typically louder and longer than the second heart sound (S2).

    A. Both statements are true.
    B. Both statements are false.
    C. The first statement is true; the second statement is false.
    D. The first statement is false; the second statement is true.

52. Which of the following stimulates the release of bile from the gallbladder?

    A. Cholecystokinin
    B. Secretin
    C. Bilirubin
    D. Chymotrypsin
    E. Pepsinogen

53. Which of the following amino acids is not synthesized from glucose?

    A. Valine
    B. Arginine
    C. Serine
    D. Glutamate
    E. Alanine

54. Which of the following muscles is not involved in swallowing?

    A. Salpingopharyngeus
    B. Levator veli palatini
    C. Palatopharyngeus
    D. Tensor veli palatini
    E. Inferior pharyngeal constrictor

55. Fluoride inhibits which of the following glycolytic enzymes?

    A. Enolase
    B. Phosphofructokinase
    C. Lactate dehydrogenase
    D. Hexokinase
    E. Aldolase

56. Glucagon secretion results in all of the following EXCEPT

    A. increased blood glucose level.
    B. increased fatty acid synthesis.
    C. increased urea synthesis.
    D. B and C.
    E. all are true glucagon secretion.

57. Parathyroid hormone (PTH) functions primarily at which segment of the nephron?

    A. Proximal convoluted tubule
    B. Descending loop of Henle
    C. Ascending loop of Henle
    D. Distal convoluted tubule
    E. Collecting duct

58. Which laboratory technique determines RNA content of a protein sample?

    A. PCR
    B. Western blot
    C. Northern blot
    D. Southern blot
    E. Southwestern blot

59. A fresh extraction socket will fill with new bone over the next few months. What type of bone formation occurs during this time period?

    A. Intramembranous
    B. Endochondral
    C. Intermembranous
    D. A and B
    E. None of the above

60. All of the following are *direct* metabolic fates of pyruvate EXCEPT

    A. oxaloacetate.
    B. acetyl-CoA.
    C. glucose.
    D. alanine.
    E. lactate.

61. All of the following are characteristics of skeletal muscle with a type II twitch speed EXCEPT

    A. it has a fast contraction speed.
    B. it has a relatively low SR content.
    C. it has a relatively low myoglobin content.
    D. it has a relatively large fiber diameter.
    E. it has a relatively high rate of ATPase activity.

62. Which of the following formulas is not correct?

    A. $MAP = CO \bullet TPR$
    B. $CO = HR \bullet SV$
    C. $R = 8\eta L/\pi r^2$
    D. $(P_{out} - P_{in}) = T/r$
    E. $F = P\pi r^4/8\eta L$

63. Epinephrine is derived from which of the following amino acids?

    A. Histidine
    B. Serine
    C. Glycine
    D. Tryptophan
    E. Phenylalanine

64. All of the following result in increased alveolar gas exchange EXCEPT

    A. decreased alveolar thickness.
    B. increased oxygen solubility.
    C. greater PaO_2 than PAO_2.
    D. increased alveolar surface area.
    E. all cause increased alveolar gas exchange.

65. Which of the following are produced after one turn of the Krebs cycle?

    A. 2 ATP, 2 NADH, 3 $FADH_2$
    B. 12 ATP, 1 GTP, 2 NADH
    C. 1 ATP, 1 NADH, 3 $FADH_2$
    D. 2 GTP, 2 NADH, 3 $FADH_2$
    E. 1 GTP, 3 NADH, 1 $FADH_2$

66. Which of the following receptors is largely responsible for detecting stretch?

    A. Free nerve endings
    B. Meissner corpuscles
    C. Ruffini corpuscles
    D. Pacinian corpuscles
    E. Merkel discs

67. ADH is produced in which structure?

    A. Hypothalamus
    B. Anterior pituitary
    C. Posterior pituitary
    D. Adrenal medulla
    E. Adrenal cortex

68. Which of the following enzymes does not match one of its functions?

    A. DNA polymerase: Synthesizes complementary DNA strand in 5′ to 3′ direction
    B. Exonuclease: Cleaves nucleotide primers
    C. Helicase: Winds the DNA molecule after replication
    D. DNA ligase: Ligates Okazaki fragments
    E. Restriction endonuclease: Cleaves DNA at specific points

69. Which of the following secretions is typically the most acidic?

    A. Bile
    B. Pancreatic
    C. Gastric
    D. Intestinal

70. The most common amino acid found in collagen is which of the following?

    A. Aspartate
    B. Proline
    C. Glycine
    D. Lysine
    E. Glutamine

71. Water is reabsorbed in all of the following segments of the nephron EXCEPT

    A. proximal convoluted tubule.
    B. descending loop of Henle.
    C. ascending loop of Henle.
    D. distal convoluted tubule.
    E. collecting duct.

72. Hematopoiesis occurs primarily in which tissue?

    A. Lymph nodes
    B. Red marrow
    C. Yellow marrow
    D. Spleen
    E. Thymus

73. The Na^+/K^+ pump functions via facilitated diffusion because it requires ATP.

    A. Both the statement and the reason are correct and related.
    B. Both the statement and the reason are correct but not related.
    C. The statement is correct, but the reason is not.
    D. The statement is not correct, but the reason is correct.
    E. Neither the statement nor the reason is correct.

74. Which of the following is the correct sequence of electrical conduction through the heart?

    A. SA node, AV node, bundle of His, Purkinje fibers, ventricular myocytes
    B. Ventricular myocytes, SA node, AV node, bundle of His, Purkinje fibers
    C. SA node, bundle of His, Purkinje fibers, AV node, ventricular myocytes
    D. AV node, SA node, bundle of His, Purkinje fibers, ventricular myocytes
    E. SA node, AV node, Purkinje fibers, bundle of His, ventricular myocytes

75. In erythrocytes, glycolysis always ends in lactate because they do not contain mitochondria.

    A. Both the statement and the reason are correct and related.
    B. Both the statement and the reason are correct but not related.
    C. The statement is correct, but the reason is not.

D. The statement is not correct, but the reason is correct.

E. Neither the statement nor the reason is correct.

76. Most skeletal muscle is innervated by what type of motor neuron?

A. α
B. β
C. γ
D. δ

77. An individual who has been taking prednisone for several months will most likely acquire which of the following?

A. Addison disease
B. Cushing disease
C. Cushing syndrome
D. Plummer disease
E. Myxedema

78. A deficiency in which of the following amino acids causes albinism?

A. Tyrosine
B. Tryptophan
C. Arginine
D. Leucine
E. Alanine

79. Which cranial nerves transmit taste to the brain?

A. VII
B. IX
C. X
D. A and B
E. All of the above

80. The Cori cycle functions by converting

A. glycogen to glucose
B. NAD^+ to NADH
C. acetyl-CoA to malonyl-CoA
D. lactate to glucose
E. pyruvate to glucose

81. All of the following will result in a right shift of the O_2-Hb dissociation curve EXCEPT

A. increased temperature.
B. decreased pH.
C. increased 2,3-biphosphoglycerate.
D. increased P_{CO_2}.
E. all will cause a right shift.

82. All preganglionic sympathetic neurons use norepinephrine as the major neurotransmitter. All postganglionic parasympathetic neurons use acetylcholine as the major neurotransmitter.

A. Both statements are true.
B. Both statements are false.
C. The first statement is true; the second statement is false.
D. The first statement is false; the second statement is true.

83. DNA synthesis occurs in which cell cycle phase?

A. Prophase
B. Metaphase
C. Anaphase
D. Telophase
E. Interphase

84. Osmosis is the simple diffusion of any liquid caused by a concentration gradient. Osmolarity is the osmotic pressure of a solution (in osmols/kg).

A. Both statements are true.
B. Both statements are false.
C. The first statement is true; the second statement is false.
D. The first statement is false; the second statement is true.

85. Which of the following is the final electron acceptor in the ETC?

A. NAD^+
B. NADH
C. O_2
D. Q
E. H_2O

86. All of the following are effects of parathyroid hormone (PTH) EXCEPT

   A. Increases renal calcium reabsorption
   B. Increases blood calcium levels
   C. Stimulates bone resorption
   D. Decreases renal phosphate reabsorption
   E. Decreases intestinal calcium absorption

87. Ventricular depolarization occurs during which portion of the ECG wave?

   A. PR interval
   B. ST segment
   C. P wave
   D. T wave
   E. QRS complex

88. All of the following events in collagen synthesis occur intracellularly EXCEPT

   A. hydroxylation of proline and lysine residues.
   B. cleavage of N- and C-terminal propeptides.
   C. glycosylation of α-chains.
   D. synthesis of α-chains.

89. Jaundice is caused by an increased blood level of

   A. bilirubin
   B. bile
   C. hemoglobin
   D. cholesterol
   E. cholecystokinin

90. In the ETC, which of the following is the terminal cytochrome?

   A. Cytochrome oxidase
   B. Cytochrome reductase
   C. Ubiquinone
   D. α-Ketoglutarate dehydrogenase
   E. NADH dehydrogenase

91. A surge of which hormone results in ovulation?

   A. Estrogen
   B. Progesterone
   C. LH

D. FSH
E. Oxytocin

92. During contraction, the length of each A band remains constant, but the H band shortens in length.

   A. Both statements are true.
   B. Both statements are false.
   C. The first statement is true; the second statement is false.
   D. The first statement is false; the second statement is true.

93. Both transcription and translation occur in the nucleus. Protein synthesis occurs in the 5' to 3' direction.

   A. Both statements are true.
   B. Both statements are false.
   C. The first statement is true; the second statement is false.
   D. The first statement is false; the second statement is true.

94. Aldosterone functions primarily at which segment of the nephron?

   A. Proximal convoluted tubule
   B. Descending loop of Henle
   C. Ascending loop of Henle
   D. Distal convoluted tubule
   E. Collecting duct

95. Which of the following statements is TRUE about myoglobin?

   A. Contains only one central zinc atom
   B. Transports oxygen in muscle tissue
   C. Can bind up to four molecules of oxygen
   D. Consists of one globin molecule
   E. Has less of an oxygen affinity compared to hemoglobin

96. Endochondral osteogenesis occurs by which of the following types of growth?

   A. Interstitial
   B. Appositional
   C. All of the above
   D. None of the above

97. Inspiration is generally an active process. Inspiration causes decreased alveolar and intrapleural pressures.

    A. Both statements are true.
    B. Both statements are false.
    C. The first statement is true; the second statement is false.
    D. The first statement is false; the second statement is true

98. Which disease is caused by a mutation of a cAMP-regulated Cl^- plasma membrane channel?

    A. Achondroplasia
    B. Cystic fibrosis
    C. Tay-Sachs disease
    D. Diabetes mellitus
    E. Multiple sclerosis

99. The motor end plate contains which type of receptor?

    A. Muscarinic
    B. Nicotinic-1
    C. Nicotinic-2
    D. Alpha-1
    E. Alpha-2

100. Which of the following is incorrect regarding the pentose phosphate pathway?

    A. Takes place in the cytosol
    B. Produces 2 ATP
    C. Converts glucose-6-phosphate to ribose-5-phosphate
    D. The rate-limiting step is the conversion of glucose-6-phosphate to 6-phosphogluconolactone
    E. Also called the hexose monophosphate shunt

101. The glossopharyngeal nerve (CN IX) provides afferent fibers to which of the following regulators?

    A. Carotid body chemoreceptors
    B. Aortic arch baroreceptors
    C. Atrial stretch receptors
    D. A and B
    E. All of the above

102. Which of the following is most important in regulating serum calcium levels?

    A. PTH
    B. Calcitonin
    C. Vitamin D
    D. Hydroxyapatite
    E. None of the above

103. Prednisone acts on which of the following enzymes?

    A. Phospholipase A_2
    B. Lipoxygenase
    C. HMG-CoA reductase
    D. Cyclooxygenase-1
    E. Cyclooxygenase-2

104. You decide to take a break after a long study session. As you get started on the treadmill, which of the following would *not* likely occur?

    A. Increased cardiac output
    B. Decreased β_1 activity
    C. Increased inotropic effect
    D. Decreased venous compliance
    E. Increased β_2 activity

105. A type I diabetic will have which change in enzymatic activity?

    A. Increased glycogen synthase
    B. Decreased lipase
    C. Increased acetyl-CoA carboxylase
    D. Increased fatty acid synthase
    E. Increased glycogen phosphorylase

106. All of the following occur in the liver EXCEPT

    A. urea cycle.
    B. gluconeogenesis.
    C. cholesterol synthesis.
    D. Entner-Doudoroff pathway.
    E. pentose phosphate pathway.

107. All of the following will create a decrease in glomerular filtration rate (GFR) EXCEPT

    A. increased hydrostatic pressure in Bowman space.
    B. decreased renal perfusion.
    C. decreased blood plasma oncotic pressure.
    D. afferent arteriole vasoconstriction.
    E. none of the above.

108. All of the following are post-transcriptional modifications EXCEPT

    A. removal of introns.
    B. removal of Okazaki fragments.
    C. addition of a 5′ cap.
    D. addition of a 3′ poly(A) tail.
    E. ligation of exons.

109. The "fight-or-flight" response is regulated by which type of cell?

    A. Dust cell
    B. Chief cell
    C. Parietal cell
    D. Chromaffin cell
    E. M cell

110. In humans, fatty acids can be converted to glucose, and glucose can be converted to fatty acids.

    A. Both statements are true.
    B. Both statements are false.
    C. The first statement is true; the second statement is false.
    D. The first statement is false; the second statement is true.

111. Postsynaptic nicotinic receptors are located on which portion of skeletal muscle?

    A. T tubule
    B. Sarcolemma
    C. Endomysium
    D. Perimysium
    E. Sarcomere

112. Taste buds are found on all of the following papillae EXCEPT

    A. fungiform.
    B. filiform.

    C. vallate.
    D. foliate.

113. Both HDL and LDL generally transport lipids to the liver. Lipoproteins contain various proportions of cholesterol, triglycerides, bile salts, and phospholipids.

    A. Both statements are true.
    B. Both statements are false.
    C. The first statement is true; the second statement is false.
    D. The first statement is false; the second statement is true.

114. All of the following will cause hypoxemia EXCEPT

    A. hyperventilation.
    B. V/Q mismatch.
    C. decreased alveolar surface area.
    D. decreased FiO_2.
    E. respiratory shunt.

115. Which of the following is the fastest mode of nerve transmission?

    A. Saltatory conduction
    B. Continuous conduction
    C. Axonotmesis
    D. Neurotmesis

116. All of the following are metabolic fates of acetyl-CoA EXCEPT

    A. glucose synthesis.
    B. cholesterol synthesis.
    C. fatty acid synthesis.
    D. ATP production.
    E. ketone body synthesis.

117. Renin ultimately results in activity of which tissue?

    A. Adrenal cortex
    B. Adrenal medulla
    C. Anterior pituitary
    D. Posterior pituitary
    E. Hypothalamus

118. Reverse transcriptase

    A. synthesizes a complementary strand of RNA from DNA.
    B. synthesizes a complementary strand of DNA from RNA.
    C. ligates each anticodon to tRNA.
    D. copies cellular RNA.
    E. copies cellular DNA.

119. Hematocrit is defined as

    A. the concentration of hemoglobin within erythrocytes.
    B. the percentage of erythrocytes in blood plasma volume.
    C. the number of erythrocytes in blood volume.
    D. the percentage of erythrocytes in blood volume.
    E. the percentage of hemoglobin in blood volume.

120. Which of the following are common methods of assessing GFR?

    A. Inulin clearance
    B. Creatinine clearance
    C. Urine production
    D. A and B
    E. All of the above

121. Which of the following has the strongest base pair bond in DNA?

    A. Guanine-cytosine
    B. Adenine-uracil
    C. Guanine-thymine
    D. Adenine-thymine
    E. Adenine-cytosine

122. Renin is secreted by cells in which segment of the nephron?

    A. Afferent arteriole
    B. Glomerulus
    C. Bowman capsule
    D. Efferent arteriole
    E. Proximal convoluted tubule

123. Under normal cellular conditions, all of the following have a higher extracellular concentration than intracellular concentration EXCEPT

    A. Na^+.
    B. Mg^{2+}.
    C. Cl^-.
    D. Ca^{2+}.
    E. HCO_3^-.

124. All of the following are secreted by pancreatic acinar cells EXCEPT

    A. pepsin.
    B. lipase.
    C. amylase.
    D. trypsin.
    E. chymotrypsin.

125. All of the following are caused by an overactive thyroid EXCEPT

    A. Grave disease.
    B. Plummer disease.
    C. Hashimoto thyroiditis.
    D. cretinism.
    E. toxic multinodular goiter.

126. Which of the following amino acids is not transaminated?

    A. Aspartate
    B. Alanine
    C. Glutamate
    D. Serine
    E. Tryptophan

127. Which type of muscle tissue behaves as a functional syncytium?

    A. Skeletal
    B. Cardiac
    C. Smooth
    D. B and C
    E. All of the above

128. Place the following organization of DNA in order of smallest to largest.

    A. Chromatin fibril, double-helix, chromosome, nucleosome
    B. Double-helix, nucleosome, chromatin fibril, chromosome
    C. Nucleosome, chromatin fibril, double-helix, chromosome
    D. Double-helix, nucleosome, chromosome, chromatin fibril

129. All of the following will increase cardiac output EXCEPT

    A. norepinephrine.
    B. SA nodal discharge.
    C. preload.
    D. contractile force.
    E. efferent vagal activity.

130. Metabolic alkalosis typically results in respiratory acidosis. The compensatory mechanism is hypoventilation.

    A. Both statements are true.
    B. Both statements are false.
    C. The first statement is true; the second statement is false.
    D. The first statement is false; the second statement is true.

131. Transamination reactions require which of the following as a cofactor?

    A. Vitamin B_2
    B. Vitamin B_6
    C. Vitamin B_{12}
    D. Vitamin C
    E. Vitamin E

132. Which of the following may be an inhibitory neurotransmitter?

    A. Acetylcholine
    B. GABA
    C. Glycine
    D. B and C
    E. All of the above

133. Sodium is impermeable to which segment of the nephron?

    A. Proximal convoluted tubule
    B. Descending loop of Henle
    C. Ascending loop of Henle
    D. Distal convoluted tubule
    E. Collecting duct

134. Which antibiotic inhibits bacterial protein synthesis?

    A. Amoxicillin
    B. Doxycycline
    C. Metronidazole
    D. Cephalexin
    E. Ciprofloxacin

135. The mandible contains only cortical bone. The maxilla contains only cancellous bone.

    A. Both statements are true.
    B. Both statements are false.
    C. The first statement is true; the second statement is false.
    D. The first statement is false; the second statement is true.

136. All of the following are true of RNA EXCEPT

    A. the backbone sugar is ribose.
    B. bases include adenine, uracil, guanine, and cytosine.
    C. it can be synthesized in the nucleolus.
    D. it is single stranded.
    E. it is abundant in smooth endoplasmic reticulum.

137. Which of the following is *not* a common second messenger in extracellular receptor signaling?

    A. cAMP
    B. Na^+
    C. Ca^{2+}
    D. IP_3
    E. DAG

138. The intrinsic and extrinsic clotting pathways meet with the activation of what factor?

    A. II
    B. IX
    C. X
    D. XI
    E. XII

139. Which amino acid is largely responsible for oxidative deamination reactions?

    A. Alanine
    B. Leucine
    C. Glutamate
    D. Methionine
    E. Valine

140. Cholecystokinin is secreted in response to duodenal disaccharides. The stimulation of gallbladder contraction is one of its major functions.

    A. Both statements are true.
    B. Both statements are false.
    C. The first statement is true; the second statement is false.
    D. The first statement is false; the second statement is true.

141. During swallowing, food may become lodged in which of the following structures?

    A. Vallecula
    B. Pyriform recess
    C. Salpingopharyngeal fold
    D. A and B
    E. All of the above

142. All of the following are true about the urea cycle EXCEPT

    A. Occurs in hepatocytes
    B. Requires aspartate
    C. Eliminates ammonia
    D. Produces urea
    E. Produces 3 ATP

143. All of the following are true of antidiuretic hormone (ADH) EXCEPT

    A. it is released from the posterior pituitary gland.
    B. it increases water reabsorption.
    C. its release is stimulated by increased thirst.
    D. it functions primarily at the collecting duct.
    E. all are true of ADH.

144. Eccrine sweat glands are controlled by cholinergic neurons. Apocrine sweat glands produce pheromones.

    A. Both statements are true.
    B. Both statements are false.
    C. The first statement is true; the second statement is false.
    D. The first statement is false; the second statement is true.

145. Each tRNA contains an anticodon. tRNA is the least prevalent RNA.

    A. Both statements are true.
    B. Both statements are false
    C. The first statement is true; the second statement is false.
    D. The first statement is false; the second statement is true.

146. Which of the following is the most important factor in determining the affinity of hemoglobin for oxygen?

    A. P_{CO_2}
    B. P_{O_2}
    C. pH
    D. Hb concentration
    E. Temperature

Biochemistry and Physiology

147. Place the following events of protein synthesis in chronological order

    A. RNA polymerase activity, small ribosomal subunit binds to mRNA, splicing of exons, anticodon binds to complementary codon, transfer of mRNA from the nucleus to cytoplasm
    B. Transfer of mRNA from the nucleus to cytoplasm, splicing of exons, small ribosomal subunit binds to mRNA, anticodon binds to complementary codon, RNA polymerase activity
    C. RNA polymerase activity, splicing of exons, transfer of mRNA from the nucleus to cytoplasm, anticodon binds to complementary codon, small ribosomal subunit binds to mRNA
    D. Transfer of mRNA from the nucleus to cytoplasm, small ribosomal subunit binds to mRNA, RNA polymerase activity, anticodon binds to complementary codon, splicing of exons
    E. RNA polymerase activity, splicing of exons, transfer of mRNA from the nucleus to cytoplasm, small ribosomal subunit binds to mRNA, anticodon binds to complementary codon

148. If the left side of the spinal cord was damaged, an individual would lose which functions?

    A. Right-side pain and temperature sense, and left-side motor function
    B. Left-side pain and temperature sense, and left-side motor function
    C. Left-side pain and temperature sense, and right-side motor function
    D. Right-side pain and temperature sense, and right-side motor function

149. The stretch reflex is mediated by muscle spindle receptors. It results in skeletal muscle relaxation.

    A. Both statements are true.
    B. Both statements are false.
    C. The first statement is true; the second statement is false.
    D. The first statement is false; the second statement is true.

150. Which of the following results from a disorder of urea synthesis?

    A. Phenylketonuria
    B. Alkaptonuria
    C. Pernicious anemia
    D. Citrullinemia
    E. Richner-Hanhart syndrome

151. Which of the following are released by the hypothalamus?

    A. TRH
    B. GHRH
    C. GnRH
    D. A and C
    E. All of the above

152. All of the following would likely result in an individual with severe anemia EXCEPT

    A. fatigue.
    B. cyanosis.
    C. hypoxia.
    D. increased cardiac output.
    E. pulmonary vasoconstriction.

153. Which of the following is not true of purines?

    A. Synthesized from ribose-5-phosphate
    B. Include adenine and guanine
    C. Catabolized to acetyl-CoA
    D. Pair with pyrimidines
    E. Cyclic structures composed of nitrogen and carbon

154. Thyroglobulin is a glycoprotein largely consisting of what amino acid?

    A. Tryptophan
    B. Arginine
    C. Lysine
    D. Proline
    E. Tyrosine

155. The immersion of cells in a hypotonic solution will result in which of the following?

    A. Cellular swelling
    B. Cellular shrinkage
    C. No change
    D. None of the above

156. Exocytosis is the process by which cells release macromolecules to the ECM. Pinocytosis is a type of exocytosis.

    A. Both statements are true.
    B. Both statements are false.
    C. The first statement is true; the second statement is false.
    D. The first statement is false; the second statement is true.

157. All of the following stimulate osteoclastic activity EXCEPT

    A. IL-1.
    B. TNF-β
    C. IL-8.
    D. PTH.
    E. RANKL.

158. Which of the following is NOT TRUE of the Entner-Doudoroff pathway?

    A. Produces 1 ATP per glucose
    B. Coverts glucose to pyruvate
    C. Occurs in hepatocytes
    D. Produces 1 NADH
    E. Produces glyceraldehyde-3-phosphate

159. Intrinsic factor binds to which of the following vitamins?

    A. Vitamin B_1
    B. Vitamin B_2
    C. Vitamin B_3
    D. Vitamin B_6
    E. Vitamin B_{12}

160. During skeletal muscle contraction, calcium binds to which of the following?

    A. Tropomyosin
    B. Actin
    C. Calmodulin
    D. Myosin
    E. Troponin

161. All of the following are water-soluble vitamins EXCEPT

    A. vitamin B_6.
    B. vitamin C.

C. folic acid.
D. vitamin E.
E. biotin.

162. Which of the following is a transient cessation of breathing?

    A. Hypoventilation
    B. Dyspnea
    C. Hypocapnia
    D. Apnea
    E. Hyperapnea

163. Beta-2 adrenergic agonists cause which of the following?

    A. Vascular smooth muscle vasoconstriction
    B. Bronchodilation
    C. Miosis
    D. Increased heart rate
    E. GI relaxation

164. All of the following are true of the genetic code EXCEPT

    A. Universal
    B. Degenerate
    C. Unambiguous
    D. Overlapping
    E. Without punctuation

165. The length of the absolute refractory period of the cardiac action potential is dictated by which of the following?

    A. Na^+ channel opening
    B. K^+ channel opening
    C. Na^+ channel closure
    D. K^+ channel closure
    E. Ca^{2+} channel opening

166. β-Oxidation converts

    A. fatty acids to acyl-CoA.
    B. triglycerides to fatty acids.
    C. acetyl-CoA to malonyl-CoA.
    D. acetyl-CoA to HMG-CoA.
    E. acyl-CoA to acetyl-CoA.

Biochemistry and Physiology

167. Central diabetes insipidus is most commonly caused by a defect in the activity of which structure?

    A. Adrenal cortex
    B. Adrenal medulla
    C. Anterior pituitary
    D. Posterior pituitary

168. The countercurrent exchange system is based on which of the following?

    A. Na^+ reabsorption
    B. H_2O reabsorption
    C. H_2O impermeability
    D. A and C
    E. All of the above

169. A deficiency in which of the following results in pernicious anemia?

    A. Cobalt
    B. Iodine
    C. Magnesium
    D. Manganese
    E. Zinc

170. Which of the following may impair odontogenesis?

    A. Cephalexin
    B. Amoxicillin
    C. Doxycycline
    D. Clindamycin
    E. None of the above

171. Which of the following metabolic enzymes require ATP?

    A. Phosphofructokinase
    B. Carbonic anhydrase
    C. Lactate dehydrogenase
    D. HMG-CoA reductase
    E. Transaminase

172. Which of the following muscles contains the food bolus in proximity of the teeth for optimal mastication?

    A. Medial pterygoid
    B. Masseter
    C. Buccinator
    D. Lateral pterygoid

173. After completing a lengthy dental procedure, you sit your patient up to rinse out. He quickly becomes dizzy and loses his balance due to orthostatic hypotension. Which of the following regulatory mechanisms is responsible for the physiologic correction several seconds later?

    A. Bainbridge reflex
    B. Chemoreceptor activity
    C. Baroreceptor activity
    D. A and C
    E. None of the above

174. Which of the following is a portion of a transcriptional promoter?

    A. TATA box
    B. Zinc finger
    C. snRNP
    D. Leucine zipper
    E. Helix-turn-helix

175. All are true of smooth muscle cells EXCEPT

    A. they have only one nucleus.
    B. they are typically very long.
    C. their myofibrils are not striated.
    D. they have an extensive SR.
    E. they do not have T tubules.

176. Which of the following metabolic reactions and their location of action are incorrect?

    A. Fatty acid synthesis: Cytosol
    B. ETC: Inner mitochondrial membrane
    C. β-Oxidation: Mitochondrial matrix
    D. Pentose phosphate pathway: Mitochondrial matrix
    E. Glycolysis: Cytosol

177. All of the following are secreted by the small intestine EXCEPT

    A. oligosaccharidases.
    B. peptidases.
    C. lipase.
    D. mucin.
    E. all are intestinal secretions.

178. Which of the following will likely occur in an individual who has just reached the peak of Mount McKinley?

    A. O_2-Hb curve shifts to the right
    B. Respiratory alkalosis
    C. Increased erythropoietin release
    D. Pulmonary vasoconstriction
    E. All of the above

179. Retinol is essential for vision because it is a constituent of rhodopsin and iodopsin.

    A. Both the statement and the reason are correct and related.
    B. Both the statement and the reason are correct but not related.
    C. The statement is correct, but the reason is not.
    D. The statement is not correct, but the reason is correct.
    E. Neither the statement nor the reason is correct.

180. The ventral horn of the spinal cord carries what fibers?

    A. Motor: skeletal muscle
    B. Motor: smooth muscle
    C. Sensory: pain and temperature
    D. Sensory: touch and pressure

181. Sodium has a much higher intracellular concentration than extracellular concentration. Blood plasma makes up about 8% of total body water.

    A. Both statements are true.
    B. Both statements are false.
    C. The first statement is true; the second statement is false.
    D. The first statement is false; the second statement is true.

182. In order to convert alanine to cholesterol, the correct sequence of intermediates is

    A. oxaloacetate, acyl-CoA, fatty acid, mevalonate, cholesterol
    B. pyruvate, acetyl-CoA, HMG-CoA, mevalonate, Cholesterol

    C. oxaloacetate, pyruvate, glycerol, HMG-CoA, cholesterol
    D. pyruvate, fatty acid, HMG-CoA, acetyl-CoA, cholesterol
    E. ketone body, HMG-CoA, mevalonate, acetyl-CoA, cholesterol

183. Gastric emptying is regulated by which of the following?

    A. CN IX
    B. CN X
    C. CN XI
    D. Spinal nerves
    E. All of the above

184. DNA polymerase synthesizes DNA from the lagging strand in the 5′ to 3′ direction. DNA polymerase synthesizes DNA from the leading strand in the 3′ to 5′ direction.

    A. Both statements are true.
    B. Both statements are false.
    C. The first statement is true; the second statement is false.
    D. The first statement is false; the second statement is true.

185. Hormones that affect females only are secreted by which of the following glands?

    A. Adrenal medulla
    B. Anterior pituitary
    C. Posterior pituitary
    D. B and C
    E. All of the above

186. According to the Frank-Starling mechanism, which of the following is the most important determinant in cardiac output?

    A. End diastolic volume
    B. Stroke volume
    C. Heart rate
    D. Oxygen consumption
    E. Systolic intraventricular pressure

187. All of the following are not true of vitamin K
EXCEPT

   A. deficiency causes a prolonged PTT.
   B. it activates clotting factors II, VIII, X,
      and XI.
   C. it is also known as tocopherol.
   D. it activates prothrombin.
   E. it is critical component of the intrinsic
      clotting pathway.

188. Calcium is stored in which of the following
muscle cell components?

   A. Sarcoplasmic reticulum
   B. Sarcomere
   C. Sarcolemma
   D. Sarcoplasm
   E. T tubules

189. *G6PD* deficiency causes hemolytic anemia
due to a decrease in NADPH production in
erythrocytes.

   A. Both the statement and the reason are
      correct and related.
   B. Both the statement and the reason are
      correct but not related.
   C. The statement is correct, but the reason is
      not.
   D. The statement is not correct, but the
      reason is correct.
   E. Neither the statement nor the reason is
      correct.

190. Bitter taste cells transmit taste stimuli by

   A. production of H^+ which closes K^+
      channels.
   B. activating IP_3 which increases intracellu-
      lar Ca^{2+}.
   C. Na^+ influx through passive ion channels.
   D. activating cAMP which closes K^+
      channels.

191. Amino acids are primarily reabsorbed in
which segment of the nephron?

   A. Proximal convoluted tubule
   B. Descending loop of Henle
   C. Ascending loop of Henle

   D. Distal convoluted tubule
   E. Collecting duct

192. All of the following are essential to TCA
cycle function EXCEPT

   A. vitamin B_1.
   B. vitamin B_2.
   C. vitamin B_3.
   D. vitamin B_5.
   E. vitamin B_6.

193. All of the following regulate bone remodeling
EXCEPT

   A. calcitonin.
   B. osteoprotegerin.
   C. parathyroid hormone.
   D. osteopontin.
   E. BMP-2.

194. All of the following are true of human mitochondrial DNA EXCEPT

   A. Circular
   B. Double stranded
   C. Contains about 1% of all cellular DNA
   D. Has lower mutation rate than nuclear
      DNA
   E. Transmitted by maternal non-Mendelian
      inheritance

195. Carbon dioxide is carried in blood as

   A. dissolved CO_2.
   B. bicarbonate.
   C. carbaminohemoglobin.
   D. A and B.
   E. all of the above.

196. Under anaerobic conditions, how many net
ATPs are produced per glucose?

   A. 0
   B. 1
   C. 2
   D. 4
   E. 6

197. Which of the following tissues have post-ganglionic sympathetic neurons that are cholinergic?

A. Sebaceous glands
B. Skeletal muscle vasculature
C. Sweat glands
D. B and C
E. All of the above

198. All of the following anatomic structures release hormones that will increase blood glucose levels EXCEPT

A. anterior pituitary gland.
B. adrenal medulla.
C. adrenal cortex.
D. pancreatic α-cells.
E. pancreatic β-cells.

199. Translation usually begins with what codon?

A. AAC
B. AUG
C. UAC
D. UAG
E. UGA

200. Sickle cell anemia is caused by what type of mutation?

A. Nonsense mutation
B. Transition mutation
C. Repeat mutation
D. Transverse mutation
E. Missense mutation

Biochemistry and Physiology

1. **The correct answer is C.** The plateau results from a very slow influx of calcium ions, balanced against the efflux of potassium ions. This period ends with the decline in calcium permeability as potassium permeability increases, resulting in repolarization.

   Answers A, B, D, and E are incorrect. See above.

2. **The correct answer is B.** The first law of thermodynamics states that the total energy of a closed system is conserved. The second law of thermodynamics states that the entropy of a closed system always increases.

   Answers A, C, and D are incorrect. See above.

3. **The correct answer is D.** Aldosterone is a steroid hormone, derived from cholesterol. Steroid hormones function by binding to intracellular receptors, forming hormone response elements (HREs). Peptide hormones are synthesized as a precursor form, transported unbound in blood, and bind to plasma membrane receptors, generating second messengers. Examples include pituitary hormones, pancreatic hormones, and parathyroid hormone.

   Answers A, B, C, and E are incorrect. See above.

4. **The correct answer is B.** Arterioles account for the largest proportion of peripheral vascular resistance. Remember that there is about a 50% drop in blood pressure as blood travels from arteries to arterioles.

   Answers A, C, D, and E are incorrect. See above.

5. **The correct answer is D.** CA is highly active in erythrocytes and nephrons.

   Answer A is incorrect. Most isoforms of CA contain a central zinc atom.

Answer B is incorrect. CA interconverts carbon dioxide and bicarbonate.

Answer C is incorrect. CA accelerates the reaction by a factor of more than a million.

Answer E is incorrect. CA II provides protons to neutralize intracellular OH^- ions after H^+ ions are pumped across osteoclastic ruffled borders.

Carbonic anhydrase

$$CO_2 + H_2O \rightleftharpoons H_2CO_3 \rightleftharpoons H^+ + HCO_3^-$$

6. **The correct answer is C.** Cardiac muscle contraction occurs via actin-linked regulation, which is dependent on calcium-troponin interactions. Remember that troponin is a thin myofilament attached to tropomyosin.

   Answers A, B, D, and E are incorrect. See above.

7. **The correct answer is B.** McArdle syndrome (type V glycogenosis) causes muscle cramping and results in decreased exercise tolerance. Muscles have abnormally high glycogen content. There is little or no lactic acid in blood after exercise.

   Answer A is incorrect. Pompe disease (type II glycogenosis) results from a deficiency of lysosomal glucosidase.

   Answer C is incorrect. Hunter syndrome is a mucopolysaccharide storage disease caused by a deficiency of L-iduronate sulfatase.

   Answer D is incorrect. Von Gierke disease (type I glycogenosis) results from a deficiency of glucose-6-phosphatase.

   Answer E is incorrect. Hurler syndrome is a mucopolysaccharide storage disease caused by a deficiency of α-L-iduronidase.

8. **The correct answer is B.** ECF comprises approximately $1/3$ of total body water. Recall

that it contains higher concentrations of Na^+, Cl^-, and bicarbonate. Intracellular fluid makes up the remaining $2/3$ of total body water. It has greater concentrations of K^+, Mg^{2+}, PO_4^{3-}, and protein.

Answers A, C, D, and E are incorrect. See above.

9. **The correct answer is B.** Only hyaline cartilage has the ability to calcify, as it is the precursor to endochondral ossification. However, not all hyaline cartilage calcifies. Hyaline cartilage is found at the articular surfaces of long bones, ribs, nose, trachea, bronchi, and larynx.

Answers A, C, D, and E are incorrect. See above.

10. **The correct answer is C.** Aminotransferases function as transaminases, converting one amino acid to another. They are not involved in DNA synthesis.

Answer A is incorrect. DNA polymerase synthesizes the new complementary strand in the $5' \rightarrow 3'$ direction.

Answer B is incorrect. Exonuclease removes the nucleotide primer at the completion of DNA synthesis.

Answer D is incorrect. Topoisomerase secures the replication fork of the DNA molecule.

Answer E is incorrect. Helicase unwinds the DNA molecule.

11. **The correct answer is B.** The parathyroid gland is not directly linked by hypothalamic regulation. Plasma Ca^{2+} is the major determinant of PTH secretion.

Answers A, C, D, and E are incorrect. See above.

12. **The correct answer is A.** Hydrolases cleave bonds by hydrolysis; lyases cleave bonds by elimination.

Answer B is incorrect. Transferases transfer functional groups; isomerases catalyze a change in molecular structure.

Answer C is incorrect. Ligases join two molecules together; oxidoreductases catalyze redox reactions.

Answers D and E are incorrect. See above.

13. **The correct answer is D.** Both GIP and secretin decrease gastric acid secretion and gastric motility. Secretin is released by a drop in pH in the duodenum, as chyme is passed through the pyloric sphincter. Gastric inhibitory peptide (GIP) is secreted by the presence of fats and glucose in the duodenum.

Answer A is incorrect. Gastrin stimulates gastric HCl secretion and increases gastric motility. It is released by the presence of peptides and amino acids within the stomach lumen.

Answers B, C, and E are incorrect. See above.

14. **The correct answer is D.** Inspiratory capacity (IC) is the maximum volume of air that can be inhaled after a normal expiration.

IC = IRV + TV.

Answer A is incorrect. Expiratory reserve volume (ERV) is the maximum amount of air that can be exhaled at the end of tidal volume.

ERV = FRC – RV.

Answers B and E are incorrect. Vital capacity (VC) is the volume of air that can be exhaled after maximum inspiration.

VC = TLV – RV, and also = TV + IRV + ERV.

Answer C is incorrect. Total lung volume (TLV) is the total volume of air in the lungs after maximum inspiration.

TLV = VC + RV, and also = IRV + TV + ERV + RV.

15. **The correct answer is E.** The Gibbs free energy change (ΔG) determines the direction of a reaction. If $\Delta G_S > \Delta G_P$, then the ΔG will be negative and the reaction will proceed spontaneously toward equilibrium. Equilibrium is attained when $\Delta G = 0$.

Answer A is incorrect. ΔG provides no information about the reaction rate.

Answer B is incorrect. Exergonic reactions will release energy; ΔG will be negative.

Answer C is incorrect. ΔG does not determine reaction equilibrium.

Answer D is incorrect. ΔG is independent of the path of the reaction.

16. **The correct answer is D.** The somatic nervous system is a subdivision of the peripheral nervous system. It consists of the 12 cranial nerves and 31 pairs of spinal nerves. Somatic motor neurons do not synapse in a peripheral ganglion (there is only one efferent neuron from the CNS to the end organ). However, somatic sensory neurons (transmitting pain, temperature, touch, etc) synapse in the dorsal root ganglion.

    Answers A, B, C, and E are incorrect. See above.

17. **The correct answer is C.** Chondroitin sulfates are the most prominent proteoglycans in cartilage and bone.

    Answer A is incorrect. Keratin sulfates are most prominent in the cornea (type I) and loose connective tissue (type II).

    Answer B is incorrect. Heparin sulfate is present mostly in basement membranes, cell surfaces, and ECM.

    Answer D is incorrect. Dermatan sulfate is widely distributed in skin and vascular tissue.

    Answer E is incorrect. Hyaluronic acid is the most unique GAG in that it consists of an unbranched chain of repeating disaccharide units. It does not form a proteoglycan and does not contain sulfur. It is widely distributed in ECM, vitreous humor, synovial fluid, and loose connective tissue.

18. **The correct answer is A.** The pulmonary circulation has less resistance than the systemic circulation. Recall that it is a much shorter cycle than the systemic circulation.

Answers B, C, D, and E are incorrect. See above.

19. **The correct answer is B.** Growth hormone (GH) exerts its effects on almost all tissues.

    Answer A is incorrect. FSH acts on testicular and ovarian tissue.

    Answer C is incorrect. ACTH acts on the adrenal gland.

    Answer D is incorrect. Prolactin acts on breast tissue.

    Answer E is incorrect. TSH acts on the thyroid gland.

20. **The correct answer is E.** A frameshift mutation involves the deletion or insertion of 1-2 base pairs, changing the entire reading frame of the DNA template, and thus the translated amino acid sequence. Remember that *point mutations* involve the substitution of one base for another. Although this may alter the amino acid sequence, it only does so for that particular codon.

    Answer A is incorrect. A nonsense mutation is a type of point mutation that results in a stop codon, terminating the polypeptide chain elongation.

    Answer B is incorrect. A repeat mutation is an amplification of the same three-nucleotide sequence. This will create consecutive strings of the same amino acid, but does not alter the entire reading frame of the DNA template.

    Answer C is incorrect. A transverse mutation is a type of point mutation in which the purine-pyrimidine orientation is changed.

    Answer D is incorrect. A missense mutation is a type of point mutation that results in the translation of a different amino acid for that particular codon (eg, valine replaces glutamate causing sickle cell anemia).

21. **The correct answer is A.** Renin is secreted by the JGA in response to a decrease in renal blood pressure and GFR. It converts

angiotensinogen to angiotensin I. Angiotensin I is then converted to angiotensin II by ACE. Angiotensin II causes vasoconstriction, and stimulates the adrenal cortex to release aldosterone, which increases sodium retention.

Answers B, C, D, and E are incorrect. See above.

22. **The correct answer is C.** Plasma membranes are asymmetrical.

   Answer A is incorrect. Plasma membranes are selectively permeable, enabling only certain molecules (water and small, nonpolar) to easily pass.

   Answer B is incorrect. Plasma membranes function as barriers.

   Answer D is incorrect. Plasma membranes contain phospholipids, glycosphingolipids, and cholesterol in varying ratios.

   Answer E is incorrect. Plasma membranes have an amphipathic lipid bilayer consisting of outer, hydrophilic head groups and inner, hydrophobic tail groups.

23. **The correct answer is C.** Almost all CT originates from mesoderm. However, some CT of the head and neck region derives from neural crest ectoderm. Recall that the calvarium, facial bones, clavicle, and jaws arise from neural crest ectoderm. Dense CT provides structural support because it has a greater fiber concentration than loose CT. However, most dense CT has an *irregular* arrangement of fibers and cells. Regular CT, consisting of an ordered arrangement of cells and fibers, is commonly found in ligaments, tendons, and aponeuroses.

   Answers A, B, and D are incorrect. See above.

24. **The correct answer is C.** The four basic tastes: sweet, sour, bitter, and salty. Each taste bud contains various taste cells surrounded by epithelial cells. So, although each taste bud may be able to sense all four of the basic tastes, there is a unique taste cell for each taste.

Answers A, B, and D are incorrect. See above.

25. **The correct answer is C.** Activation energy is the energy needed to initiate a reaction. Therefore, an increase in activation energy will slow the reaction rate. Enzymes function by lowering the activation energy of a reaction.

   Answer A is incorrect. A rise in temperature will increase reaction rate. However, an extreme increase in temperature can cause enzyme denaturation.

   Answer B is incorrect. An increase in enzyme concentration will increase reaction rate.

   Answer D is incorrect. An increase in substrate concentration will increase reaction rate.

   Answer E is incorrect. See above.

26. **The correct answer is E.** The Z line is a dark band that bisects each I band. The portion of a myofibril located between two Z lines is defined as a sarcomere.

   Answer A is incorrect. The A band is a dark band consisting of myosin filaments (centrally) and actin filaments (laterally). It is bisected by the M line.

   Answer B is incorrect. The H band is a lighter band that bisects the A band.

   Answer C is incorrect. The I band is a light band that consists only of actin.

   Answer D is incorrect. The M line bisects both the A band and the sarcomere.

27. **The correct answer is D.** Mannose is an aldose monosaccharide.

   Answer A is incorrect. Sucrose is a disaccharide of glucose + fructose.

   Answer B is incorrect. Maltose is a disaccharide of glucose + glucose.

   Answer C is incorrect. Lactose is a disaccharide of glucose + galactose.

28. **The correct answer is E.** The intrinsic pathway is initiated by the activation of factor XII

(Hageman factor) from collagen, platelets, and fibrin. Recall that the extrinsic clotting pathway is initiated by tissue factor (tissue thromboplastin) as a response to contact with injured tissue.

Answers A, B, C, and D are incorrect. See above.

29. **The correct answer is C.** Segmentation (mixing) is most common in the small intestine, decreasing its rate as you progress further down the GI tract. It involves rhythmic contractions which serve to chop chyme, mixing it with digestive enzymes, and keeping it in contact with the gut wall for maximum absorption. In the duodenum, it occurs at a rate of 11-12 cycles per minute.

    Answer A is incorrect. Tonic contractions occur at sphincters throughout the GI tract, and last much longer than segmentation.

    Answer B is incorrect. Peristalsis is a series of coordinated contractions that propels chyme down the GI tract.

    Answers D and E are incorrect. See above.

30. **The correct answer is B.** Zymogens are enzymatically inactive precursors of proteolytic enzymes. Protcases cleave the proenzyme propeptides, activating the enzyme. Calmodulin is an already active enzyme that binds Ca^{2+}, activating the actin-myosin complex of smooth muscle. It also serves other microfilament-mediated functions such as cell motility, conformational changes, mitosis, exocytosis, and endocytosis.

    Answer A is incorrect. Factor I (fibrinogen) is cleaved by thrombin to form fibrin.

    Answer C is incorrect. Trypsinogen is cleaved by enteropeptidase to form trypsin.

    Answer D is incorrect. Factor X is cleaved by tissue factor complex to form factor Xa.

    Answer E is incorrect. Procollagen is cleaved by endopeptidases to form tropocollagen.

31. **The correct answer is D.** Hyperventilation is initiated due to an increase in P_{CO_2}. The increased rate of breathing "blows off" excess CO_2. Thus, hyperventilation results in a decrease of P_{CO_2} to its normal physiologic range.

    Answer A is incorrect. The increased respiratory rate causes a $\uparrow P_{O_2}$.

    Answer B is incorrect. The resultant decrease in CO_2 causes hypocapnia.

    Answer C is incorrect. The resultant decrease in P_{CO_2} causes vasoconstriction, leading to $\downarrow$ cerebral blood flow.

    Answer E is incorrect. Respiratory alkalosis occurs due to the $\uparrow$ pH.

32. **The correct answer is A.** Aminoacyl-tRNA synthetase adds each amino acid to tRNA.

    Answer B is incorrect. tRNA carries the anticodon to each mRNA.

    Answer C is incorrect. Although there are two ribosomal subunits that are involved in protein synthesis, they are of different sizes.

    Answer D is incorrect. Protein synthesis occurs in both prokaryotic (containing 70S ribosomes) and eukaryotic cells (containing 80S ribosomes).

    Answer E is incorrect. Translation occurs in the 5' to 3' direction.

33. **The correct answer is B.** By blocking sodium channels, the absolute refractory period is prolonged (APs cannot be generated), and transient anesthesia occurs.

    Answers A, C, D, and E are incorrect. See above.

34. **The correct answer is C.** You need to understand Starling forces to correctly answer this question. Hydrostatic pressure is the "push" created by a fluid (moving that fluid from one space to another). Oncotic pressure, on the other hand, is the "pull" force exerted by proteins and large molecules (which do not diffuse). Recall that edema is excess fluid in the interstitial space. The only answer choice which creates a gradient that moves fluid from the vasculature to the surrounding connective tissue is decreased capillary oncotic pressure.

Answers A, B, D, and E are incorrect. See above.

35. **The correct answer is B.** Competitive inhibitors increase K_m without any change in V_{max}. Noncompetitive inhibitors decrease V_{max} without any change in K_m.

    Answers A, C, and D are incorrect. See above.

36. **The correct answer is D.** All of these drugs are bisphosphonates, which are potent inhibitors of osteoclasts. Several case reports and reviews have associated their use with a rare condition called osteonecrosis of the jaws (ONJ), in which portions of the maxilla or mandible become exposed and necrotic. Intravenous bisphosphonates (pamidronate and zolendronate) are often used to treat bone cancers (such as multiple myeloma); while oral bisphosphonates (alendronate, risedronate, and ibandronate) are used to treat osteopenia and osteoporosis.

    Answers A, B, C, and E are incorrect. See above.

37. **The correct answer is B.** Amylases cleave α-1,4-glycosidic linkages. Isomaltase cleaves α-1,6-glycosidic linkages.

    Answer A is incorrect. α-Amylase is secreted by both the parotid gland and the pancreas.

    Answers C and D are incorrect. Amylases catalyze the hydrolysis of starch to dextrins, and a mixture of glucose, maltose, and isomaltose.

38. **The correct answer is C.** Hyperparathyroidism (↑ PTH) results in increased bone resorption and loss of bone density. On periapical radiographs, you may find a loss of a normal trabecular pattern, widened PDL spaces, absence of a lamina dura, and radiolucent cystlike spaces (brown tumors).

    Answers A, B, D, and E are incorrect. See above.

39. **The correct answer is B.** Remember that TPR is the vascular resistance of the systemic circulation. TPR = (MAP − CVP)/CO. Thus,

TPR is indirectly proportional to CO. It is also highly regulated by the sympathetic nervous system ($α_1$ activation ↑ TPR, $β_2$ activation ↓ TPR), and thermal changes (extreme cold ↑ TPR).

Answers A, C, and D are incorrect. See above.

40. **The correct answer is E.** Both vitamin H (biotin) and vitamin B_5 (pantothenic acid) are cofactors for acetyl-CoA carboxylase, which converts acetyl-CoA → malonyl-CoA during fatty acid synthesis.

    Answer A is incorrect. Vitamin E (tocopherol) is a potent antioxidant.

    Answer B is incorrect. Vitamin B_1 (thiamine) is a cofactor for pyruvate dehydrogenase (converts pyruvate → acetyl-CoA), α-ketoglutarate dehydrogenase (converts α-ketoglutarate → succinyl-CoA in TCA cycle), and ketoacid dehydrogenase (metabolism of leucine, isoleucine, and valine).

    Answer C is incorrect. Vitamin B_6 (pyridoxine) is a cofactor in transamination reactions.

    Answer D is incorrect. Vitamin B_{12} (cobalamin) is a cofactor for methionine synthase (converts homocysteine → methionine) and methylmalonyl-CoA isomerase (converts methylmalonyl-CoA → succinyl-CoA).

41. **The correct answer is D.** Calmodulin is an integral part of myosin-linked regulation during smooth muscle contraction. Calcium (from the SR or extracellular sources) binds calmodulin, which then activates a myosin light-chain kinase.

    Answers C and E are incorrect. It is the myosin light-chain kinase that transfers a P_i from ATP to myosin, enabling interaction with actin, and thus contracting the muscle fibers.

42. **The correct answer is A.** Simple Michaelis-Menten kinetics is *not* followed in most allosteric enzyme reactions.

    Answer B is incorrect. Both the allosteric and catalytic binding sites on enzymes are unique.

Biochemistry and Physiology

Answer C is incorrect. Many allosteric reactions involve feedback regulation (either negatively or positively).

Answer D is incorrect. Allosteric effects can be on K_m or on V_{max}. For some reactions, substrate concentration kinetics are competitive in the sense that K_m is increased without a change in V_{max}. However, other reactions follow noncompetitive substrate concentration kinetics in that V_{max} is lowered without affecting K_m.

Answer E is incorrect. See above.

43. **The correct answer is D.** Both FSH and LH function in both males and females. FSH stimulates sperm production (in testicular Sertoli cells) and graafian follicle development (in ovaries). LH promotes testosterone production (in testicular Leydig cells) and estrogen production (in ovaries).

    Answers A, B, and C are incorrect. See above.

44. **The correct answer is D.** Blood is slightly alkaline. Its pH is tightly regulated by the bicarbonate to CO_2 ratio.

    Answers A, B, C, and E are incorrect. See above.

45. **The correct answer is A.** The tumor suppressor, p53, is a DNA binding transcription factor that plays a key role in G_1 and G_2 checkpoint control. An increased level of p53 activates a series of genes that delay the cell cycle. If DNA damage is too severe, the affected cell undergoes apoptosis.

    Answers B, C, D, and E are incorrect. See above.

46. **The correct answer is E.** Remember that the pancreas is both an endocrine and an exocrine gland. Insulin, glucagon, and somatostatin are released from the endocrine portion (pancreatic islets) directly into the bloodstream. Only the pancreatic exocrine products (lipase, amylase, trypsinogen, etc) are secreted via ducts. Thus, if the question had asked about these secretions, the answer would be "D," merocrine and acinar.

Answers A, B, C, and D are incorrect. See above.

47. **The correct answer is C.** Although the vast majority of oxygen is transported in blood by hemoglobin, a small amount is dissolved in the blood.

    Answer A is incorrect. Recall that CO_2 is carried mostly by serum bicarbonate.

    Answers B, D, and E are incorrect. See above.

48. **The correct answer is D.** Collagen is not a component of plasma cell membranes.

    Answer A is incorrect. Sphingomyelin and phosphoglycerides are the two major phospholipids commonly found in plasma membranes.

    Answer B is incorrect. Cholesterol is commonly found in plasma membranes.

    Answer C is incorrect. G proteins are transmembrane GTPase receptors.

    Answer E is incorrect. Arachidonic acid accounts for 5%-15% of the fatty acids in phospholipids of plasma membranes.

49. **The correct answer is C.** Pain and temperature afferent neurons are carried in the anterolateral pathway (lateral spinothalamic tract) of white matter. After synapsing in the dorsal root ganglion, recall that these fibers decussate in the dorsal horn (gray matter) before entering the ascending column (contralateral ascension).

    Answers A and E are incorrect. The dorsal column pathway transmits touch and pressure afferent neurons (ipsilateral ascension). When they enter the medulla, they synapse with neurons in the dorsal column nuclei, decussate, and enter the thalamus as part of the medial lemniscal pathway. The neurons in the thalamus then extend into the cortex.

    Answer B is incorrect. Light touch afferents are carried in the anterolateral pathway (anterior spinothalamic tract) of white matter.

Answer D is incorrect. The corticospinal tract transmits efferent motor neurons that control fine, skilled movements of skeletal muscle.

50. **The correct answer is D.** The rate-limiting step in glycolysis is the conversion of fructose-6-phosphate to fructose-1,6-biphosphate via phosphofructokinase (PFK). This step requires the hydrolysis of 1 ATP.

    Answer A is incorrect. Each molecule of glucose is converted to 2 molecules of pyruvate.

    Answer B is incorrect. Glycolysis is also called Embden-Meyerhof pathway.

    Answer C is incorrect. Glycolysis occurs in the cytosol.

    Answer E is incorrect. The metabolism of one glucose molecule produces 4 ATP. Remember, though, that 2 ATP are hydrolyzed via hexokinase and PFK. Therefore, glycolysis results in the direct net production of 2 ATP.

51. **The correct answer is D.** The first heart sound (S1 – "lub") is caused by the closure of the AV (mitral and tricuspid) valves, and indicates the start of systole (ventricular contraction). The second heart sound (S2 – "dub") is caused by the closure of the semilunar (aortic and pulmonic) valves, and indicates the beginning of diastole (ventricular filling). S1 is generally louder and longer than S2.

    Answers A, B, and C are incorrect. See above.

52. **The correct answer is A.** Cholecystokinin stimulates contraction of the gallbladder and relaxation of the sphincter of Oddi. This, in turn, releases bile into the small intestine.

    Answers B, C, D, and E are incorrect. See above.

53. **The correct answer is A.** Valine is an essential amino acid and cannot be synthesized from dietary intake of glucose. Remember the mnemonic for the essential amino acids: Private Tim Hall.

    Answer B is incorrect. Arginine is a nonessential amino acid.

Answer C is incorrect. Serine is a nonessential amino acid.

Answer D is incorrect. Glutamate is a nonessential amino acid.

Answer E is incorrect. Alanine is a nonessential amino acid.

54. **The correct answer is A.** The salpingopharyngeus elevates the nasopharynx and opens the auditory tube. It is generally not involved in swallowing.

    Answer B is incorrect. The levator veli palatini raises the palate.

    Answer C is incorrect. The palatopharyngeus raises the pharynx and larynx.

    Answer D is incorrect. The tensor veli palatini tenses the palate.

    Answer E is incorrect. All of the pharyngeal constrictors contract in waves (to propel food downward).

55. **The correct answer is A.** Enolase converts 2-phosphoglycerate → phosphoenolpyruvate.

    Answer B is incorrect. PFK converts fructose-6-phosphate → fructose-1,6-biphosphate. This is the rate-limiting reaction of glycolysis.

    Answer C is incorrect. Lactate dehydrogenase converts pyruvate → lactate.

    Answer D is incorrect. Hexokinase converts glucose → glucose-6-phosphate. This is the first step in glycolysis.

    Answer E is incorrect. Aldolase converts fructose-1,6-biphosphate → dihydroxyacetone phosphate + glyceraldehyde-3-phosphate.

56. **The correct answer is E.** Glucagon is released from pancreatic alpha cells in response to states of hypoglycemia. It significantly increases glycogenolysis, fatty acid synthesis, amino acid synthesis, and urea synthesis. Remember that its effects are opposite of insulin.

    Answers A, B, C, and D are incorrect. See above.

57. **The correct answer is D.** The regulation of Ca^{2+} reabsorption by PTH occurs at the distal convoluted tubule. Recall that Na^+ and Cl^- are also reabsorbed in this portion of the nephron.

    Answers A, B, C, and E are incorrect. See above.

58. **The correct answer is C.** The Northern blot allows visualization of RNA fragments.

    Answer A is incorrect. PCR (polymerase chain reaction) amplifies DNA sequences.

    Answer B is incorrect. The Western blot allows visualization of protein fragments.

    Answer D is incorrect. The Southern blot allows visualization of DNA fragments.

    Answer E is incorrect. The Southwestern blot allows visualization of protein and DNA interactions.

59. **The correct answer is A.** Recall that the maxilla and mandible (except the condyles) are developed by intramembranous ossification. Extraction sites heal in the same manner.

    Answer C is incorrect. There is no such thing as intermembranous ossification.

    Answers B, D, and E are incorrect. See above.

60. **The correct answer is C.** Although pyruvate can be converted back to glucose, it must first be converted to glucose-6-phosphate. Remember that gluconeogenesis is not a direct reversal of glycolysis, and is under strict hormonal control.

    Answer A is incorrect. Pyruvate is converted to oxaloacetate via pyruvate carboxylase.

    Answer B is incorrect. Pyruvate is converted to acetyl-CoA via pyruvate dehydrogenase.

    Answer D is incorrect. Pyruvate is converted to alanine via alanine aminotransferase.

    Answer E is incorrect. Pyruvate is converted to lactate via lactate dehydrogenase.

61. **The correct answer is B.** A type II skeletal muscle twitch produces fast and powerful contractions. Since there will need to be an ample supply of Ca^{2+}, the SR content will be relatively high.

    Answers A, C, D, and E are incorrect. See above.

62. **The correct answer is C.** Resistance is inversely proportional to the radius to the fourth power. So, the equation should be: $R = 8\eta L/\pi r^4$. This is an important concept in fluid dynamics.

    Answer A is incorrect. Mean arterial pressure is defined as cardiac output times total peripheral resistance.

    Answer B is incorrect. Cardiac output is defined as heart rate times stroke volume.

    Answer D is incorrect. Laplace law.

    Answer E is incorrect. Poiseuille law.

63. **The correct answer is E.** Epinephrine is derived from phenylalanine.

    Answer A is incorrect. Histamine is derived from histidine.

    Answer B is incorrect. Signal transduction enzymes are derived from serine.

    Answer C is incorrect. Creatine and heme is derived from glycine.

    Answer D is incorrect. Serotonin is derived from tryptophan.

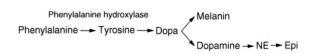

64. **The correct answer is C.** An increase in alveolar gas exchange occurs when there is a partial pressure gradient from high to low. Recall that oxygen diffuses from alveoli to the blood. Thus, P_{AO_2} (partial alveolar oxygen pressure)

must be greater than P_aO_2 (partial pulmonary artery oxygen pressure).

Answers A, B, D, and E are incorrect. Increased alveolar gas exchange is also a function of alveolar barrier thickness, gas solubility, and alveolar surface area.

65. **The correct answer is E.** The Krebs cycle produces 1 GTP, 3 NADH, and 1 $FADH_2$ per turn. Remember that, in the metabolism of one glucose molecule, the Krebs cycle will turn twice (once per pyruvate) yielding 2 GTP, 6 NADH, and 2 $FADH_2$. Assuming all reducing equivalents are transferred to the ETC, one turn of the Krebs cycle will produce 12 ATP.

Answers A, B, C, and D are incorrect. See above.

66. **The correct answer is C.** Ruffini corpuscles are encapsulated stretch receptors. They are located in the dermis of hairy skin.

Answer A is incorrect. Free nerve endings detect primarily pain, but also touch, pressure, and temperature. They are unencapsulated, and located in skin, cornea, alimentary tract, connective tissue, haversian systems, and dental pulp.

Answer B is incorrect. Meissner corpuscles are encapsulated mechanoreceptors, allowing two-point discrimination. They are located in the dermal papillae of skin.

Answer D is incorrect. Pacinian corpuscles are encapsulated vibration and pressure receptors. They are located in the dermis, subcutaneous tissue, ligaments, and joints.

Answer E is incorrect. Merkel discs are unencapsulated touch receptors. They are located in hairless skin, including fingertips.

67. **The correct answer is A.** Careful! Remember that ADH (and oxytocin) is produced in the hypothalamus, but stored and secreted from the posterior pituitary gland.

Answers B, C, D, and E are incorrect. See above.

68. **The correct answer is C.** Helicase unwinds the DNA molecule prior to replication.

Answer A is incorrect. DNA polymerase synthesizes a complementary DNA strand in the 5' to 3' direction.

Answer B is incorrect. Exonuclease cleaves nucleotide primers.

Answer D is incorrect. DNA ligase joins Okazaki fragments.

Answer E is incorrect. Restriction endonuclease cleaves DNA at specific points.

69. **The correct answer is C.** Gastric secretions (including HCl) are by far the most acidic, with a pH range of 1.0 to 3.5. Intestinal secretions are mainly mucous, so their pH ranges from 7.5 to 8.0. Bile has a pH of about 7.8. The pH of pancreatic secretions rang from 8.0 to 8.3.

Answers A, B, and D are incorrect. See above.

70. **The correct answer is C.** The typical amino acid sequence of each α-chain is gly-x-y.

Answers A, B, D, and E are incorrect. See above.

71. **The correct answer is C.** The ascending loop of Henle is impermeable to H_2O. Here, Na^+, Cl^-, and K^+ are reabsorbed.

Answers A, B, D, and E are incorrect. See above.

72. **The correct answer is B.** Hematopoiesis, blood cell formation, occurs primarily in red bone marrow, as it contains pluripotential stem cells. It is also to site of B-cell maturation.

Answer A is incorrect. Lymph nodes house T cells and B cells.

Answer C is incorrect. Yellow marrow contains mostly fat cells.

Biochemistry and Physiology

Answer D is incorrect. The spleen is the site of fetal erythropoiesis. In adults, lymphocyte proliferation and erythrocyte scavenging occur here.

Answer E is incorrect. The thymus is the site of T-cell maturation.

73. **The correct answer is E.** The Na^+/K^+ pump functions via primary active transport, which requires the direct participation of ATP. For each ATP hydrolyzed, 3 Na^+ ions are moved outside the cell, and 2 K^+ ions are brought into the cell. Digitalis and other cardiac glycosides inhibit the Na^+/K^+ ATPase by binding to the extracellular domain.

Answers A, B, C, and D are incorrect. See above.

74. **The correct answer is A.** The SA node is the pacemaker of the heart. The correct sequence leading to ventricular contraction is SA node → AV node → bundle of His → Purkinje fibers → ventricular myocytes.

Answers B, C, D, and E are incorrect. See above.

75. **The correct answer is A.** Erythrocytes do not contain mitochondria. All of the pyruvate formed from glycolysis is converted to lactate via lactate dehydrogenase. Further oxidation of pyruvate (in the Krebs cycle) and $NADH/FADH_2$ (in the ETC) is impossible since these reactions occur in mitochondria. Remember that lactic acid is converted back to glucose via the Cori cycle in hepatocytes.

Answers B, C, D, and E are incorrect. See above.

76. **The correct answer is A.** The majority of skeletal muscle contains extrafusal fibers, which are innervated by α-motor neurons. Remember that intrafusal skeletal muscle fibers are innervated by γ-motor neurons.

Answers B, C, and D are incorrect. See above.

77. **The correct answer is C.** Cushing syndrome is often caused by a long-term use of exogenously administered glucocorticoids. It may also result from an increase in endogenous cortisol release as a result of a cortisol-secreting adrenocortical tumor. Cushing syndrome is characterized by central obesity with abdominal striae, moon face, buffalo hump, proximal muscle wasting, and hypertension.

Answer A is incorrect. Addison disease is caused by adrenocortical insufficiency.

Answer B is incorrect. Cushing disease is caused by an increase in endogenous cortisol secretion secondary to excess ACTH release (often from a pituitary tumor).

Answer D is incorrect. Plummer syndrome is hyperthyroidism resulting in toxic multinodular goiter.

Answer E is incorrect. Myxedema is adult-onset hypothyroidism.

78. **The correct answer is A.** Tyrosine is converted to acetyl-CoA, but can also be converted to melanin. The lack of melanin expression causes albinism.

Answer B is incorrect. Tryptophan is converted to acetyl-CoA, but can also be converted to serotonin.

Answer C is incorrect. Arginine is converted to α-ketoglutarate, but can also be converted to nitric oxide (NO).

Answer D is incorrect. Leucine is converted to acetyl-CoA.

Answer E is incorrect. Alanine is converted to pyruvate.

79. **The correct answer is E.** CN VII (via the chorda tympani nerve) carries taste sensation from the anterior $2/3$ of the tongue. CN IX conveys taste fibers from the posterior $1/3$ of the tongue. CN X carries taste sensation from the area around the epiglottis.

Answers A, B, C, and D are incorrect. See above.

80. **The correct answer is D.** Lactic acid is converted back to glucose via the Cori cycle in the liver. It provides quick ATP production during *anaerobic* glycolysis in muscle and erythrocytes.

    Answer A is incorrect. Glycogen is catabolized to glucose through a series of enzymatic reactions. Remember that glycogen phosphorylase is under strict hormonal regulation.

    Answer B is incorrect. NAD^+ is reduced to NADH as a coenzyme in numerous dehydrogenase reactions.

    Answer C is incorrect. Acetyl-CoA is converted to malonyl-CoA via acetyl-CoA carboxylase in the cytosol of hepatocytes during fatty acid synthesis.

    Answer E is incorrect. Pyruvate can be converted to glucose-6-phosphate (then glucose) via gluconeogenesis reactions. Remember that these reactions are tightly regulated by several hormones.

81. **The correct answer is E.** Remember that a right shift favors the release of O_2 in the tissues due to an acidic environment (eg, exercising muscle). Thus, a right shift occurs when there is ↓ pH, caused by ↑ CO_2, lactic acid buildup, 2,3-DPG formation (from glycolysis), and temperature. A left shift, on the other hand, favors oxygen uptake in the lungs.

    Answers A, B, C, and D are incorrect. See above.

82. **The correct answer is D.** All preganglionic autonomic neurons (sympathetic and parasympathetic) are cholinergic. All postganglionic parasympathetic neurons are also cholinergic. All postganglionic sympathetic neurons are adrenergic except for those innervating eccrine sweat glands and skeletal muscle vasculature.

Answers A, B, and C are incorrect. See above.

83. **The correct answer is E.** Interphase consists of G_1, S, and G_2. DNA synthesis occurs during the S (synthesis) phase, which takes about 7 hours to complete.

    Answer A is incorrect. In prophase, the chromatin coils within the nucleus and the mitotic spindle forms.

    Answer B is incorrect. In metaphase, the chromosomes line up at the equatorial plate of the mitotic spindle.

    Answer C is incorrect. In anaphase, the chromosomes split to opposite poles of the cell.

    Answer D is incorrect. In telophase, cytokinesis occurs, dividing the cytoplasm into two daughter cells.

84. **The correct answer is D.** Osmosis is the simple diffusion of *water* caused by a concentration gradient. Osmolality is the osmotic pressure of water (in osmols/kg). Recall that osmotic pressure is defined as the pressure developed as a result of net osmosis into a solution (it depends on the number of solute particles present).

    Answers A, B, and C are incorrect. See above.

85. **The correct answer is C.** Oxygen is the final electron receptor in complex IV.

    Answer A is incorrect. See below.

    Answer B is incorrect. NADH is reoxidized back to NAD^+ via NADH dehydrogenase.

    Answer D is incorrect. Q (ubiquinone) is a coenzyme that links flavoproteins to cytochrome *b* in complex III.

    Answer E is incorrect. Water is the final end product of the ETC.

86. **The correct answer is E.** PTH, secreted by parathyroid chief (principal) cells, functions

to increase serum calcium levels. In order to do so, more calcium must be retained (and less excreted). Thus, PTH will ↑ renal and intestinal Ca^{2+} reabsorption, and ↓ renal PO_4^{3-} reabsorption. Since excess calcium is also taken from hydroxyapatite, bone resorption occurs.

Answers A, B, C, and D are incorrect. See above.

87. **The correct answer is E.** Both ventricular depolarization and atrial repolarization occur within the QRS complex.

Answer A is incorrect. The PR interval is the length of time between atrial depolarization and ventricular depolarization.

Answer B is incorrect. The ST segment is the length of time the action potential is in ventricular muscle.

Answer C is incorrect. The P wave represents atrial depolarization.

Answer D is incorrect. The T wave represents ventricular repolarization.

88. **The correct answer is B.** Endopeptidases cleave the N- and C- terminal propeptides of procollagen, forming tropocollagen, extracellularly. Tropocollagen then aggregates to form collagen fibrils.

Answer A is incorrect. Occurs in the rER.

Answer C is incorrect. Occurs in the Golgi.

Answer D is incorrect. Occurs in the rER.

89. **The correct answer is A.** Bilirubin is derived from catabolized hemoglobin. It is normally carried to the liver, conjugated, and excreted into the intestine as a component of bile. Elevated blood levels of bilirubin cause jaundice, a yellowish discoloration of the skin and sclera. Jaundice is a common sign of liver disease (hepatitis or cirrhosis), but may also be caused by hemolytic anemia and choledocholithiasis.

Answers B, C, D, and E are incorrect. See above.

90. **The correct answer is A.** Cytochrome oxidase is the final cytochrome in complex IV. It combines the final reducing equivalents with molecular oxygen to form water and ATP. Because it has a high affinity for O_2, it functions continuously until all of the oxygen has been depleted.

Answer B is incorrect. Cytochrome reductase is in complex III.

Answer C is incorrect. Ubiquinone (Q) is a coenzyme that links flavoproteins to cytochrome b in complex III.

Answer D is incorrect. α-Ketoglutarate dehydrogenase converts α-ketoglutarate → succinyl-CoA in the Krebs cycle.

Answer E is incorrect. NADH dehydrogenase oxidizes NADH → NAD^+. The resulting reducing equivalents are passed on to Q.

91. **The correct answer is C.** Although estrogen stimulates LH release, it is a surge of LH that promotes ovulation. Recall that ovulation occurs about 14 days prior to menses (regardless of cycle length).

Answers A, B, D, and E are incorrect. See above.

92. **The correct answer is A.** The A band is a dark band consisting of myosin filaments (centrally) and actin filaments (laterally). It will remain the same length during contraction. Both the H band and I band decrease in length as the sarcomere contracts.

Answers B, C, and D are incorrect. See above.

93. **The correct answer is D.** Transcription occurs in the nucleus, but translation occurs in the cytoplasm (in ribosomes). Both DNA and protein syntheses (translation) occur in the $5' \rightarrow 3'$ direction.

Answers A, B, and C are incorrect. See above.

94. **The correct answer is E.** Na^+ reabsorption is regulated in the collecting duct by aldosterone. H_2O reabsorption is tightly regulated here by ADH. Recall that urine concentrates as it descends the collecting duct (as more and more water is reabsorbed).

    Answers A, B, C, and D are incorrect. See above.

95. **The correct answer is D.** Both hemoglobin and myoglobin contain only one globin molecule.

    Answer A is incorrect. Myoglobin contains only one heme, which has a central iron atom.

    Answer B is incorrect. Myoglobin generally stores oxygen in muscle tissue.

    Answer C is incorrect. Myoglobin can only bind one molecule of oxygen since it contains only one heme.

    Answer E is incorrect. Myoglobin has a significantly higher oxygen affinity compared to hemoglobin.

96. **The correct answer is C.** Endochondral osteogenesis can occur by both appositional and interstitial growth. During appositional growth, new bone matrix is added once osteoprogenitor cells contact existing bony spicules, and differentiate into osteoblasts. In interstitial growth, mesenchymal cells first differentiate and deposit a cartilage matrix. The cartilage matrix then calcifies, and bone matrix is deposited in the same manner as in appositional growth.

    Answers A, B, and D are incorrect. Intramembranous osteogenesis develops only by appositional growth.

97. **The correct answer is A.** Inspiration requires muscular effort, and is thus an active process. Expiration, on the other hand, is generally a passive process resulting from lung recoil (except in certain respiratory diseases such as emphysema). The decrease in alveolar and intrapleural pressures creates a gas flow down-gradient from the mouth to the alveoli. The opposite happens during expiration.

    Answers B, C, and D are incorrect. See above.

98. **The correct answer is B.** CF is a recessive genetic disease affecting Caucasians in North America and certain parts of northern Europe. The abnormality of membrane Cl^- permeability results in the increased viscosity of many bodily secretions, especially those of the respiratory tract.

    Answer A is incorrect. Achondroplasia is caused by a mutation of a FGF receptor, resulting in impaired maturation of cartilage in the developing growth plate. Dwarfism commonly results.

    Answer C is incorrect. Tay-Sachs disease is an autosomal recessive disorder caused by a deficiency of hexosaminidase A, leading to an accumulation of gangliosides. It is rapidly fatal.

    Answer D is incorrect. Diabetes mellitus is a chronic disorder of carbohydrate, fat, and protein metabolism, resulting in hyperglycemia. It can be inherited (often as a defect in insulin production/secretion), or acquired.

    Answer E is incorrect. Multiple sclerosis is an autoimmune disease caused by an overactive T-cell response against myelin. It is the most common demyelinating disease of the CNS.

99. **The correct answer is C.** Nicotinic-2 receptors are cholinergic receptors located at the neuromuscular junction. Stimulation results in muscle contraction.

    Answer A is incorrect. Muscarinic receptors are cholinergic receptors located on postganglionic parasympathetic effector organs, as well as sweat glands and skeletal muscle vasculature which are under postganglionic sympathetic control.

Answer B is incorrect. Nicotinic-1 receptors are cholinergic receptors located on postganglionic autonomic (parasympathetic and sympathetic) neurons.

Answer D is incorrect. Alpha-1 receptors are adrenergic receptors located on vascular smooth muscle.

Answer E is incorrect. Alpha-2 receptors are adrenergic receptors located at presynaptic nerve terminals, platelets, adipocytes, and the GI tract wall.

100. **The correct answer is B.** The pentose phosphate pathway does not produce any ATP.

    Answer A is incorrect. It occurs in the cytosol of several (but not all) cells including liver, adipose, adrenal cortex, thyroid, mammary gland, and erythrocytes.

    Answer C is incorrect. Its function is to convert glucose-6-phosphate $\rightarrow$ ribose-5-phosphate, forming ribose (for nucleotide synthesis) and NADPH (for fatty acid and steroid synthesis).

    Answer D is incorrect. The rate-limiting step is the conversion of glucose-6-phosphate $\rightarrow$ 6-phosphogluconolactone via *G6PD*.

    Answer E is incorrect. The PPP is also called the hexose monophosphate shunt.

    Glucose-6-phosphate + 2 NADP$^+$ + H$_2$O $\rightarrow$
    Ribose-5-phosphate + 2 NADPH + 2 H$^+$ + CO$_2$

101. **The correct answer is A.** Both carotid body chemoreceptors and carotid sinus baroreceptors receive afferent fibers from CN IX. The atrial stretch receptors, aortic body chemoreceptors, and aortic arch baroreceptors receive their afferent fibers from the vagus nerve (CN X).

Answers B, C, D, and E are incorrect. See above.

102. **The correct answer is A.** Compared to PTH, calcitonin plays a minor role in regulating serum calcium levels.

    Answer B is incorrect. Calcitonin is more important during bone development.

    Answer C is incorrect. Vitamin D is essential for the GI absorption of calcium.

    Answer D is incorrect. Hydroxyapatite is the crystalline mineral content of bone, which serves as a source of calcium and phosphorus: $Ca_{10}(PO_4)_6(OH)_2$.

    Answer E is incorrect. See above.

103. **The correct answer is A.** Corticosteroids inhibit PLA$_2$, blocking the synthesis of arachidonic acid.

    Answer B is incorrect. 5-LOX converts arachidonic acid to leukotrienes. 15-LOX converts arachidonic acid to lipoxins.

    Answer C is incorrect. HMG-CoA reductase converts HMG-CoA to mevalonate. Statins inhibit HMG-CoA reductase.

    Answer D is incorrect. COX-1 constitutively converts arachidonic acid to prostaglandins to maintain renal blood flow, vasomotor tone, and mucosal integrity in the stomach. Aspirin and NSAIDs inhibit both COX-1 and COX-2.

    Answer E is incorrect. COX-2 converts arachidonic acid to prostaglandins during inflammation. Aspirin and NSAIDs inhibit both COX-1 and COX-2. Selective COX-2 inhibitors include celecoxib and meloxicam.

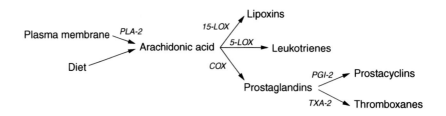

104. **The correct answer is B.** During exercise, there is a significant increase in α_1-, β_1-, and β_2-adrenergic function. β_1 receptor activation in the heart will increase HR, SV (from $\uparrow$ inotropic effect), and thus CO. The increase in preload will decrease venous compliance. β_2 stimulation will cause central vasodilation. Activation of α_1 receptors will result in peripheral vasoconstriction and increased arterial pressure.

Answers A, C, D, and E are incorrect. See above.

105. **The correct answer is E.** Type I diabetes often results from a defect in insulin production, secretion, or receptor function, leading to increased blood glucose. Remember that insulin promotes glycogen synthesis. Thus, a decrease in insulin allows for increased glycogen phosphorylase activity, leading to an increase in blood glucose.

Answer A is incorrect. Insulin positively regulates glycogen synthase activity.

Answer B is incorrect. Insulin negatively regulates lipase activity.

Answer C is incorrect. Insulin positively regulates acetyl-CoA carboxylase activity.

Answer D is incorrect. Insulin positively regulates fatty acid synthase.

106. **The correct answer is D.** Recall that the Entner-Doudoroff pathway is the main glycolytic pathway in aerobic bacteria. The liver has a myriad of functions, including mineral and vitamin storage; carbohydrate, protein, and lipid metabolism; cholesterol synthesis; detoxification; phagocytosis of foreign antigens; and bile production.

Answers A, B, C, and E are incorrect. See above.

107. **The correct answer is C.** A decrease in plasma oncotic pressure creates a gradient of flow from the vasculature to Bowman space, increasing GFR. The opposite is true of an increased hydrostatic pressure in Bowman space. Decreased blood flow ($\downarrow$ renal perfusion and afferent arteriole vasoconstriction) to the glomerulus will result in a decreased GFR. Efferent arteriole vasodilation will also lower GFR.

Answers A, B, D, and E are incorrect. See above.

108. **The correct answer is B.** Okazaki fragments are the series of complementary DNA strands synthesized from the lagging strand during DNA synthesis. They are not formed during transcription or translation.

Answer A is incorrect. The removal of introns (noncoding segments) is a part of RNA splicing after transcription.

Answer C is incorrect. The 5' cap is added post-transcription to enable translation initiation and to prevent binding of the 5' end by exonucleases.

Answer D is incorrect. The 3' poly(A) tail is added post-transcription to prevent binding of the 3' end by exonucleases.

Answer E is incorrect. The ligation of exons (coding segments) is a part of RNA splicing after transcription.

109. **The correct answer is D.** The catecholamines (epinephrine and norepinephrine) regulate the "fight-or-flight" response. They are released by chromaffin cells of the adrenal medulla.

Answer A is incorrect. Dust cells are alveolar macrophages.

Answer B is incorrect. Gastric chief cells secrete pepsinogen. Additionally, parathyroid chief (principal) cells release PTH.

Answer C is incorrect. Gastric parietal cells release HCl and intrinsic factor.

Answer E is incorrect. M cells are located in the Peyer patches of the ileum. They absorb antigens into the underlying lymphatic tissue.

Biochemistry and Physiology

110. **The correct answer is D.** There is no pathway in humans to convert fatty acids to glucose; however, glucose is converted to fatty acids using acetyl-CoA as an intermediate.

   Answers A, B, and C are incorrect. See above.

111. **The correct answer is B.** Remember that each motor unit consists of a motor neuron, synaptic cleft, and the associated muscle fibers. When an action potential arrives at the NMJ, acetylcholine is released from the axon terminus and binds to the nicotinic receptors on the plasma membrane of skeletal muscle cells.

   Answer A is incorrect. T tubules transmit the action potential from the sarcolemma to the sarcoplasmic reticulum of two adjacent sarcomeres.

   Answer C is incorrect. The endomysium is a CT layer that surrounds each muscle fiber.

   Answer D is incorrect. The perimysium is a CT layer that surrounds each fascicle.

   Answer E is incorrect. The sarcomere is the functional unit of each myofibril.

112. **The correct answer is B.** Filiform papillae do not contain taste buds. The most taste buds are found on vallate papillae. In addition to papillae, they can also be found in the epithelium of the soft palate, posterior pharynx, and epiglottis.

   Answers A, C, and D are incorrect. See above.

113. **The correct answer is C.** IDL, LDL, and HDL generally carry triglycerides and cholesterol to the liver. Chylomicrons and VLDL generally carry lipids to the extrahepatic tissues. Lipoproteins contain varying proportions of cholesterol, cholesterol esters, triglycerides, and phospholipids, but not bile salts.

   Answers A, B, and D are incorrect. See above.

114. **The correct answer is A.** Hypoxemia ($PO_2 < 85$ mm Hg), is induced by hypoventilation. This can result from a decreased respiratory drive, or the decreased ability for chest excursion.

   Answer B is incorrect. An unequal ventilation and perfusion ratio will result in a segment of the lung that is ventilated, but not perfused.

   Answer C is incorrect. Diffusion limitations include decreased alveolar surface area, a thicker blood-gas barrier, and a decreased ability for hemoglobin to carry oxygen.

   Answer D is incorrect. Less inspired oxygen will certainly cause hypoxemia.

   Answer E is incorrect. A shunt will result in a segment of the lung that is perfused, but not aerated.

115. **The correct answer is A.** Saltatory conduction occurs in myelinated nerves. Because there is decreased membrane capacitance, action potentials "jump" from one node of Ranvier to another.

   Answer B is incorrect. Continuous conduction occurs in unmyelinated nerves. Action potentials travel along the entire membrane surface. This type of conduction is much slower (about 1 m/s).

   Answer C is incorrect. Axonotmesis is a form of nerve injury in which the axon is damaged, but the connective sheath remains intact.

   Answer D is incorrect. Neurotmesis is a form of nerve injury in which the entire nerve trunk is severed.

116. **The correct answer is A.** Acetyl-CoA cannot be directly converted back to glucose.

   Answer B is incorrect. Acetyl-CoA can form cholesterol through HMG-CoA via HMG-CoA lyase.

   Answer C is incorrect. Acetyl-CoA can form fatty acids through malonyl-CoA via acetyl-CoA carboxylase.

Answer D is incorrect. Acetyl-CoA can lead to ATP production through the Krebs cycle and then oxidative phosphorylation.

Answer E is incorrect. Acetyl-CoA can form ketone bodies through HMG-CoA via HMG-CoA reductase.

117. **The correct answer is A.** Renin, released from the renal JGA, converts angiotensinogen to angiotensin I. ACE converts angiotensin I to angiotensin II, which then stimulates the adrenal cortex to secrete aldosterone. Recall that aldosterone will increase sodium and water reabsorption ($\uparrow Na^+$ and water plasma levels), and decrease potassium reabsorption ($\downarrow K^+$ plasma levels).

Answers B, C, D, and E are incorrect. See above.

118. **The correct answer is B.** Reverse transcriptase forms a complementary strand of DNA from the original RNA.

Answer A is incorrect. RNA polymerase synthesizes a complementary strand of RNA from DNA.

Answer C is incorrect. Aminoacyl-tRNA synthetase adds each amino acid to tRNA.

Answer D is incorrect. RNA polymerase synthesizes a complementary strand of RNA from the original DNA.

Answer E is incorrect. DNA polymerase synthesizes a complementary strand of DNA from the original DNA.

119. **The correct answer is D.** Hematocrit (HCT) is the percentage of erythrocytes in a sample of blood. The normal value for males is about 47% and 42% for females.

Answer A is incorrect. The mean corpuscular hemoglobin (MCH) index measures the concentration of hemoglobin in a sample of erythrocytes in picograms (pg).

Answer B is incorrect. Recall that plasma is whole blood volume minus formed elements (cells and platelets).

Answer C is incorrect. The number of RBCs in a sample of blood is counted in millions per microliter (μl).

Answer E is incorrect. The amount of hemoglobin (Hb) in a sample of blood is measured in gram per deciliter (g/dl).

120. **The correct answer is D.** Inulin is the "gold standard" for measuring GFR because it is cleared from the plasma unhindered, solely by glomerular filtration. However, inulin needs to be infused, and is later measured by taking a blood sample. Due to this inconvenience, endogenous creatinine clearance is often used. Although creatinine is secreted as well as filtered, the difference is usually small. The amount of urine production will not provide information on what is being filtered at the glomerulus.

Answers A, B, C, and E are incorrect. See above.

121. **The correct answer is A.** Guanine binds cytosine via three H-bonds in DNA.

Answer B is incorrect. Adenine binds uracil via 2 H-bonds in RNA.

Answer C is incorrect. Guanine does not pair with thymine.

Answer D is incorrect. Adenine binds thymine via 2 H-bonds in DNA.

Answer E is incorrect. Adenine does not pair with cytosine.

122. **The correct answer is A.** Renin is secreted by juxtaglomerular cells, which are modified smooth muscle cells of the afferent arterioles. The juxtaglomerular apparatus (JGA) consists of the macula densa, juxtaglomerular cells, and extraglomerular mesangial cells.

Answers B, C, D, and E are incorrect. See above.

Biochemistry and Physiology

123. **The correct answer is B.** Mg^{2+} has a higher intracellular concentration: 30 mmol/L versus 1.5 mmol/L.

    Answer A is incorrect. Na^+ has a higher extracellular concentration: 140 mmol/L versus 10 mmol/L.

    Answer C is incorrect. Cl^- has a higher extracellular concentration: 100 mmol/L versus 4 mmol/L.

    Answer D is incorrect. Ca^{2+} has a higher extracellular concentration: 2.5 mmol/L versus 0.1 μmol/L.

    Answer E is incorrect. HCO_3^- has a higher extracellular concentration: 27 mmol/L versus 10 mmol/L.

124. **The correct answer is A.** The presence of HCl converts pepsinogen to pepsin in the stomach. Recall that pepsinogen is secreted by gastric chief cells; and HCl is released by gastric parietal cells.

    Answers B, C, D, and E are incorrect. See above.

125. **The correct answer is D.** Cretinism is adolescent-onset hypothyroidism.

    Answers A, B, C, and E are incorrect. All result from hyperthyroidism.

126. **The correct answer is D.** Only lysine, serine, and threonine are not transaminated.

    Answers A, B, C, and E are incorrect. See above.

127. **The correct answer is D.** Both cardiac and smooth muscle act as a functional syncytium. Recall that most of these cells relay the action potential via gap junctions. Thus, even though not all cells are directly innervated, the entire muscle functions as though they are.

    Answers A and E are incorrect. See above.

128. **The correct answer is B.** Arranged in order of smallest to largest: DNA double-helix (2 nm) < nucleosome (10 nm) < chromatin fibril (30 nm) < chromosome (1400 nm).

    Answers A, C, and D are incorrect. See above.

129. **The correct answer is E.** Vagus nerve (CN X) activity decreases SA nodal discharge and the rate of depolarization through the heart. Thus, cardiac output will eventually decrease.

    Answers A, B, C, and D are incorrect. See above.

130. **The correct answer is A.** Metabolic alkalosis leads to an increase in blood pH due to any cause (eg, vomiting) other than a decrease in P_{CO_2}. The compensatory hypoventilation ↑ P_{CO_2}, leading to ↓ pH. Remember that the opposite occurs with metabolic acidosis.

    Answers B, C, and D are incorrect. See above.

131. **The correct answer is B.** Vitamin B_6 (pyridoxine) is a required cofactor for all transamination reactions.

    Answer A is incorrect. Vitamin B_2 (riboflavin) is a component of FAD and FMN.

    Answer C is incorrect. Vitamin B_{12} (cobalamin) is a coenzyme in the conversion of methylmalonyl-CoA to succinyl-CoA.

    Answer D is incorrect. Vitamin C is a coenzyme for the hydroxylation of praline and lysine in collagen synthesis.

    Answer E is incorrect. Vitamin E is a potent antioxidant.

132. **The correct answer is E.** Glycine and GABA are strictly inhibitory. Acetylcholine may be inhibitory at some postganglionic parasympathetic end organs.

    Answers A, B, C, and D are incorrect. See above.

133. **The correct answer is B.** The descending loop of Henle is impermeable to Na^+. Water

is primarily reabsorbed in this portion of the nephron.

Answers A, C, D, and E are incorrect. See above.

134. **The correct answer is B.** Doxycycline (and the tetracyclines) inhibits bacterial protein synthesis by binding to 30S ribosomal subunits, blocking aminoacyl-tRNA binding.

Answer A is incorrect. Amoxicillin (and the penicillins) inhibits cell wall peptidoglycan cross-linking.

Answer C is incorrect. Metronidazole inhibits bacterial DNA synthesis.

Answer D is incorrect. Cephalexin (and the cephalosporins) inhibits cell wall peptidoglycan cross-linking.

Answer E is incorrect. Ciprofloxacin (and the fluoroquinolones) inhibits bacterial DNA gyrase (topoisomerase).

135. **The correct answer is B.** The maxilla and mandible contain both cortical and cancellous bone. However, mandibular bone often has thicker cortical bone than the maxilla.

Answers A, C, and D are incorrect. See above.

136. **The correct answer is E.** rRNA is the major component of ribosomes, which are found on rough ER.

Answer A is incorrect. The backbone of RNA is ribose.

Answer B is incorrect. RNA bases include adenine, uracil, guanine, and cytosine.

Answer C is incorrect. rRNA is synthesized in the nucleolus. tRNA and mRNA are synthesized in the nucleus.

Answer D is incorrect. RNA is single stranded.

137. **The correct answer is B.** Sodium is critical in maintaining the resting potential of plasma membranes, but is not a second messenger.

Answers A, C, D, and E are incorrect. See above.

138. **The correct answer is C.** Both the intrinsic and extrinsic clotting pathways converge with the activation of factor X.

Answers A, B, D, and E are incorrect. See above.

139. **The correct answer is C.** Oxidative deamination serves as an alternative to the transamination of amino acids. It results in the formation of α-ketoacids (for energy) and ammonia (for urea formation). In humans, the vast majority of oxidative deamination derives from glutamate.

Answers A, B, D, and E are incorrect. See above.

140. **The correct answer is D.** Cholecystokinin is secreted by the duodenum in response to the presence of fat and amino acids. In addition to stimulating digestive enzyme release by the pancreas, it also promotes gallbladder contraction, which then results in the secretion of bile.

Answers A, B, and C are incorrect. See above.

141. **The correct answer is D.** The vallecula is a small depression located within the median glossoepiglottic fold. The pyriform recess is a trough that lies between the lateral glossoepiglottic fold and the lateral wall of the laryngeal pharynx.

Answer C is incorrect. The salpingopharyngeal fold is located in the nasopharynx.

Answers A, B, and E are incorrect. See above.

142. **The correct answer is E.** The urea cycle does not produce ATP.

Answer A is incorrect. It occurs in the cytosol and mitochondrial matrix of hepatocytes.

Answer B is incorrect. It requires aspartate.

Answer C is incorrect. It eliminates ammonia in the form of urea.

Answer D is incorrect. See above.

$$CO_2 + NH_4^+ + 3\ ATP + Aspartate + 2H_2O \rightarrow$$
$$Urea + 2\ ADP + 2\ P_i + AMP + PP_i + Fumarate$$

143. **The correct answer is E.** ADH (also called vasopressin) functions to retain water by increasing its reabsorption. It is secreted by the posterior pituitary.

    Answers A, B, C, and D are incorrect. See above.

144. **The correct answer is A.** Eccrine sweat glands secrete sweat to regulate body temperature. They are innervated by postganglionic sympathetic cholinergic fibers. Remember: All postganglionic sympathetic neurons are adrenergic except for those innervating eccrine sweat glands and skeletal muscle vasculature. Apocrine sweat glands secrete a serous fluid containing pheromones. These sweat glands are innervated by postganglionic sympathetic adrenergic neurons.

    Answers B, C, and D are incorrect. See above.

145. **The correct answer is C.** Each tRNA carries the anticodon to the mRNA-ribosomal complex, where it binds to its complementary codon. It is the *most* prevalent RNA. mRNA is the least prevalent RNA.

    Answer A, B, and D are incorrect. See above.

146. **The correct answer is B.** The PO_2 determines the affinity of hemoglobin for oxygen binding by causing a conformational change in the Hb molecule.

    Answers A, C, D, and E are incorrect. See above.

147. **The correct answer is E.** In chronological order: RNA polymerase activity, splicing of exons, transfer of mRNA from the nucleus to cytoplasm, small ribosomal subunit binding to mRNA, anticodon binding to complementary codon. Remember that transcription occurs in the nucleus, but translation occurs in the cytoplasmic ribosomes.

    Answers A, B, C, and D are incorrect. See above.

148. **The correct answer is A.** Remember that a lesion on one side of the spinal cord causes ipsilateral motor (corticospinal) loss, and contralateral pain and temperature (spinothalamic) loss.

    Answers B, C, and D are incorrect. See above.

149. **The correct answer is C.** The muscle spindles of the stretch reflex detect muscle length and tension. However, this reflex results in contraction, not relaxation. Remember, the stretch reflex maintains muscle tone.

    Answers A, B, and D are incorrect. See above.

150. **The correct answer is D.** Citrullinemia is caused by a defect in argininosuccinate synthase activity, the enzyme that converts citrulline → argininosuccinate in the urea cycle, causing elevated plasma and CSF citrulline levels.

    Answer A is incorrect. Phenylketonuria (PKU) is caused by a defect in phenylalanine hydroxylase, the enzyme that converts phenylalanine → tyrosine. PKU has a frequency of 1:10,000 and causes severe mental retardation.

    Answer B is incorrect. Alkaptonuria is caused by a defect in homogentisate oxidase, the enzyme that converts homogentisate → maleylacetoacetate in tyrosine catabolism. It causes urine to turn black due to the oxidation of the excreted homogentisic acid.

    Answer C is incorrect. Pernicious anemia is caused by a deficiency of vitamin B_{12} (cobalamin).

Answer E is incorrect. Richner-Hanhart syndrome (type II tyrosinemia) is caused by a defect in tyrosine aminotransferase, the enzyme that converts tyrosine → hydroxyphenylpyruvate.

151. **The correct answer is E.** The hypothalamus releases thyrotropin-releasing hormone (TRH), growth hormone-releasing hormone (GHRH), gonadotropin-releasing hormone (GnRH), and corticotrophin-releasing hormone (CRH), somatostatin, among others.

   Answers A, B, C, and D are incorrect. See above.

152. **The correct answer is B.** Cyanosis does not typically occur in severe anemia since it would take more than 5 g of deoxygenated hemoglobin per 100 mL of blood in order to clinically detect.

   Answers A, C, D, and E are incorrect. All are typical of an individual with severe anemia.

153. **The correct answer is C.** In humans, purines are catabolized to uric acid. Pyrimidines are catabolized to water-soluble metabolites such as CO_2, NH_3, and β-alanine.

   Answer A is incorrect. Purines are synthesized from ribose-5-phosphate.

   Answer B is incorrect. Adenine and guanine are the two purines.

   Answer D is incorrect. Purines pair with pyrimidines in DNA and RNA.

   Answer E is incorrect. Purines are cyclic structures composed of nitrogen and carbon.

154. **The correct answer is E.** Thyroglobulin is a glycoprotein that contains many tyrosine residues, which are incorporated into the two major thyroid hormones. It is synthesized by thyroid follicular cells, and stored in follicular colloid.

   Answers A, B, C, and D are incorrect. See above.

155. **The correct answer is A.** A hypotonic solution is one in which the solute < solvent.

Thus, there is a greater cellular uptake of solvent leading to cellular swelling.

   Answers B, C, and D are incorrect. See above.

156. **The correct answer is C.** Exocytosis is the process by which cells release large molecules to the ECM. Endocytosis is the process by which cells take in large molecules. Pinocytosis and phagocytosis are two types of endocytosis.

   Answers A, B, and D are incorrect. See above.

157. **The correct answer is C.** IL-8 is a chemotactic factor for PMNs. It has no effect on bone metabolism.

   Answers A, B, D, and E are incorrect. IL-1, IL-6, and TNF-β stimulate osteoclast maturation. Parathyroid hormone (PTH) and receptor-activated nuclear kappa-b ligand (RANKL) induce osteoclast activity. Recall that RANKL binds to RANK receptors on the osteoclast cell membrane, initiating resorption.

158. **The correct answer is C.** The Entner-Doudoroff pathway is the glycolytic pathway in aerobic bacteria. It converts glucose → pyruvate + glyceraldehyde-3-phosphate. It yields 1 ATP, 1 NADH, and 1 NADPH per glucose molecule.

   Answers A, B, D, and E are incorrect. See above.

159. **The correct answer is E.** Intrinsic factor is a glycoprotein secreted in the stomach that is essential for the absorption of vitamin B_{12} (cobalamin) in the small intestine.

   Answers A, B, C, and D are incorrect. See above.

160. **The correct answer is E.** Calcium binds to troponin C, which is attached to tropomyosin. Both are bound to the actin, forming a

Biochemistry and Physiology

functional filament. Once calcium is bound, tropomyosin undergoes a conformational change, allowing the actin filament to interact with myosin.

Answers A, B, C, and D are incorrect. See above.

161. **The correct answer is D.** Remember the four fat-soluble vitamins: A, D, E, and K.

    Water-soluble. **Answers A, B, C, and E are incorrect.** These are water-soluble.

162. **The correct answer is D.** Apnea is the transient cessation of breathing. In individuals who suffer from sleep apnea, respiration can stop for relatively long periods of time (often 30 to 60 seconds).

    Answer A is incorrect. Hypoventilation is ↓ alveolar ventilation, which leads to ↑ P_{CO_2}.

    Answer B is incorrect. Dyspnea is a difficulty in breathing.

    Answer C is incorrect. Hypocapnia is ↓ CO_2 in arterial blood, secondary to ↑ ventilation.

    Answer E is incorrect. Hyperapnea is abnormally deep and rapid breathing.

163. **The correct answer is B.** Beta-2 adrenergic receptors are located on skeletal muscle (causing vasodilation) and bronchial smooth muscle (causing bronchodilation).

    Answer A is incorrect. Activation of alpha-1 adrenergic receptors causes vascular smooth muscle vasoconstriction.

    Answer C is incorrect. Activation of alpha-1 adrenergic receptors causes miosis.

    Answer D is incorrect. Activation of beta-1 adrenergic receptors causes increased heart rate and contractility.

    Answer E is incorrect. Activation of alpha-2 adrenergic receptors causes presynaptic nerve inhibition and GI tract relaxation.

164. **The correct answer is D.** The genetic code is *nonoverlapping*, meaning that it does not involve any overlap of codons.

    Answer A is incorrect. It is virtually universal, meaning that, for the most part, each codon codes for only one specific amino acid.

    Answer B is incorrect. It is degenerate, meaning that the same codon will decode the same amino acid.

    Answer C is incorrect. It is unambiguous, meaning that only a specific amino acid is indicated for any codon.

    Answer E is incorrect. It is without punctuation, meaning that the message is read in a continuing sequence of nucleotides until a stop codon is reached.

165. **The correct answer is C.** The absolute refractory period is the period in which a second AP cannot be generated regardless of how much the cell membrane is depolarized. During this time, sodium gates are closed and have not been reset. Remember that depolarization occurs with the rapid influx of Na^+ ions.

    Answers A, B, D, and E are incorrect. See above.

166. **The correct answer is E.** β-Oxidation converts acyl-CoA → acetyl-CoA in fatty acid metabolism.

    Answer A is incorrect. Fatty acids are converted to acyl-CoA by acyl-CoA synthetase. Carnitine serves as a cofactor in this reaction.

    Answer B is incorrect. Triglycerides are converted to fatty acids by various lipases.

    Answer C is incorrect. Acetyl-CoA is converted to malonyl-CoA by acetyl-CoA carboxylase. Biotin and vitamin B_5 serve as cofactors in this reaction.

    Answer D is incorrect. Acetyl-CoA is condensed with acetoacetyl-CoA to form HMG-CoA by HMG-CoA synthase.

167. **The correct answer is D.** Diabetes insipidus is generally caused by a decrease in ADH, which is secreted from the posterior pituitary. However, DI can also result from a lessened renal tubule response to ADH (but ADH secretion is normal).

Answers A, B, and C are incorrect. See above.

168. **The correct answer is D.** The countercurrent exchange system occurs due to the reabsorption of Na^+ in the thick ascending loop of Henle. Recall that this segment of the nephron is impermeable to water. This creates a gradient in the collecting duct to allow for more concentrated urine in the renal cortex compared to the medulla.

Answers A, B, C, and E are incorrect. See above.

169. **The correct answer is A.** Cobalt is a major constituent of vitamin B_{12} (cobalamin). A deficiency of vitamin B_{12} results in pernicious anemia.

Answer B is incorrect. Iodine is a major constituent of T_3 and T_4. Its deficiency results in cretinism or myxedema.

Answer C is incorrect. Magnesium is a major constituent of chlorophyll.

Answer D is incorrect. Manganese is a cofactor for several enzymes.

Answer E is incorrect. Zinc is a major constituent of MMPs. Its deficiency results in altered collagen metabolism.

170. **The correct answer is C.** Tetracyclines, because they chelate divalent cations, can be incorporated into mineralizing tissues (including bone, dentin, cementum, and enamel) during their development. This can result in brownish-gray banding within enamel. Because of this, these antibiotics should not be given to pregnant mothers or children under the age of 8 (about the time the permanent second molars complete calcification).

Answers A, B, D, and E are incorrect. Penicillins, cephalosporins, and clindamycin are relatively safe to administer during pregnancy, and in children.

171. **The correct answer is A.** PFK is the rate-limiting step in glycolysis, converting fructose-6-phosphate $\rightarrow$ fructose-1,6-biphosphate. It requires 1 ATP.

Answer B is incorrect. Carbonic anhydrase interconverts CO_2 and bicarbonate.

Answer C is incorrect. Lactate dehydrogenase converts pyruvate $\rightarrow$ lactic acid.

Answer D is incorrect. HMG-CoA reductase converts HMG-CoA $\rightarrow$ mevalonate.

Answer E is incorrect. Transaminases cleave the α-amino nitrogen of most amino acids.

172. **The correct answer is C.** The buccinator is the accessory muscle of mastication, innervated by CN VII. It compresses the cheeks against the teeth, keeping food inside the mouth.

Answers A, B, and D are incorrect. These are muscles of mastication that control mandibular movement.

173. **The correct answer is C.** A sudden drop in upper-body blood pressure when sitting up is sensed by baroreceptors, such as those in the carotid sinus or aortic arch. There is a resulting decrease in parasympathetic activity with concomitant increase in sympathetic activity. This ultimately increases heart rate, cardiac output, and blood pressure.

Answers A, B, D, and E are incorrect. See above.

174. **The correct answer is A.** The TATA box is a portion of the DNA promoter region.

Answer B is incorrect. The zinc finger is a motif that mediates the binding of regulatory proteins to DNA.

Biochemistry and Physiology

Answer C is incorrect. snRNP is involved in mRNA splicing.

Answer D is incorrect. The leucine zipper is a motif that mediates the binding of regulatory proteins to DNA.

Answer E is incorrect. The helix-turn-helix is a motif that mediates the binding of regulatory proteins to DNA.

175. **The correct answer is D.** Smooth muscle cells have a poorly developed sarcoplasmic reticulum. Recall that relaxation occurs when Ca^{2+} is taken up by the SR. With a less extensive SR, smooth muscle can maintain contraction for longer periods of time.

    Answers A, B, C, and E are incorrect. See above.

176. **The correct answer is D.** The PPP occurs in the cytosol.

    Answer A is incorrect. Fatty acid synthesis occurs in the cytosol.

    Answer B is incorrect. The ETC occurs in the inner mitochondrial membrane.

    Answer C is incorrect. β-oxidation occurs in the mitochondrial matrix.

    Answer E is incorrect. Glycolysis occurs in the cytosol.

177. **The correct answer is C.** Lipase is secreted by the pancreas. It is the only enzyme of the GI tract that can catabolize triacylglycerols.

    Answers A, B, D, and E are incorrect. See above.

178. **The correct answer is E.** In high altitudes, there is a significant decrease in the fraction of inspired oxygen ($\downarrow FiO_2$). This causes alveolar hypoxia ($\downarrow PaO_2$) and arterial hypoxemia ($\downarrow PaO_2$). As a result, there will be pulmonary vasoconstriction (because of alveolar hypoxia), increased erythropoietin release (which $\uparrow$ RBC production), respiratory alkalosis (because of $\uparrow$ respiratory rate), an O_2-Hb curve shift to the right (because of $\uparrow$ glycolysis), and increased renal bicarbonate excretion (to compensate for respiratory alkalosis).

    Answers A, B, C, and D are incorrect. See above.

179. **The correct answer is A.** Vitamin A (retinol) is the major constituent of the visual proteins: rhodopsin (in rods) and iodopsin (in cones). A deficiency of retinol results in night blindness and xerophthalmia.

    Answers B, C, D, and E are incorrect. See above.

180. **The correct answer is A.** The ventral horns (of gray matter) contain efferent motor nerves that innervate skeletal muscle. Recall that the dorsal horns (of gray matter) carry sensory fibers (received from the dorsal root ganglia).

    Answer B is incorrect. Motor function to smooth muscle is carried by the autonomic nervous system (SNS and PNS).

    Answer C is incorrect. The anterolateral pathway (of white matter) carries afferent pain and temperature fibers. Recall that these nerves decussate when they enter the spinal cord.

    Answer D is incorrect. The dorsal column pathway (of white matter) carries afferent touch and pressure fibers. Remember that these nerves decussate in the medulla.

181. **The correct answer is D.** Na^+ concentration is much higher extracellularly. K^+, on the other hand, has a significantly greater intracellular concentration. Blood plasma constitutes about 25% of the ECF, which comprises approximately $1/3$ total body water. Thus, plasma makes up roughly 8% of total body water.

    Answers A, B, and C are incorrect. See above.

182. **The correct answer is B.** The steps to form cholesterol from alanine include the following:

(1) Alanine is transaminated to pyruvate. (2) Pyruvate is oxidized to acetyl-CoA. (3) Acetyl-CoA is converted to HMG-CoA. (4) HMG-CoA is reduced to mevalonate. (5) Mevalonate is converted to cholesterol through a series of reactions.

Answers A, C, D, and E are incorrect. See above.

183. **The correct answer is B.** The vagus nerve (CN X) regulates gastric emptying. It is the major nerve of the PNS, originating in the medulla.

Answers A, C, D, and E are incorrect. See above.

184. **The correct answer is C.** DNA polymerase always forms a complementary strand of DNA in the 5′ → 3′ direction, regardless of which strand it uses. It forms a continuous complementary strand from the leading strand, but forms several Okazaki fragments from the lagging strand.

Answers A, B, and D are incorrect. See above.

185. **The correct answer is D.** Oxytocin stimulates uterine contraction and breast milk ejection. It is secreted by the posterior pituitary. Prolactin promotes breast milk production. It is secreted by the anterior pituitary.

Answers A, B, C, and E are incorrect. See above.

186. **The correct answer is A.** The most important determinant of CO is venous return (end diastolic volume). An increase in EDV results in an increase in preload, which leads to an increase in contraction force, stroke volume, and ultimately cardiac output.

Answers B, C, D, and E are incorrect. See above.

187. **The correct answer is D.** Vitamin K activates prothrombin and the vitamin K–dependent clotting factors: II, VII, IX, and X.

Answer A is incorrect. Vitamin K deficiency affects prothrombin, resulting in a prolonged PT.

Answer B is incorrect. Vitamin K activates clotting factors II, VII, IX, and X.

Answer C is incorrect. Phylloquinone, menaquinones, and menadione have the biologic activity of vitamin K.

Answer E is incorrect. Vitamin K (and its clotting factors) is a critical component of the extrinsic clotting pathway.

188. **The correct answer is A.** The SR is an extensive network of channels throughout the cytoplasm that stores calcium. All muscle types have SR, but it is much less developed in smooth muscle.

Answer B is incorrect. The sarcomere is the functional unit of the myofibril.

Answer C is incorrect. The sarcolemma is the plasma membrane of muscle cells.

Answer D is incorrect. The sarcoplasm is the cytoplasm of muscle cells.

Answer E is incorrect. T tubules transmit the action potential from the sarcolemma to the sarcoplasmic reticulum. Only skeletal and cardiac muscle cells have T tubules.

189. **The correct answer is A.** The NADH produced from the pentose phosphate pathway (PPP) is normally used to rid cells of free radicals and H_2O_2. A defect in *G6PD* reduces the amount of NADH produced, thereby increasing the amount of oxidizing agents within erythrocytes and causing hemolytic anemia.

Answers B, C, D, and E are incorrect. See above.

190. **The correct answer is B.** Bitter taste cells initiate nerve conduction via second messengers. Intracellular Ca^{2+} levels are increased by activation of IP_3 at the cell membrane receptor.

Answer A is incorrect. This is the pathway in sour taste cells.

Answer C is incorrect. This is the pathway in salty taste cells.

Answer D is incorrect. This is the pathway in sweet taste cells.

191. **The correct answer is A.** All larger molecules such as glucose, amino acids, and proteins are reabsorbed in the proximal convoluted tubule. H_2O, Na^+, Cl^-, K^+, and bicarbonate are also reabsorbed here.

    Answers B, C, D, and E are incorrect. See above.

192. **The correct answer is E.** Vitamin B_6 (pyridoxine) is a coenzyme in transamination reactions.

    Answer A is incorrect. Vitamin B_1 (thiamine) is a coenzyme in the decarboxylation of α-ketoglutarate in the Krebs cycle.

    Answer B is incorrect. Vitamin B_2 (riboflavin) is a component of FAD, an important dehydrogenase cofactor in the Krebs cycle.

    Answer C is incorrect. Vitamin B_3 (niacin) is a component of NAD, an important dehydrogenase cofactor in the Krebs cycle.

    Answer D is incorrect. Vitamin B_5 (pantothenic acid) is a component of coenzyme A, the cofactor attached to active carboxylate residues in the Krebs cycle.

193. **The correct answer is D.** Osteopontin (bone sialoprotein I) is an extracellular structural protein of bone. It is synthesized by osteoblasts, osteocytes, odontoblasts, and other tissue cells. Its secretion is regulated by vitamin D.

    Answer A is incorrect. Calcitonin, secreted by parafollicular cells of the thyroid gland, inhibits osteoclastic activity (preventing resorption).

    Answer B is incorrect. Osteoprotegerin (OPG), secreted by osteoblasts, functions as an inhibitory signal to osteoclasts (preventing resorption).

    Answer C is incorrect. Parathyroid hormone (PTH), released by chief cells of the parathyroid gland, stimulates osteoclastic activity (stimulating resorption).

    Answer E is incorrect. Bone morphogenetic proteins (BMPs) belong to the transforming growth factor (TGF) superfamily of protein growth factors. Both BMP-2 and BMP-7 stimulate osteoblast differentiation, increasing bone formation.

194. **The correct answer is D.** Mitochondrial DNA has 5-10 times the mutation rate of nuclear DNA.

    Answer A is incorrect. It is circular.

    Answer B is incorrect. It is double stranded.

    Answer C is incorrect. It contains about 1% of all cellular DNA.

    Answer E is incorrect. It is transmitted by non-Mendelian inheritance.

195. **The correct answer is E.** Most carbon dioxide is transported in the blood as bicarbonate (in both serum and erythrocytes). A small portion is also dissolved in the blood. About 20% of CO_2 is carried by carbaminohemoglobin, which contains an amino group (not Fe^{2+}).

    Answers A, B, C, and D are incorrect. See above.

196. **The correct answer is C.** One molecule of glucose is converted to two molecules of pyruvate in glycolysis. Under anaerobic conditions, though, pyruvate is reduced to lactic acid instead of being oxidized to acetyl-CoA. There are only 2 net ATP produced in glycolysis (4 gross ATP are produced, but 2 are used in the hexokinase and PFK reactions).

    Answers A, B, D, and E are incorrect. See above.

197. **The correct answer is D.** All postganglionic sympathetic neurons are adrenergic except for eccrine sweat glands and skeletal muscle blood vessels (cholinergic).

Answers A, B, C, and E are incorrect. See above.

198. **The correct answer is E.** Pancreatic β-cells produce insulin, which decreases blood glucose (by promoting glycogen formation and fatty acid synthesis).

Answer A is incorrect. The anterior pituitary produces ACTH, which stimulates glucocorticoid production in the adrenal cortex, and increases blood glucose.

Answer B is incorrect. The adrenal medulla produces epinephrine and norepinephrine, both of which increase blood glucose.

Answer C is incorrect. The adrenal cortex produces cortisol, which increases blood glucose.

Answer D is incorrect. Pancreatic α-cells produce glucagon, which increases blood glucose.

199. **The correct answer is B.** AUG, which codes for methionine, is a start codon.

Answer A is incorrect. AAC codes for asparagine.

Answer C is incorrect. UAC codes for tyrosine.

Answer D is incorrect. UAG is a stop codon.

Answer E is incorrect. UGA is a stop codon.

200. **The correct answer is E.** In sickle cell anemia, a missense mutation causes valine to be replaced by glutamate.

Answer A is incorrect. A nonsense mutation is a type of point mutation that results in a stop codon, terminating the polypeptide chain elongation.

Answer B is incorrect. A transition mutation is a type of point mutation in which a purine is replaced by another purine, or a pyrimidine is replaced by another pyrimidine.

Answer C is incorrect. A repeat mutation is an amplification of the same three-nucleotide sequence.

Answer D is incorrect. A transverse mutation is a type of point mutation in which the purine-pyrimidine orientation is changed.

Biochemistry and Physiology

CHAPTER 3

Microbiology and Pathology

Questions 1-4 pertain to the following clinical vignette:

A 30-year-old male presents to your office for routine dental care. The patient complains of frequent night sweats and generalized malaise. On physical exam, you note multiple enlarged, swollen, rubbery nodes upon palpation of the cervical and submandibular regions. After weeks of increase in size of the affected nodes, you decide to refer the patient for a nodal biopsy.

1. Which of the following diseases show the presence of Reed-Sternberg cells on cytological exam?

   A. Non-Hodgkin lymphoma
   B. Acute lymphocytic leukemia
   C. Chronic myelogenous leukemia
   D. Hodgkin lymphoma
   E. Multiple myeloma

2. Each of the following are signs/symptoms one would find in a patient with non-Hodgkin lymphoma EXCEPT

   A. night sweats.
   B. malaise.
   C. fatigue.
   D. weight gain.
   E. solid tumor masses.

3. Each of the following regarding Burkitt lymphoma is true EXCEPT

   A. close association with Epstein Barr virus.
   B. high-grade T-cell malignancy.
   C. cytogenic chromosomal change seen is t(8; 14).
   D. it is a form of non-Hodgkin lymphoma.
   E. lymph nodes are often spared.

4. Which of the following diseases show Pautrier microabscesses on histological exam?

   A. Ewing sarcoma
   B. Osteosarcoma
   C. Mycosis fungoides
   D. Multiple myeloma
   E. Chronic lymphocytic leukemia

5. Each of the following is true of cell-mediated immunity EXCEPT

   A. it is responsible for type IV hypersensitivity reactions.
   B. it defends against parasites.
   C. it is important in transplant rejection.
   D. it involves NK cells and macrophages.
   E. it involves predominantly B cells.

Questions 6-10 pertain to the following clinical vignette:

A 17-year-old male presents to your office for extraction of all four third molars. The patient denies any significant medical history, and you proceed with the procedure. While starting an intravenous line, the patient's arm is accidentally cut, and he begins bleeding excessively.

6. Which of the following secondary hemostatic disorders is this patient MOST likely affected by

   A. von Willebrand disease
   B. Hemophilia A
   C. Bernard-Soulier syndrome
   D. Thrombocytopenia
   E. Hemophilia C

7. Each of the following with regard to von Willebrand disease is correct EXCEPT

   A. it is a qualitative platelet defect.
   B. vWF allows adhesion of platelets to collagen.
   C. it affects both the platelet plug and coagulation cascade.
   D. vWF functions independent of factor VIII.
   E. it is an autosomal dominant disorder.

8. Which of the following is TRUE regarding vitamin K deficiency?

   A. Increased activity of clotting factors II, VII, IX, X
   B. Decreased PT
   C. No change in PTT
   D. Caused by malabsorption of fat
   E. Abnormal platelet count

9. Each of the following regarding wound repair is true EXCEPT

   A. secondary intention wound healing occurs when a sizeable gap exists between margins.
   B. a large extraction socket heals by primary intention.
   C. the inflammatory stage occurs immediately after tissue injury.
   D. contact inhibition occurs when migrating epithelial wound margins meet.
   E. healing by primary intention occurs at a faster rate than secondary intention.

10. Each of the following is a topical antibiotic EXCEPT

   A. neomycin.
   B. bacitracin.
   C. polymyxin B.
   D. ofloxacin.
   E. all of the above are topical antibiotics.

11. Which of the following bacteria is a gram-positive cocci that commonly causes skin infection and abscess formation?

   A. *Staphylococcus aureus*
   B. *Streptococcus bovis*
   C. *Streptococcus viridans*
   D. *Staphylococcus saprophyticus*
   E. *Actinomyces israelii*

12. Each of the following antibiotics is correctly matched with its mode of action EXCEPT

   A. macrolide—inhibits protein synthesis by binding 50S ribosomal subunit.
   B. cephalosporin—inhibits cell wall synthesis by blocking peptidoglycan cross-linking.
   C. penicillin—inhibits cell wall synthesis by blocking peptidoglycan cross-linking.
   D. tetracycline—inhibits protein synthesis by binding 30S ribosomal subunit.
   E. clindamycin—inhibits DNA gyrase.

13. Which of the following is TRUE regarding the viral growth curve?

   A. Eclipse period is when both virions and nucleic acid grow exponentially.
   B. Virions and viral nucleic acid have nearly an identical growth curve during the rise period.
   C. The rise period occurs first once a virus enters a cell.
   D. One virus normally takes days to double.
   E. During the rise period, there is a decreased number of virions.

14. Which of the following bacteria is most strongly associated with sex-steroid-induced gingivitis?

   A. *Lactobacillus casei*
   B. *Prevotella intermedia*
   C. *Streptococcus mutans*
   D. *Actinomyces viscosus*
   E. *Lactobacillus acidophilus*

15. Which of the following components of the complement system mediates opsonization?

   A. C5a
   B. C6
   C. C8
   D. C9
   E. C3b

Questions 16 and 17 pertain to the following clinical vignette:

A 55-year-old woman presents to your office complaining of burning mouth, dry eyes, and a rash on her midface. On exam, you note multiple carious lesions and a lack of saliva. You decide to order a blood draw and labs for certain immunologic markers prior to beginning routine dental care.

16. Suppose that lab results show the presence of antinuclear antibodies. Which of the following diseases would one expect this to be indicative of?

   A. Reiter syndrome
   B. Behcet syndrome
   C. Scleroderma
   D. Ankylosing spondylitis
   E. Sjögren syndrome

Microbiology and Pathology

17. What is the most common autoimmune disorder in the United States?

    A. Sjögren syndrome
    B. Rheumatoid arthritis
    C. Lupus
    D. Polyarteritis nodosa
    E. Dermatomyositis

18. Which of the following is FALSE with regard to the Stephan curve?

    A. Nonfermentable carbohydrates cause a rapid decrease in salivary pH.
    B. It takes up to 40 minutes to recover normal salivary pH after eating sugar.
    C. Sucrose ingestion can greatly affect salivary pH.
    D. Normal salivary pH is around 7.0.
    E. Enamel begins to demineralize at a pH of 5.5.

19. Which of the following plaque control agents has the highest alcohol content?

    A. Total (sodium fluoride triclosan)
    B. Gel-Kam (stannous fluoride)
    C. Listerine (phenolic/essential oil compound)
    D. Peridex (chlorhexidine gluconate)
    E. Scope (cetylpyridinium chloride)

20. Which of the following is TRUE about the bacterial growth curve?

    A. Cell growth plateaus during the stationary phase.
    B. The initial phase is signified by increased cell death.
    C. There is an exponential increase in bacterial growth during the log phase.
    D. There is increased metabolic activity during the lag phase.
    E. The lag phase is characterized by a lack of required bacterial nutrients.

Questions 21 and 22 pertain to the following clinical vignette:

Suppose a patient presents to you with tall and thin stature, abnormally long legs and arms, and spiderlike fingers. They also mention that they suffer from cystic medial necrosis of the aorta.

21. Which of the following diseases does this patient most likely have?

    A. Cystic fibrosis
    B. von Hippel-Lindau disease
    C. Tay-Sachs disease
    D. Fabry disease
    E. Marfan syndrome

22. Which of the following genes would you suspect to be mutated with this condition?

    A. VHL
    B. Fibrillin
    C. BRCA-1
    D. N-myc
    E. BRCA-2

Questions 23-25 pertain to the following clinical vignette:

A 20-year-old male presents as a referral for extraction of a necrotic tooth. You decide that the tooth cannot be immediately extracted due to an active infection, and you place the patient on a regimen of penicillin for 1 week. The patient calls your office the next day complaining of a bulls-eye rash on the back of his hand and forearm.

23. What do you believe this patient is suffering from?

    A. Impetigo
    B. Type IV hypersensitivity
    C. Bullous pemphigoid
    D. Pemphigus vulgaris
    E. Erythema multiforme

24. What type of hypersensitivity reaction do you believe this lesion to be from?

    A. Type I
    B. Type II
    C. Type III
    D. Type IV
    E. Not a hypersensitivity reaction

25. Which of the following is TRUE regarding pemphigus vulgaris and bullous pemphigoid?

    A. Both lesions have very different clinical presentations.
    B. They are both mediated by IgM.

C. Histology is of no diagnostic help when differentiating between the two.
D. Only pemphigus vulgaris has Tzanck cells.
E. Immunofluorescence shows the same features between the two.

26. Which of the following bacteria possesses hyaluronidase and is known to cause glomerulonephritis?

A. *Bordetella pertussis*
B. *Streptococcus pyogenes*
C. *Haemophilus influenzae*
D. *Helicobacter pylori*
E. *Francisella tularensis*

27. Which of the following is FALSE regarding bacterial classification?

A. Gram-positive microorganisms contain LTA in their cell walls.
B. Obligate anaerobes typically grow well in oxygenated environments.
C. Spores are produced by gram-positive rods only.
D. Only one bacterium is differentiated by the acid-fast stain.
E. Bacteria designated as cocci are microscopically round.

Questions 28-32 pertain to the following clinical vignette:

A 12-year-old male presents to your office for regular dental cleanings. While taking a health history, his mother tells you that he had a "bad sore throat which went away, then a fever returned a few weeks with small bumps on his knee and wrist." You are suspicious of this illness, and decide to further investigate via physician referral.

28. Upon receiving physician workup, you see that (more specifically) the patient experienced polyarthritis, erythema marginatum, chorea, carditis, and subcutaneous nodules. What illness are these symptoms indicative of?

A. Rheumatic fever
B. Measles
C. Pneumonia

D. Mumps
E. Parvovirus

29. Which of the following hypersensitivity reactions occur with this illness?

A. Type I
B. Type II
C. Type III
D. Type IV
E. Not a hypersensitivity reaction

30. Each of the following are included in the grouping of Aschoff bodies EXCEPT

A. Anitschkow cells.
B. multinucleated giant cells.
C. Aschoff myocytes.
D. focal interstitial myocardial inflammation.
E. lines of Zahn.

31. Which of the following Streptococcal strains are seen in rheumatic fever?

A. Group A beta-hemolytic
B. Group C
C. Group B beta-hemolytic
D. Alpha-hemolytic
E. Group D beta-hemolytic

32. According to the Jones Criteria, how many major and minor criteria are met from the following symptoms—arthritis, fever, ECG changes, arthralgias?

A. 3 major, 1 minor
B. 2 major, 2 minor
C. 1 major, 3 minor
D. 4 major
E. 4 minor

33. Which of the following is FALSE concerning necrotic changes?

A. Ischemia is seen with coagulative necrosis.
B. Fatty acids are released with liquefactive necrosis.
C. Myocardial infarcts cause liquefactive necrosis.
D. Caseous necrosis is seen in tuberculosis infection.
E. Granulomas are considered as being characteristic of caseous necrosis.

Microbiology and Pathology

34. Which of the following is secreted by B cells?

    A. IL-4
    B. INF-γ
    C. IL-2
    D. TGF-β
    E. TNF-α

35. Each of the following cellular injuries is matched up correctly with its causative chemical EXCEPT

    A. methanol—blindness.
    B. cyanide—renal tubular necrosis.
    C. lead—basophilic stippling of red blood cells.
    D. mercury—pneumonitis.
    E. carbon tetrachloride—fatty liver.

36. Each of the following is true regarding periodontal health EXCEPT

    A. the epitactic concept states that calculus formation is independent of proteins.
    B. materia alba is largely composed of desquamated cells and is easily washed away.
    C. subgingival plaque is largely composed of gram-negative bacteria.
    D. chlorhexidine gluconate is the most effective antiplaque mouthrinse.
    E. supragingival plaque is largely composed of gram-positive bacteria.

37. Which of the following types of periodontal disease commonly presents with punched-out interproximal papillae, fetor oris, and marginal gingival pseudomembrane formation?

    A. Chronic periodontitis
    B. Aggressive periodontitis
    C. Plaque-induced gingivitis
    D. Necrotizing ulcerative gingivitis
    E. Candidiasis

Questions 38-40 pertain to the following clinical vignette:

A patient presents to you for extraction of several teeth. Upon examining intraorally, you notice diffuse mucosal pigmentation of the gingiva, tongue, hard palate, and buccal mucosa. When questioning the patient, he mentions that he has been fatigued lately and very weak. You decide to send for a physician's consultation on the patient as well as labs prior to treatment.

38. The above symptoms coupled with the following labs (decreased cortisol, increased serum sodium, increased serum potassium), you would expect which of the following?

    A. Cushing disease
    B. Addison disease
    C. Primary hyperparathyroidism
    D. Cushing syndrome
    E. Plummer disease

39. What does the ACTH stimulation test accomplish?

    A. Differentiates between primary and secondary hyperparathyroidism
    B. Differentiates between hyper- and hypothyroidism
    C. Differentiates between Cushing disease and syndrome
    D. Differentiates between primary and secondary Addison disease
    E. Differentiates between acromegaly and dwarfism

40. Which of the following would be an adequate treatment for Addison disease?

    A. Administer cortisol
    B. Administer aldosterone
    C. Administer androgens
    D. Administer growth hormone
    E. Administer parathyroid hormone

41. Which of the following diseases presents with cystic bone lesions, nephrocalcinosis, and metastatic calcifications?

    A. Hyperparathyroidism
    B. Grave disease
    C. Hyperthyroidism
    D. Hypoparathyroidism
    E. Addison disease

42. Chvostek and Trousseau sign test for which of the following?

    A. Chronic hypocalcemia
    B. Acute hypercalcemia
    C. Acute hypocalcemia
    D. Acute hypercalcemia
    E. Hyperphosphatemia

43. Each of the following is true of adrenal gland neoplasia EXCEPT

    A. pheochromocytoma causes an increase in catecholamine release.
    B. eurofibromatosis and von Hippel-Lindau disease are related to neuroblastoma.
    C. the N-myc gene is found mutated in neuroblastoma.
    D. metastatic spread to the liver is a sequelae of neuroblastoma.
    E. the symptoms of pheochromocytoma include paroxysmal HTN and hyperglycemia.

44. Which of the following endogenous pigments is formed via auto-oxidation, accumulates in Kupffer cells, and is indicative of hepatocellular injury?

    A. Ceroid
    B. Lipofuscin
    C. Hemosiderin
    D. Melanin
    E. Bilirubin

45. Each of the following are true regarding immune defense EXCEPT

    A. acquired immunity includes cell- and antibody-mediated defense.
    B. innate immunity exhibits immunological memory.
    C. active and passive defense are different ways to classify acquired immunity.
    D. lysozymes are an example of innate immunity.
    E. B lymphocytes are an example of acquired immunity.

46. Each of the following is found within the PMNs cytoplasmic granules EXCEPT

    A. neuraminidase.
    B. hydrolase.
    C. myeloperoxidase.
    D. lactoferrin.
    E. interferon.

47. A young patient presents to you with the following symptoms: multiple white lesions on the buccal mucosa and a nonpruritic maculopapular brick-red rash. Which family of viruses do you believe to be suspect?

    A. Rhabdovirus
    B. Paramyxovirus
    C. Papovirus
    D. Reovirus
    E. Calicivirus

48. Each of the following is an RNA enveloped virus EXCEPT

    A. poliovirus.
    B. rubella virus.
    C. human T-cell leukemia virus.
    D. human immunodeficiency virus.
    E. hepatitis C virus.

49. Each of the ADA-standardized guidelines for antibiotic prophylaxis below are correct dosages EXCEPT

    A. adult unable to take oral medication: ampicillin 2 g IM or IV 30 minutes prior to procedure.
    B. children allergic to penicillins: cephalexin 50 mg/kg PO 1 hour prior to procedure.
    C. adults allergic to penicillins: clindamycin 2 g PO 1 hour prior to procedure.
    D. adult standard prophylaxis: penicillin 2 g PO 1 hour prior to procedure.
    E. children allergic to penicillin: clindamycin 20 mg/kg PO 1 hour prior to procedure.

Microbiology and Pathology

50. Which of the following is FALSE regarding bacterial vaccines?

    A. Antitoxin vaccine is a form of active immunity.
    B. Immunity from cholera is provided via killed vaccine.
    C. Active immunity includes whole bacteria, capsular polysaccharides, or toxoids.
    D. Antitoxin vaccine contains antibodies to bacterial exotoxins.
    E. Passive immunity includes preformed antibody preparations which elicit immunity.

51. Which of the following is TRUE with regard to cellular dysplasia?

    A. It is nonmalignant cellular growth.
    B. It involves atypical cells with invasion.
    C. It is disorganized and structureless maturation and spatial arrangement of cells.
    D. It can be caused by chronic irritation.
    E. There is increased mitosis and pleomorphism.

52. Each of the tumor markers are correctly matched to their associated cancer EXCEPT

    A. CEA—adenocarcinoma.
    B. LSA—lymphomas.
    C. AFP—neuroblastoma.
    D. hCG—choriocarcinoma.
    E. desmin—rhabdomyosarcoma.

Questions 53-54 pertain to the following clinical vignette:

Suppose a 35year-old male patient has been taking excessive doses of NSAIDs due to odontogenic pain. The patient is now experiencing extreme pain of the peritoneum. The patient did note one bout of hematemesis a few days ago.

53. Based on the above case presentation, which of the following illnesses would you suspect?

    A. Peptic ulcer disease
    B. Duodenal ulcers
    C. Gastroesophageal reflux disease
    D. Hiatal hernia
    E. Inflammatory bowel disease

54. Which of the following conditions is caused by backflux of acid and a weak lower esophageal sphincter?

    A. Achalasia
    B. Mallory-Weiss syndrome
    C. Hiatal hernia
    D. Intestinal lymphangiectasia
    E. Gastroesophageal reflux disease

55. Each of the following is characteristic of basal cell carcinoma EXCEPT

    A. it is locally aggressive.
    B. it is malignant.
    C. it is the most common skin cancer.
    D. it appears as a pearly papule.
    E. it is the most common form of cancer in the United States.

56. Which of the following is TRUE regarding the diagnosis and treatment of basal cell carcinoma?

    A. Because it is not malignant, the stage of treatment is not vital.
    B. It rarely metastasizes.
    C. It is not disfiguring when left alone.
    D. It presents as neoplastic epidermoid cells.
    E. Surgical excision is rarely effective in early stages.

Questions 57-60 pertain to the following clinical vignette:

A 9-year-old patient presents to your office for consultation. The patient begins to sneeze upon your entrance into the room, and says his chest is tight and he is wheezing. Not knowing any medical history about this patient (and having the mother down the hallway in the restroom), you quickly contemplate what to do.

57. Based on the given information, what would you suspect this patient is suffering from?

    A. Chronic bronchitis
    B. Emphysema
    C. Asthma
    D. Asbestosis
    E. Anthracosis

58. Each of the following is true regarding chronic bronchitis EXCEPT

    A. it is caused by mucous hypersecretion in the bronchi and smaller airways.
    B. symptoms include a productive cough and wheezing.
    C. there is a decreased Reid index.
    D. you would expect to find an increased P_{O_2}.
    E. they are known as "blue bloaters."

59. Aortic dissection is characterized by all of the following EXCEPT

    A. rupture can cause pericardial tamponade.
    B. the carotid artery may become occluded, leading to stroke.
    C. it can be life threatening.
    D. blood "dissects" between the intima and adventitia of the aorta.
    E. the mitral valve often becomes damaged.

60. A pregnant woman (22 weeks) with diabetes and normal blood pressure readings suddenly develops frequent readings of 144/92. Which of the following complications would you be concerned of?

    A. Malignant hypertension.
    B. Aortic aneurysm.
    C. Primary hypertension.
    D. Preeclampsia.
    E. Cardiac tamponade.

61. Each of the following endocrine disorders can contribute to secondary hypertension EXCEPT

    A. Cushing syndrome.
    B. diabetes.
    C. pheochromocytoma.
    D. hypoaldosteronism.
    E. hyperthyroidism.

62. Which of the following bacteria is implicated in the majority of subacute bacterial endocarditis?

    A. *Streptococcus viridians*
    B. *Streptococcus epidermidis*
    C. *Staphylococcus aureus*
    D. *Streptococcus sanguis*
    E. *Streptococcus mutans*

63. Regarding different types of endocarditis, each of the following are true EXCEPT

    A. Libman-Sacks form of endocarditis is caused by intrinsic bacteremia.
    B. dental seeding and intravenous drug use cause the infective form.
    C. the mitral valve is most often affected in the Libman-Sacks form.
    D. the rheumatic form occurs in areas of greatest hemodynamic stress.
    E. the mitral valve is most often affected in rheumatic form.

64. The specific accumulation of serious fluid in the pericardial space is referred to as

    A. hemopericardium.
    B. acute pericarditis.
    C. constrictive pericarditis.
    D. hydropericardium.
    E. myocarditis.

65. Consider a patient who is unaware of the cardiac condition he is suffering from. You note splinter hemorrhages under his finger nails. What is this clinical sign indicative of?

    A. Cardiac tamponade
    B. Endocarditis
    C. Primary hypertension
    D. Coronary artery disease
    E. Angina

66. Which of the following is FALSE regarding antigenicity?

    A. Most antigens are proteins.
    B. Haptens illicit immune response on their own.
    C. Adjuvants enhance the immune response to antigen.
    D. The binding site for an antigen is an epitope.
    E. They induce an immune response by binding to antibody.

Microbiology and Pathology

67. With regard to immune defense, macrophages

    A. are formed within the thymus.
    B. lack the ability to produce cytokines.
    C. present antigen via class II MHC.
    D. lack the ability to phagocytose within connective tissue.
    E. cannot be activated by bacterial components.

68. An important defense of the body against parasitic infection is mediated by

    A. eosinophils.
    B. basophils.
    C. mast cells.
    D. PMNs.
    E. dendritic cells.

69. Each of the following is an antigen presenting cell EXCEPT

    A. monocytes.
    B. B cells.
    C. macrophages.
    D. Langerhans cells.
    E. PMNs.

Questions 70-74 pertain to the following clinical vignette:

A 3-year-old patient presents to your pediatric dental practice with an emergency of odontogenic origin. Clinically, you notice deformation of his ear and lip. The mother mentions that he was born with a syndrome that also affects his immune system, but cannot remember the name.

70. Which of the following disorders do you believe this child has?

    A. Common variable immunodeficiency
    B. Wiskott-Aldrich syndrome
    C. SCID
    D. Bruton X-linked agammaglobulinemia
    E. DiGeorge syndrome

71. Each of the following presents with a defect in B cell function EXCEPT

    A. Bruton X-linked agammaglobulinemia.
    B. Wiskott-Aldrich syndrome.

    C. isolated IgA deficiency.
    D. Job syndrome.
    E. ataxia telangiectasia.

72. Each of the following is seen with DiGeorge syndrome EXCEPT

    A. hypercalcemia.
    B. thymic hypoplasia.
    C. microdeletion of chromosome 22.
    D. palatal clefting.

73. Which of the following is TRUE of a type IV hypersensitivity reaction?

    A. It is mediated by B cells.
    B. It is an immediate response.
    C. It involves the binding of class II MHC to a TCR.
    D. An example of this reaction is seen with hemolytic anemia.
    E. An example of this reaction is seen with atopic allergy.

74. Which of the following types of graft is from genetically different individuals of the same species?

    A. Xenograft
    B. Allograft
    C. Autograft
    D. Isograft
    E. None of the above

75. The antibody which can cross the placenta is

    A. IgA.
    B. IgG.
    C. IgD.
    D. IgE.
    E. IgM.

76. Immunoglobulin A is secreted via exocrine glands and

    A. mediates type I hypersensitivity.
    B. activates complement.
    C. its response is uncertain.
    D. is the main antimicrobial defense of the primary response.
    E. prevents mucosal membrane attachment of microbes.

77. Each of the following is true of an antibody's general structure EXCEPT

    A. activation of complement via the alternative pathway.
    B. its Fab regions determine the idiotype.
    C. its Fc regions determine the isotype.
    D. the constant regions bind APC or C3b.
    E. the variable regions bind specific antigen.

78. Trisomy 18 is seen in which of the following syndromes?

    A. Patau
    B. Klinefelter
    C. Down
    D. Turner
    E. Edward

79. Regarding pathological development, which of the following is NOT teratogenic?

    A. Cytomegalovirus
    B. Rubella
    C. Toxoplasmosis
    D. Herpes simplex virus
    E. Influenza

80. Which of the following is TRUE of impetigo?

    A. Noncontagious
    B. Primarily affects the elderly
    C. Caused by *Staphylococcus aureus* or *Streptococcus pyogenes*
    D. Invades deep into the skin structure
    E. Very low cure rate

81. Each of the following is commonly found in patients afflicted with cystic fibrosis EXCEPT

    A. malfunction of the Cl^- transporter.
    B. meconium ileus.
    C. pathology of chromosome 9.
    D. pancreatic exocrine insufficiency.
    E. bronchiectasis.

82. Suppose a patient presents with café au lait spots, which of the following is NOT commonly associated with this clinical finding?

    A. Neurofibromatosis (type 1)
    B. Tuberous sclerosis
    C. Fanconi anemia
    D. McCune-Albright syndrome
    E. Vitiligo

83. What type of thrombus typically forms after a myocardial infarct or from atrial fibrillation?

    A. Mural
    B. Agonal
    C. Red
    D. White
    E. Fibrin

84. Each of the following is a characteristic of the nonprogressive/early stage of shock EXCEPT

    A. it is considered compensated.
    B. the body is maintaining perfusion to vital organs.
    C. increased total peripheral resistance.
    D. metabolic acidosis.
    E. increase in sympathetic nervous output.

85. Which of the following is TRUE of septic shock?

    A. Causes vasodilation.
    B. Due to exotoxin release.
    C. Caused by gram-positive bacteria.
    D. Caused by injury to the CNS.
    E. It is a type I hypersensitivity reaction.

86. If a patient is stricken with Caisson disease, one would expect to find

    A. solid mass occluding a vessel.
    B. fatty emboli from a broken bone.
    C. air embolizing within the circulation.
    D. a blood clot.
    E. emboli caused by amniotic fluid.

Microbiology and Pathology

87. Each of the following is true regarding hyperemia EXCEPT

   A. increased arteriolar dilation in active hyperemia.
   B. chronic passive hyperemia of the liver is caused directly by left-sided heart failure.
   C. passive hyperemia causes a decrease in venous return.
   D. inflammation and blushing is a clinical finding of active hyperemia.
   E. obstruction and increased back pressure is a clinical finding of chronic hyperemia.

88. A dietary deficiency of vitamin B_{12} causes which of the following?

   A. Aplastic anemia
   B. Sickle cell anemia
   C. Pernicious anemia
   D. Plummer-Vinson syndrome
   E. Folate deficiency anemia

89. Which of the following is TRUE of polycythemia?

   A. True polycythemia has a decrease in RBC mass and decrease in total blood volume.
   B. Primary polycythemia has no genetic predisposition.
   C. Spurious polycythemia (Gaisböck syndrome) is a form of relative polycythemia.
   D. In secondary polycythemia, erythropoietin levels are decreased.
   E. In primary polycythemia, erythropoietin levels are increased.

Questions 90-95 pertain to the following clinical vignette:

A 59-year-old female presents to your office for root canal therapy for tooth No. 9. She mentions that an experience of increased thirst, blurred vision, and frequent urination. You take a fingerstick and note that her blood glucose level is 180 mg/dL.

90. Which of the following diseases do you suspect this patient has?

   A. Hyperthyroidism
   B. Type II diabetes mellitus
   C. Hypothyroidism
   D. Addison disease
   E. Type I diabetes mellitus

91. Nephrogenic diabetes insipidus is characterized by all of the following EXCEPT

   A. sensitized kidney tubules to ADH.
   B. a genetic (sex-linked) predilection to men.
   C. normal ADH production and secretion.
   D. large volumes of dilute urine are produced.
   E. can be caused by lithium.

92. Each of the following have different values in type I diabetes mellitus and type II diabetes mellitus EXCEPT

   A. symptoms.
   B. cause.
   C. genetic predisposition.
   D. treatment.
   E. age of onset.

93. Hyperglycemia is characterized by blood glucose levels greater than

   A. 100 mg/dL.
   B. 90 mg/dL.
   C. 125 mg/dL.
   D. 75 mg/dL.
   E. 50 mg/dL.

94. Each of the following is true of ketoacidosis EXCEPT

   A. it is caused by starvation or severe insulin deficiency.
   B. it is most common in type II diabetes.
   C. it is caused by an accumulation of ketone bodies.
   D. it is acetoacetic acid and beta-hydroxybutyric acid are synthesized from free fatty acids.
   E. it can be life threatening.

95. Which of the following best describes the term glycosylated hemoglobin?

   A. Value used to assess the short-term control of diabetes.
   B. Reversible glycosylation of specific hemoglobin molecules.

C. Accurately measures glucose levels over the past 2-3 days.
D. Normal levels range from 4%-7%.
E. The reaction is based on enzymatic glycosylation.

96. Bence-Jones proteins are found in the urine of patients stricken with which of the following illnesses?

A. Non-Hodgkin lymphoma
B. Burkitt lymphoma
C. Multiple myeloma
D. Chronic myelogenous leukemia
E. Acute myelogenous leukemia

97. Each of the following findings is consistent with multiple myeloma EXCEPT

A. increased platelet count.
B. decreased white blood cell count.
C. decreased red blood cell count.
D. increased plasma cell count.
E. increase in osteolytic lesions.

98. Which of the following illnesses can directly lead to development of type II diabetes?

A. Amyloidosis
B. Pheochromocytoma
C. Small cell carcinoma
D. Neuroblastoma
E. Rheumatoid arthritis

99. Each of the following is a characteristic of an eosinophilic granuloma EXCEPT

A. it is benign and common in males in the 3rd decade of life.
B. the maxilla is most commonly affected.
C. mobile teeth and periodontal inflammation are symptoms.
D. it is typically asymptomatic.
E. it is caused by abnormal histiocytes.

100. Each of the following illnesses is a histiocytosis X disease EXCEPT

A. Letterer-Siwe disease.
B. Hand-Schüller-Christian disease.
C. Haberman disease.
D. eosinophilic granuloma.
E. none of the above.

101. The hyperacute phase of tissue graft rejection is most directly mediated by which of the following?

A. T cells attacking foreign class I MHC
B. Preformed antibody to graft antigen
C. Necrosis of graft vasculature via antibody
D. T cells attacking foreign class II MHC
E. PMN attack of graft antigen

102. Which of the following is TRUE with regard to blood typing?

A. Anti-B antibody is considered blood type B.
B. Blood type O has both A and B antigens.
C. Patients with erythrocyte antigen A has anti-A plasma antibody.
D. Plasma antibody A and B are seen in patients with blood type O.
E. Blood type AB is the universal recipient.

103. Hemagglutination occurs when

A. blood type A is given to a patient with anti-B plasma antibodies.
B. blood type AB is given to a patient with anti-A plasma antibodies.
C. blood type B is given to a patient with anti-A plasma antibodies.
D. blood with erythrocyte antigen A is given to a patient anti-B plasma antibody.
E. blood with erythrocyte antigen B is given to a patient with anti-A plasma antibody.

104. Malfunction of oxidative phosphorylation is seen in poisoning with

A. lead.
B. carbon monoxide.
C. cyanide.
D. mercury.
E. none of the above.

105. Each of the following enzymes is elevated after a myocardial infarct and heart damage EXCEPT

A. CK-MB.
B. troponin T.
C. myoglobin.
D. creatine phosphokinase.
E. alkaline phosphatase.

106. Each of the following conditions can lead to tissue hypoxia EXCEPT

    A. carbon monoxide poisoning.
    B. decreased tissue perfusion.
    C. decreased blood oxygenation.
    D. vascular ischemia.
    E. none of the above.

107. Which of the following is a type of irreversible cell injury?

    A. Karyorrhexis.
    B. Ribosomal detachment from endoplasmic reticulum.
    C. Chromatin clumping.
    D. Cellular and organelle swelling.
    E. Bleb formation.

108. Each of the following cellular reactions is correctly matched EXCEPT

    A. aplasia →complete lack of cells.
    B. hypertrophy →increase in number of cells.
    C. metaplasia →cellular change from one type to another.
    D. atrophy →decrease in cellular mass.
    E. hypoplasia →decrease in number of cells.

109. Which of the following is transmitted by ingestion of undercooked pork?

    A. *Taenia saginata*
    B. *Taenia solium*
    C. *Trichinella spialis*
    D. *Enterobius vermicularis*
    E. *Giardia lamblia*

110. Regarding the parasites' phylogeny, each of the following is true EXCEPT

    A. sporozoans are a type of Protozoa.
    B. parasites are comprised of Protozoa and Metazoa.
    C. Nemathelminthes are a type of Protozoa.
    D. "flatworms" is another name for Platyhelminthes.
    E. Trematoda and Cestoda are subgroups of Platyhelminthes.

111. Which of the following is transmitted through inhalation?

    A. *Cryptosporidium parvum*
    B. *Pneumocystis carinii*
    C. *Entamoeba histolytica*
    D. *Toxoplasma gondii*
    E. *Trichomonas vaginalis*

112. Which of the following troche-form antifungal drugs is effective via inhibition of ergosterol synthesis?

    A. Clotrimazole
    B. Ketoconazole
    C. Fluconazole
    D. Nystatin
    E. Amphotericin B

Questions 113-115 pertain to the following clinical vignette:

Suppose that a patient presents to you for comprehensive dental care. When taking a medical history, he begins complaining of frequent itching of his scalp, groin, and feet. You note that he has nail fungus on his toes. Although you are his dentist, it is still your responsibility to refer him to the correct medical practitioner.

113. Which of the following diseases do you suspect this patient has?

    A. Histoplasmosis.
    B. Coccidioidomycosis.
    C. Blastomycosis.
    D. Dermatophytosis.
    E. Mucormycosis.

114. Treatment could include each of the following EXCEPT

    A. miconazole.
    B. clotrimazole.
    C. trimethoprim.
    D. tolnaftate.
    E. griseofulvin.

115. Which of the following is TRUE of fungi?

    A. They are gram positive.
    B. Cell walls are composed of ergosterol.
    C. They are obligate anaerobes.

D. They are prokaryotic.

E. Their asexual form of reproduction is via spores.

Questions 116-121 pertain to the following clinical vignette:

A 45-year-old male patient presents to your office for extraction of multiple teeth. He appears jaundiced to you, and mentions that he is often fatigued with a generalized muscle ache. The patient frequently has fevers, a loss of appetite, and feels bouts of nausea. He is sexually active with multiple partners, and has not ever had any sort of testing done. You decide to order labs prior to proceeding with his treatment.

116. With the symptoms noted in the clinical vignette, which of the following diseases would you suspect is evident?

A. HIV

B. Syphilis

C. Hepatitis C

D. Gonorrhea

E. Chlamydia

117. A lab finding of HBsAg is consistent with which disease?

A. Acute hepatitis C infection

B. Acute hepatitis A infection

C. Acute hepatitis B infection

D. Chronic hepatitis E infection

E. Chronic hepatitis B infection

118. For which type of hepatitis is there a commonly administered vaccine for healthcare workers?

A. Hepatitis A

B. Hepatitis B

C. Hepatitis C

D. Hepatitis D

E. Hepatitis E

119. The picornavirus is responsible for which form of hepatitis?

A. Hepatitis A

B. Hepatitis B

C. Hepatitis C

D. Hepatitis D

E. Hepatitis E

120. Which of the following forms of sterilization is adequate for killing hepatitis B?

A. Autoclaving

B. Ethylene oxide gas

C. Chemical vapor

D. Formaldehyde

E. Glutaraldehyde

121. Which of the following is TRUE of using glutaraldehyde 2% as a sterilization technique?

A. The technique takes very little time.

B. It is not associated with hypersensitivity.

C. It alkylates nucleic acids and proteins.

D. It denatures proteins.

E. It is the preferred method of sterilizing liquid solutions.

122. An endemic infection is BEST described as

A. an infection occurring more frequently than normal within a population.

B. an infection occurring worldwide.

C. an infection which occurs within different countries.

D. an infection occurring at a minimal level within a population.

E. none of the above.

123. Ludwig angina involves all of the following fascial spaces EXCEPT

A. sublingual.

B. submandibular.

C. submental.

D. parapharyngeal.

E. none of the above.

124. Which of the following is defined as a fluid-filled sac lined by true epithelium?

A. Granuloma.

B. Abscess.

C. Cellulitis.

D. Cyst.

E. All of the above.

Microbiology and Pathology

125. Which of the following infectious states is characterized as having active growth of microorganisms with or without symptoms?

    A. Chronic
    B. Acute
    C. Latent
    D. Subclinical
    E. Carrier

126. The correct temperature for autoclaving/ sterilization with moist heat is

    A. 121°C for 15-20 minutes.
    B. 320°F for 2 hours.
    C. 170°C for 1 hour.
    D. 250°F for 4 hours.
    E. 132°C for 20-30 minutes.

127. The greatest risk of bloodborne infection amongst healthcare workers is

    A. Hepatitis B.
    B. HSV.
    C. HIV.
    D. HPV.
    E. Hepatitis C.

128. Which of the following is TRUE regarding tuberculosis infection?

    A. Secondary form is widely disseminated.
    B. Ghon complex is characteristic of the primary and secondary form.
    C. It is a viral infection.
    D. It is contracted via bloodborne transmission.
    E. It does not involve lymph nodes.

129. Hemoptysis is a clinical symptom of each of the following diseases EXCEPT

    A. pneumonia.
    B. tuberculosis.
    C. emphysema.
    D. bronchitis.
    E. idiopathic pulmonary hemosiderosis.

130. Ascites is characteristic of each of the following diseases EXCEPT

    A. pancreatitis.
    B. pneumonia.

C. congestive heart failure.
D. constrictive pericarditis.
E. nephrotic syndrome.

131. Which of the following is TRUE regarding syndromes of malabsorption?

    A. It can result in steatorrhea.
    B. Celiac disease is most likely caused by infection of some sort.
    C. There is a correlation between increased length of breastfeeding and Whipple disease.
    D. Malabsorption is due to nutrients not being absorbed by the large intestine.
    E. Sore tongue is a clinical complication of Whipple disease.

132. Which of the following is TRUE of caries pathogenesis?

    A. Glucans and fructans inhibit the adherence of plaque to the tooth surface.
    B. Lactic acid buildup causes an increase in salivary pH.
    C. The most detrimental effect on salivary pH is frequency of carbohydrate intake.
    D. Sucrose is a byproduct of glucan metabolism. The quantity of carbohydrate intake is not detrimental to salivary pH.

133. Each of the following typically comprises the majority of dental calculus EXCEPT

    A. calcium.
    B. hydroxyapatite.
    C. carbohydrate.
    D. desquamated cells.
    E. by-products of viral replication.

134. Each of the following is true of free radical injury EXCEPT

    A. it can lead to cross-linking of proteins.
    B. it is generated from redox reactions.
    C. it can induce autocatalytic reactions.
    D. it is formed from catalase.
    E. it is induced by activated oxygen species.

135. Which of the following is TRUE of pathologic calcification?

    A. Metastatic calcification occurs in damaged heart valves.
    B. Metastatic calcification is due in part to increased phosphate concentration.
    C. Serum calcium is normal in dystrophic calcification.
    D. Dystrophic calcification occurs with normal tissue.
    E. Eggshell calcification cannot be seen on chest x-ray.

136. Which of the following definitions is NOT correct regarding classical signs of acute inflammation?

    A. Calor →due to decreased tissue perfusion
    B. Tumor →due to tissue edema
    C. Rubor →due in part to vasodilation
    D. Function laesa →due to pain and swelling
    E. Dolor →due to inflammatory mediators

137. Each of the following is true of acute inflammation EXCEPT

    A. PMNs are the first leukocyte to respond.
    B. granuloma formation includes formation of pus from neutrophils, necrotic cells, and exudates.
    C. regeneration is the first stage of wound repair following inflammation.
    D. chronic inflammation differs from acute in that monocytes and macrophages are present.
    E. elimination of infectious agents and ridding of necrotic tissue occur in the initial response to tissue injury.

138. Which of the following autosomal chromosomal abnormalities occur most frequently?

    A. Edward syndrome
    B. Patau syndrome
    C. Klinefelter syndrome
    D. Down syndrome
    E. Turner syndrome

139. Which of the following is TRUE regarding pathological primary hypertension?

    A. There is hypertrophy of capillaries.
    B. Decreased wall-to-lumen ratio.
    C. Increased arteriolar and capillary density.
    D. Decreased smooth muscle growth.
    E. Decreased cross-sectional area of capillaries and arterioles.

140. Each of the following is a risk factor for atherosclerosis EXCEPT

    A. smoking.
    B. hypertension.
    C. premenopause.
    D. nephrosclerosis.
    E. diabetes.

141. Which of the following is TRUE of right sided heart failure?

    A. Isolated right heart failure is common.
    B. Typically occurs independent of left heart failure.
    C. Can be a sequelae of cor pulmonale.
    D. Typical symptoms include rales and cardiac enlargement.
    E. A S3 of S4 (gallop rhythm) is heard when present.

142. A decrease in alpha-1 antitrypsin is seen in which of the following diseases?

    A. Asthma
    B. Chronic bronchitis
    C. Emphysema
    D. Pneumonia
    E. Tuberculosis

143. A patient with a history of alcoholism presents with a lung abscess. Which of the following bacteria would you most suspect is the causative agent?

    A. *Klebsiella*
    B. *Staphylococcus*
    C. *Streptococcus*
    D. *Bacillus*
    E. *Clostridium*

144. Which of the following bacteria will show characteristic sulfur granules on histological study?

    A. *Listeria monocytogenes*
    B. *Staphylococcus aureus*
    C. *Actinomyces israelii*
    D. *Clostridium botulinum*
    E. *Clostridium tetani*

145. Each of the following can be caused by *Neisseria* infection EXCEPT

    A. septic arthritis.
    B. Waterhouse-Friderichsen syndrome.
    C. meningitis.
    D. gonorrhea.
    E. pseudomembranous colitis.

146. Infection by which species of *Clostridium* after ingestion of reheated meats causes symptoms of necrotizing fasciitis and myonecrosis?

    A. *Dificile*
    B. *Perfringens*
    C. *Tetani*
    D. *Botulinum*
    E. None of the above

147. Which of the following bacteria is correctly matched with the disease it causes?

    A. *Shigella* → dysentery
    B. *Escherichia* → typhoid fever
    C. *Klebsiella* → peptic ulcers
    D. *Vibrio* → urinary tract infection
    E. *Helicobacter* → cholera

148. Which of the following is TRUE of syphilis infection?

    A. The secondary form is characterized by gumma formation.
    B. It is treated with penicillin.
    C. It is caused by *Mycobacterium* infection.
    D. The primary form includes a highly infectious maculopapular rash.
    E. The tertiary stage is characterized by a painless ulcer.

149. The smallest bacterium is

    A. *Chlamydia trachomatis.*
    B. *Mycobacterium tuberculosis.*
    C. *Mycoplasma pneumoniae.*
    D. *Rickettsia rickettsii.*
    E. *Borrelia burgdorferi.*

150. Each of the following diseases is caused by infection of Picornavirus EXCEPT

    A. aseptic meningitis.
    B. herpangia.
    C. polio.
    D. hepatitis B.
    E. common cold.

151. Which of the following is TRUE of coronary artery disease?

    A. Increased blood flow to myocardium.
    B. Increased oxygen and nutrients to myocardium.
    C. Hypotension is a risk factor.
    D. The classic symptom is angina.
    E. Ischemia is a rare consequence of it.

152. Each of the following is seen in a patient with a myocardial infarct EXCEPT

    A. pain radiating to the right arm.
    B. sweating.
    C. ECG changes.
    D. angina.
    E. leakage of cardiac enzymes.

153. Which of the following definitions is correctly matched to its form of angina?

    A. Stable angina → intermittent chest pain at rest
    B. Prinzmetal angina → vasospasm
    C. Prinzmetal angina → most common type
    D. Unstable angina → most common type
    E. Stable angina → precipitated by exertion

Questions 154-158 pertain to the following clinical vignette:

A 70-year-old male patient presents for endodontic therapy. He mentions to you that he is a 30 pack-year smoker since he was 20 years of age. While in your chair, he demonstrates labored breathing and when he coughs, it seems dry and nonproductive. The patient shows you a note from his physician stating that he has an increased total lung capacity, increased residual volume, and decreased FEV_1/FVC.

154. Which of the following diseases do you suspect this patient has?

    A. Chronic bronchitis
    B. Asthma
    C. Emphysema
    D. Pneumonia
    E. Tuberculosis

155. Asthma is precipitated by each of the following mechanism EXCEPT

    A. increased sympathetic stimulation.
    B. cox inhibitors.
    C. direct bronchodilator release.
    D. increased vagal stimulation.
    E. type I hypersensitivity reaction.

156. The term "blue bloater" is given to patients stricken with which of the following conditions?

    A. Emphysema
    B. Asthma
    C. Chronic bronchitis
    D. Pneumonia
    E. Bronchiectasis

157. Each of the following is a possible complication of chronic bronchitis EXCEPT

    A. peripheral edema.
    B. chronic productive cough.
    C. right ventricular overload.
    D. noncaseating granulomas.
    E. bronchogenic carcinoma.

158. Each of the following is a mechanism of airway obstruction EXCEPT

    A. increased elastic recoil.
    B. increased mucous.
    C. airway hyperreactivity.
    D. increased elastic recoil.
    E. none of the above.

159. Which of the following is TRUELY matched with its definition?

A. Precipitation →ABO blood typing
B. Radioimmunoassay →detection of antigen in histologic section
C. Immunofluorescence →detection of serum antigen
D. Agglutination →antibody cross-linking with soluble antigen
E. ELISA →substrate-activated enzyme reaction labeling antigen-antibody complex

160. Which of the following is TRUE of T cells?

    A. TH-1 cells secrete IL-4 and -5.
    B. CD8 lymphocytes respond to class II MHC proteins.
    C. Memory T cells do not respond to reexposure.
    D. TH-2 cells signal B cells to differentiate into plasma cells.
    E. CD4 lymphocytes are considered cytotoxic lymphocytes.

161. Tissue regeneration occurs in each of the following EXCEPT

    A. liver.
    B. cartilage.
    C. skeletal muscle.
    D. bone.
    E. intestinal mucosa.

162. Which of the following is TRUE of histamine function?

    A. Causes vasodilation.
    B. Causes bronchodilation.
    C. It has no effect in type I hypersensitivity reactions.
    D. It is secreted by leukocytes.
    E. It activates complement.

163. Regarding inflammatory mediators, each of the following is correctly matched up with its precursor EXCEPT

A. serotonin →tryptophan.
B. complement protein → hepatocytes.
C. nitric oxide →histidine.
D. bradykinin →kininogen.
E. leukotrienes →arachidonic acid.

Microbiology and Pathology

164. TGF-β is secreted by each of the following EXCEPT

    A. monocytes.
    B. fibroblasts.
    C. T cells.
    D. B cells.
    E. macrophages.

165. Each of the following is part of the cellular stage of acute inflammation EXCEPT

    A. diapedesis.
    B. margination.
    C. chemotaxis.
    D. vasodilation.
    E. adhesion.

166. Which of the following is TRUE of subgingival plaque?

    A. It is located coronal to the gingival margin.
    B. It is not affected by diet and saliva.
    C. It is predominately gram-positive facultative cocci.
    D. The calculus it forms is due to saliva.
    E. It does not attach to gingival epithelial sources.

167. Which of the following is TRUE of bacteriophages?

    A. There are three pathways of replication.
    B. The lytic cycle includes a prophage.
    C. The host cell is not destroyed in the lysogenic cycle.
    D. They are viruses.
    E. DNA is incorporated into the host-cell chromosome in the lytic cycle.

168. Which of the following cannot be prevented with a vaccine?

    A. Infectious mononucleosis
    B. Primary varicella
    C. Smallpox
    D. Hepatitis B
    E. Hepatocellular carcinoma

169. Each of the following is true of human immunodeficiency virus EXCEPT

    A. it contains only one strand of RNA.
    B. gp120 mediates attachment to CD4.
    C. gp41 mediates fusion to the host cell.
    D. p24 and p7 combine to form the nucleocapsid.
    E. it contains reverse transcriptase.

170. Which of the following is TRUE of cephalosporins?

    A. They inhibit protein synthesis.
    B. They contain beta lactam rings.
    C. They are bacteriostatic.
    D. There is only one generation of the drug available.
    E. There is 90% cross-hypersensitivity with penicillins.

171. Haemophilus influenzae can cause each of the following illnesses EXCEPT

    A. otitis media.
    B. epiglottitis.
    C. meningitis in children.
    D. upper respiratory tract infection.
    E. enterocolitis.

Questions 172-175 pertain to the following clinical vignette:

An 8-year-old female presents to your office for regular dental care. On physical exam, you note that she has delayed eruption of several teeth and dentin and enamel defects. The caries rate also seems high.

172. Which of the following diseases do you suspect this patient has?

    A. Osteomalacia
    B. Paget disease
    C. Fibrous dysplasia
    D. Osteoporosis
    E. Osteitis fibrosa cystic

173. Each of the following is a cause of vitamin D deficiency EXCEPT

    A. decreased dietary intake.
    B. malabsorption.
    C. increased phosphate intake.
    D. decreased sunlight exposure.
    E. kidney failure.

174. The laboratory findings of anemia, increased alkaline phosphatase, and increased urinary hydroxyproline are seen in

A. Paget disease.
B. fibrous dysplasia.
C. osteoporosis.
D. osteochondrosis.
E. osteopetrosis.

175. Each of the following classifications of fractures is correctly matched with its definition EXCEPT

A. greenstick →bone cracks through one side only.
B. comminuted →bone is crushed into many pieces.
C. open →bone pierces skin.
D. complete →bone bends but does not break.
E. single →bone breaks only in one place.

Questions 176-179 pertain to the following clinical vignette:

A 79-year-old female presents to your office requesting a consultation about dental implants. While reviewing her medical history, you notice that her hand is shaking as she sits in your chair. You ask her if she is nervous, and she denies. As she is leaving the room after the consultation, you become aware that she has a shuffling gait as she is walking.

176. Which of the following diseases do you suspect this patient is suffering from?

A. Multiple sclerosis
B. Myasthenia gravis
C. Alzheimer disease
D. Parkinson disease
E. Eaton-Lambert syndrome

177. Which of the following is NOT part of the triad of symptoms seen with multiple sclerosis?

A. Scanning speech
B. Dementia
C. Intention tremor
D. Nystagmus
E. None of the above

178. Each of the following is true of a stroke EXCEPT

A. it is due to an infarct of the cerebrum or another part of the brain.
B. it can be caused by a thrombus of embolism of the carotid artery.
C. symptoms vary based on what part of the brain is affected.
D. sudden paralysis and numbness of the body on the ipsilateral side of the stroke is common.
E. hemorrhage of the brain can cause a stroke.

179. Which of the following signs and symptoms are incorrectly matched with their causative disease?

A. Alzheimer disease →Lewy bodies
B. Parkinson disease →depigmentation of the substantia nigra
C. Werdnig-Hoffman disease →tongue fasciculations
D. Poliomyelitis →lower motor neuron damage
E. Huntingdon disease →chorea and dementia

180. Each of the following tumors is matched up with their definition EXCEPT

A. choristoma →normal tissue misplaced within another organ.
B. myxoma →malignant tumor derived from connective tissue.
C. teratoma →neoplasm comprised of all three embryonic germ cell layers.
D. adenoma →neoplasm of glandular epithelium.
E. papilloma →tumor from surface epithelium.

181. Each of the following causes of mutagenesis is correctly matched with its mechanism of action EXCEPT

A. ultraviolet light →produces free radicals that can attack DNA bases.
B. dimers →interfere with DNA replication.
C. chemicals →may alter an existing DNA base.
D. viruses →frameshift mutations.
E. viruses →frameshift deletions.

182. The clinical signs of peau d'orange and enlarged axillary lymph nodes are evident in which of the following neoplasias?

   A. Squamous cell carcinoma
   B. Lung cancer
   C. Colorectal cancer
   D. Breast cancer
   E. Uterine cancer

183. Which of the following cells has the lowest radiosensitivity?

   A. Lymphocytes
   B. Reproductive cells
   C. Nerve cells
   D. Epithelial cells
   E. Bone marrow

184. Which of the following is a highly malignant cerebellar tumor that is also of primitive neuroectodermal origin?

   A. Glioblastoma multiforme
   B. Medulloblastoma
   C. Low-grade astrocytoma
   D. Craniopharyngioma
   E. Ependymoma

185. Which of the following cancers has the highest incidence in men?

   A. Colorectal
   B. Urinary tract
   C. Prostate
   D. Lung
   E. Leukemia

Questions 186-189 pertain to the following clinical vignette:

A 64-year-old male presents to you complaining of a painful growth on his midface. It appears somewhat pearly with overlying telangiectatic vessels. He mentions that it sometimes bleeds and it doesn't seem to ever heal. You decide to perform a biopsy.

186. Which of the following do you suspect this lesion is?

   A. Dermatofibroma
   B. Basal cell carcinoma

   C. Squamous cell carcinoma
   D. Actinic keratosis
   E. Melanoma

187. Which of the following skin neoplasms is benign?

   A. Pigmented nevus
   B. Squamous cell carcinoma
   C. Melanoma
   D. Keratocanthoma
   E. None of the above

188. Each of the following is true regarding squamous cell carcinoma of the skin EXCEPT

   A. keratin pearls are seen histologically.
   B. there are increased laminin receptors seen in malignant epithelial cells.
   C. a normal treatment regimen requires chemotherapy.
   D. it can be caused by sun damage and radiation.
   E. it typically presents as a scaling, indurated, ulcerative nodule.

189. Which of the following is FALSE regarding melanoma of the skin?

   A. It is a malignancy of melanocytes of nevus cells.
   B. The most common form is superficial spreading type.
   C. It is the most deadly form of skin cancer.
   D. The clinical course may include very rapid spread.
   E. The initial phase of growth is vertical followed by radial.

190. Which of the following is TRUE regarding Ewing sarcoma?

   A. Histology alone is not specific for diagnosis.
   B. It is not sensitive to radiation therapy.
   C. It occurs in the 5th-6th decades of life.
   D. It originates in skeletal muscle.
   E. It is benign.

191. Each of the following is a possible cause of disseminated intravascular coagulation EXCEPT

   A. major trauma.
   B. malignancy.

C. gram-negative sepsis.

D. amniotic fluid embolism.

E. type I hypersensitivity reaction.

192. Which of the following is FALSE regarding iron deficiency?

A. It can be caused by chronic blood loss.

B. Clinical symptoms include pallor, fatigue, and shortness of breath.

C. It results in macrocytic anemia.

D. It can lead to Plummer-Vinson syndrome.

E. Poor diet can be a cause.

193. Each of the following is a cause of vitamin B_{12} deficiency EXCEPT

A. pernicious anemia.

B. duodenal resection.

C. gastric resection.

D. specific dietary deficiency.

E. none of the above.

194. Which of the following lab findings would be seen with nephrotic syndrome?

A. Hyperalbuminemia

B. Hypolipidemia

C. Hypocholesterolemia

D. Optimally functioning renal glomeruli

E. Proteinuria

195. In general, which of the following is TRUE of the systemic response to infection?

A. *Giardia* infections are largely associated with neutrophilia.

B. *Rubella* infections are largely associated with lymphocytosis.

C. It rarely results in fever.

D. Leukocytosis is a rare result of bacterial, parasitic, and viral infection.

E. *Clostridium* infections are largely associated with eosinophilia.

196. Which of the following is TRUE regarding the physiology of edema?

A. There is a decrease in capillary permeability.

B. There is an increase in interstitial fluid colloid osmotic pressure.

C. There is a decrease in plasma colloid osmotic pressure.

D. There is a decrease in capillary hydrostatic pressure.

E. Fluid moves into the intravascular space.

197. Which of the following is TRUE regarding the pathophysiology of shock?

A. There is a decrease in urinary output.

B. The patient becomes hypertensive.

C. There is an increase in blood flow.

D. There is an increase in cardiac output.

E. There is an increase in stroke volume.

198. Each of the following can lead to cirrhosis of the liver EXCEPT

A. hemochromatosis.

B. biliary obstruction.

C. Wilson disease.

D. viral hepatitis.

E. portal hypertension.

199. Each of the following is true of hemolytic anemia EXCEPT

A. the first sign is yellow sclera.

B. hyperbilirubinemia is a common laboratory finding.

C. there is a decrease in unconjugated bilirubin in the blood.

D. conjugated bilirubin forms from albumin and unconjugated bilirubin.

E. hemoglobinuria is a common laboratory finding.

200. Which of the following is TRUE of sickle cell anemia?

A. The homozygotic form is less severe.

B. The spleen is rarely affected.

C. Caucasians are most commonly affected.

D. It is an inherited autosomal dominant disease.

E. Patients with sickle-cell trait are heterozygotic.

Microbiology and Pathology

1. **The correct answer is D.** Reed-Sternberg cells are pathognomonic for Hodgkin lymphoma. These cells are true neoplastic cells found within lymph nodes of affected persons, and are also malignant.

   Answer A is incorrect. Non-Hodgkin lymphoma is a disease with similar symptoms to Hodgkin, but lacking the presence of Reed-Sternberg cells. Diagnosis is based on clinical symptoms and histology.

   Answer B is incorrect. Acute lymphocytic leukemia is a malignancy of the bone marrow. It is characterized by overexpression of immature white blood cells.

   Answer C is incorrect. Chronic myelogenous leukemia is a form of cancer affecting myelogenous cells of the bone marrow. Presence of the Philadelphia chromosome is diagnostic.

   Answer E is incorrect. Multiple myeloma is a cancer which is characterized by unregulated proliferation of plasma cells.

2. **The correct answer is D.** Weight gain is not commonly seen in patients suffering from non-Hodgkin lymphoma.

   Answer A is incorrect. Night sweats are seen in patients with non-Hodgkin lymphoma.

   Answer B is incorrect. Malaise is a symptom seen in patients with non-Hodgkin lymphoma.

   Answer C is incorrect. Fatigue is a symptom seen in patients with non-Hodgkin lymphoma.

   Answer E is incorrect. Solid tumor masses in the cervical and supraclavicular region of the neck.

3. **The correct answer is B.** Burkitt lymphoma is not a high grade T-cell malignancy.

   Answer A is incorrect. EBV also is thought to play a significant role in Burkitt lymphoma, especially in African nations (95% of cases).

Answer C is incorrect. With this disease, a chromosomal change is seen at t(8; 14), and is noted on genetic studies.

Answer D is incorrect. Burkitt lymphoma is a form of NHL, and is signified by defective B cells. The illness is also closely related to ALL.

Answer E is incorrect. Lymph nodes are often spared with this disease.

4. **The correct answer is C.** Mycosis fungoides is a form of NHL which is characterized by eczematoid-type skin lesions with regional erythema. The lesions eventually progress to tumors. Histologically, one would find atypical CD4 cells with cerebriform nuclei and Pautrier microabscesses, which are small pockets of tumor cells within the epidermis.

   Answer A is incorrect. Ewing sarcoma is a cancer of bone frequently found in teenagers. Its clinical presentation and radiographic analysis are diagnostic.

   Answer B is incorrect. Osteosarcoma is a malignant bone disease which is diagnosed histologically based on the presence of affected osteoid.

   Answer D is incorrect. Multiple myeloma is a cancer which is due to uncontrolled proliferation of plasma cells and is diagnosed histologically.

   Answer E is incorrect. Chronic lymphocytic leukemia (CLL) is a cancer which affects the bone marrow. Proliferation of B cells is most commonly involved.

5. **The correct answer is E.** Cell-mediated immunity is a part of the host defense which involves T lymphocytes, NK cells, and macrophages, but is not predominately B-cell mediated.

   Answer A is incorrect. Cell-mediated immunity is responsible for type IV hypersensitivity reactions. This involves T-cell immunological attack.

Answer B is incorrect. Cell-mediated immunity helps the body defend against parasites, as well as intracellular bacteria, viruses, and fungi.

Answer C is incorrect. Cell-mediated immunity is important in transplant rejection. Dysfunction of this sect of the host defense can lead to granulomatous infection, tumor suppression, rejection of organs posttransplant, and graft-vs-host reaction.

Answer D is incorrect. Cell-mediated immunity involves NK cells and macrophages.

6. **The correct answer is B.** This patient is most likely suffering from Hemophilia A. This form of Hemophilia is seen in males (X-linked) commonly under the age of 25. With this disease, one would experience excessive bleeding from minor wounds (superficial cuts, etc.) as well as hematomas, hemarthroses, and epistaxis.

Answer A is incorrect. von Willebrand disease (primary and secondary hemostatic disorder) has a common predilection between males and females (autosomal dominant).

Answer C is incorrect. Bernard-Soulier disease is a disorder characterized by dysfunction of primary hemostasis.

Answer D is incorrect. Thrombocytopenia is a disorder characterized by dysfunction of primary hemostasis.

Answer E is incorrect. Hemophilia C (secondary hemostatic disorder) is not sex linked and there is far less severe bleeding.

It is important to note that disorders of primary hemostasis deal with the platelet plug, whereas secondary hemostatic disorders affect coagulation.

7. **The correct answer is D.** von Willebrand disease is bleeding and it functions independent of factor VIII.

Answer A is incorrect. von Willebrand disease is a qualitative platelet disorder, thus the overall number of platelets is not affected.

Answer B is incorrect. von Willebrand disease involves dysfunction of the vWF glycoprotein, which allows adhesion of platelets to collagen.

Answer C is incorrect. von Willebrand disease affects the platelet plug and the coagulation cascade. Under normal conditions, vWF (which is located on platelets) allows adhesion of platelets to collagen. This is how primary hemostasis (platelet plug) is achieved. vWF also has binding sites for factor VIII, thus, involvement in secondary hemostasis (coagulation cascade).

Answer E is incorrect. von Willebrand disease is an autosomal dominant disorder.

8. **The correct answer is D.** Vitamin K deficiency is caused by malabsorption of fat. This is commonly due to pancreatic and GI dysfunction.

Answer A is incorrect. There is a decreased activity of clotting factors II, VII, IX, and X. With a lack of vitamin K, there is a subsequent lack in production of coagulation factors II, VII, IX, and X.

Answer B is incorrect. There is an increase in PT. It measures the extrinsic pathway of coagulation.

Answer C is incorrect. There is a change in PTT. It measures both intrinsic and common pathways of coagulation.

Answer E is incorrect. The platelet count is found to be normal.

With this problem with secondary hemostasis, one would expect to see an increase in PT, increase in PTT, and no change in platelet quantity.

9. **The correct answer is B.** A large extraction socket does not heal by primary intention. Rather, it heals by secondary intention. A normal extraction site is an example of healing by secondary intention. Wound healing is a process which begins as soon as tissue is damaged. There are three stages to wound repair, all of which possess some overlap: inflammatory stage (immediately after tissue injury) fibroplastic stage (3-4 days after injury and lasts for 2-3 weeks, characterized by

completion of epithelial migration, angiogenesis, and increased collagen formation), and remodeling stage (begins 2-3 weeks after injury and continues indefinitely; collagen remodeling and wound contraction with scar formation occurs).

Answer A is incorrect. Secondary intention wound healing occurs when a sizeable gap exists between margins. The two methods of wound healing include primary intention (when wound margins are closely approximated, resulting in faster healing, examples include well-reduced bone fracture or incision margin) and secondary intention (gap between wound margins, slower healing, examples includes large burns/ulcers and extraction sockets).

Answer C is incorrect. The inflammatory stage occurs immediately after tissue injury. It lasts 3-5 days, characterized by fibrin clot formation and commencing of epithelial migration.

Answer D is incorrect. Contact inhibition occurs when migrating epithelial wound margins meet.

Answer E is incorrect. Healing by primary intention occurs at a faster rate than secondary intention.

10. **The correct answer is D.** Ofloxacin is an example of a fluoroquinone. It is not used in topical form.

Answer A is incorrect. Neomycin is an antibiotic used via topical application. It is an aminoglycoside.

Answer B is incorrect. Bacitracin is an antibiotic used via topical application. It functions to inhibit cell-wall synthesis.

Answer C is incorrect. Polymyxin B is an antibiotic used via topical application. It functions by altering cell-membrane permeability.

11. **The correct answer is A.** *Staphylococcus aureus* is a gram-positive coccus which causes abscess formation, gastroenteritis, endocarditis, toxic shock syndrome, and scalded skin syndrome.

The major virulence factors include protein A, β-lactamase, and enterotoxin.

Answer B is incorrect. *Streptococcus bovis* is a gram-positive coccus. Infection causes endocarditis.

Answer C is incorrect. *Streptococcus viridans* is a gram-positive coccus. Infection causes caries and endocarditis.

Answer D is incorrect. *Staphylococcus saprophyticus* is a gram-positive coccus. Infection causes urinary tract infections.

Answer E is incorrect. *Actinomyces israelii*, although it does cause abscesses, is a gram-positive bacillus. It produces sulfur granules.

12. **The correct answer is E.** Clindamycin does not inhibit DNA gyrase. It is bacteriostatic by inhibiting protein synthesis via binding of 50S ribosomal subunits in organisms.

Answer A is incorrect. Macrolides are bacteriostatic and have narrow (erythromycin) and more broad (azithromycin) spectrum formulations. They inhibit protein synthesis by binding 50S ribosomal subunit.

Answer B is incorrect. Cephalosporins are bacteriocidal. They inhibit cell-wall synthesis by blocking peptidoglycan cross-linking.

Answer C is incorrect. Penicillin is bacteriocidal. It inhibits cell-wall synthesis by blocking peptidoglycan cross-linking.

Answer D is incorrect. Tetracycline is a broad spectrum, bacteriostatic antibiotic. It inhibits protein synthesis by binding 30S ribosomal subunit.

13. **The correct answer is B.** Virions and viral nucleic acid have nearly an identical growth curve during the rise period.

Answer A is incorrect. The eclipse period is when one virion enters a cell and there is an immediate decrease in their quantity.

Answer C is incorrect. The rise period is when there is an exponential increase in nucleic acid and virions. It occurs prior to virus release.

Answer D is incorrect. One virus can double within hours. It is possible that one virus may replicate for a yield of up to hundreds of new virions.

Answer E is incorrect. During the rise period, there is an increased number of virions.

14. **The correct answer is B.** *Prevotella intermedia* is often found in high proportions where gingivitis is caused by sex steroid fluctuation. These fluctuations are commonly seen with pregnancy, puberty, menstrual cycle, and oral contraceptive use. *P. intermedia* use these steroids as growth factors.

Answers A, C, D, and E are incorrect. *Lactobacillus casei, Streptoccus mutans, Actinomyces viscosus,* and *Lactobacillus acidophilus* are commonly found as part of oral environment flora, but are not strongly correlated to sex-steroid-induced gingivitis.

15. **The correct answer is E.** Opsonization, which functions to enhance phagocytosis, is mediated by C3b. This component of the complement system binds to the Fc site of immunoglobulin (which in turn binds antigen), thus, allowing phagocytes to bind this complex and destroy the invader.

Answer A is incorrect. C5a is a part of the complement system. It functions to mediate chemotaxis.

Answer B is incorrect. C6 is a part of the complement system. It combines with other complement factors to form the membrane attack complex.

Answer C is incorrect. C8 is a part of the complement system. It combines with other complement factors to form the membrane attack complex.

Answer D is incorrect. C9 is a part of the complement system. It combines with other complement factors to form the membrane attack complex.
    Note that complement factors C5a, and C6, C8, and C9 (combined with C5b and C7) form the membrane attack complex. This disrupts cell membrane permeability.

16. **The correct answer is E.** Sjögren syndrome has the classic clinical triad of xerostomia (dry mouth), keratoconjunctivitis (dry eyes), and systemic lupus erythematous (characteristic butterfly rash on face). Sjögren most often affects women around the age of 50 years. Rheumatoid arthritis may also be present. Ultimately, exocrine glands are infiltrated by lymphocytes and become fibrotic and atrophied. This leads to decreased secretions and the above symptoms, as well as rampant caries from increased acidogenic bacteria in the oral cavity.

Answer A is incorrect. Reiter syndrome is an autoimmune condition characterized by arthritis, conjunctivitis, and urethritis.

Answer B is incorrect. Behcet syndrome is an immune disease characterized by symptoms of ulcers, skin and eye inflammation, and arthritis, to name a few.

Answer C is incorrect. Scleroderma is a disease characterized by localized and systemic deposits of collagen. It can occur in the skin, as well as other organs of the body.

Answer D is incorrect. Ankylosing spondylitis is a chronic disease which involves arthritis of the spine. It can be seen radiographically when spinal fusion occurs.

17. **The correct answer is B.** Rheumatoid arthritis is the most common autoimmune disorder. It is a chronic inflammatory disorder which affects joints and surrounding tissue by proliferative inflammation of synovial membranes. Organ systems may also become affected. Middle age females have nearly a 2.5x predilection for the disease. Genetically, persons more likely to be stricken with this illness possess HLA-DR4 markers.

Answer C is incorrect. Lupus is an autoimmune disorder found in peoples worldwide, but it is not the most common.

Answer D is incorrect. Polyarteritis nodosa is an autoimmune disorder found in peoples worldwide, but it is not the most common.

Microbiology and Pathology

Answer E is incorrect. Dermatomyositis is an autoimmune disorder found in peoples worldwide, but it is not the most common.

Collagen vascular diseases include rheumatoid arthritis, SLE, polyarteritis nodosa, dermatomyositis, and scleroderma. All collagen vascular diseases are characterized by inflammatory damage to connective tissue and blood vessels, as well as the deposition of fibrinoid material in these regions.

18. **The correct answer is A.** Fermentable carbohydrates cause a rapid decrease in salivary pH. The Stephan Curve shows the relationship between salivary pH over a span of roughly one hour. Once a fermentable carbohydrate (ie, sucrose) is ingested, it is synthesized by oral microflora to produce lactic acid.

Answer B is incorrect. It takes up to 40 minutes to recover normal salivary pH after eating sugar. Recovery can occur as early as 15 minutes.

Answer C is incorrect. Sucrose ingestion can greatly affect salivary pH. Within minutes of eating sugar, oral bacteria can cause rapid enamel demineralization.

Answer D is incorrect. Normal salivary pH is around 7.0. Acid causes a rapid decrease in the salivary pH (within minutes) below the threshold of enamel demineralization (pH of 5.5).

19. **The correct answer is C.** Listerine contains the highest alcohol content of all chemical plaque control agents. It contains a phenolic/essential oil compound and 26.9% alcohol. This product inhibits plaque buildup and concomitant gingivitis.

Answer A is incorrect. Total (sodium fluoride/triclosan) contains 0.3% triclosan. It does not contain alcohol.

Answer B is incorrect. Gel-Kam (stannous fluoride) does not contain alcohol.

Answer D is incorrect. Peridex (0.12% chlorhexidine gluconate) typically contains about 11.6% alcohol.

Answer E is incorrect. Scope (cetylpyridinium chloride) contains about 10% alcohol.

20. **The correct answer is B.** The initial stage (lag phase) is characterized by increased metabolic activity and a slight upswing in the curve. The bacterial growth curve is broken up into four stages (lag, log, stationary, death).

Answer A is incorrect. The stationary phase is signified by a plateau on the graph and demonstrates a balance in the number of new and dead cells which is caused by a lack of required nutrients.

Answer C is incorrect. The log phase begins an exponential growth and division of bacteria which is shown by an increase in the curve.

Answer D is incorrect. There is increased metabolic activity during the lag phase.

Answer E is incorrect. The lag phase is characterized by a lack of required bacterial nutrients.

The final stage, the death phase, shows an exponential increase in bacterial death and is shown as a decrease on the growth curve.

21. **The correct answer is E.** Marfan syndrome is an uncommon hereditary connective tissue disorder in which patients present with the above clinical features. They suffer from cystic medial necrosis of the aorta which puts the patient at an increased risk of aortic incompetence and dissecting aortic aneurysms. They also have a distensible mitral valve. Along with these skeletal and cardiovascular abnormalities, these patients also suffer from ocular lens dislocation.

Answer A is incorrect. Cystic fibrosis is a progressive disease which is due to malfunction of chloride channels throughout the body. It results in excessive, thick mucous production. It is autosomal recessive.

Answer B is incorrect. von-Hippel Lindau disease is an autosomal dominant disorder which is characterized by cysts and adenomas of the liver, kidney, adrenals, and pancreas.

Answer C is incorrect. Tay-Sachs disease is an x-linked disorder which involves lysosomal storage. It is autosomal recessive.

Answer D is incorrect. Fabry disease is an x-linked disorder which involves lysosomal storage. It is autosomal dominant.

22. **The correct answer is B.** Fibrillin is commonly found mutated in patients with Marfan syndrome. This gene causes connective tissue disorders in patients. The mutation, though, is quite uncommon.

Answer A is incorrect. VHL is a gene found mutated in von Hippel-Lindau disease.

Answer C is incorrect. BRCA-1 is a gene mutated in breast cancer.

Answer D is incorrect. N-myc is a gene mutated in neuroblastoma.

Answer E is incorrect. BRCA-2 is a gene mutated in breast cancer.

23. **The correct answer is E.** This patient most likely has erythema multiforme. This skin lesion is caused by medications (sulfa, penicillins, barbiturates), infections, HSV, and mycoplasma. Damage occurs to blood vessels of the skin by way of immune complex formation. Clinically, one would find a "target," "bulls-eye," or "iris" skin lesion on the locations listed above. Systemic complications are not present.

Answer A is incorrect. Impetigo is a bacterial skin infection common in children with itchy blisters.

Answer B is incorrect. Type IV hypersensitivity can cause a skin rash and other allergic responses.

Answer C is incorrect. Bullous pemphigoid is an immunologic skin lesion characterized by oral and skin lesions due to IgG autoantibodies against epidermal intercellular cement substance.

Answer D is incorrect. Pemphigus vulgaris is an immunologic skin lesion characterized by oral and skin lesions due to IgG autoanti-

bodies against epidermal intercellular cement substance.

Bullous pemphigoid and pemphigus vulgaris are differentiated by immunofluorescence and histology.

24. **The correct answer is C.** Erythema multiforme causes a type III hypersensitivity reaction. Type III reactions are due to antigen and antibody forming complexes and depositing themselves in areas such as vessel walls, thus allowing complement to be activated and damage to adjacent tissue.

Answer A is incorrect. Type I reactions are anaphylactic and caused by IgE binding to mast cells with subsequent cross-linking of antibody and allergen. This activates the mast cell to release histamine and cause systemic reactivity.

Answer B is incorrect. Type II reactions are cytotoxic hypersensitivity, with IgG binding to antigen on a red blood cell with eventual complement destruction being an example.

Answer D is incorrect. Type IV reactions are delayed/cell mediated and involve T-helper cells binding via MHC protein and TCR to antigen and macrophage to cause release of inflammatory mediators.

Answer E is incorrect. It is a hypersensitivity reaction.

25. **The correct answer is D.** Pemphigus vulgaris has Tzanck cells histologically.

Answer A is incorrect. Both pemphigus vulgaris and bullous pemphigoid are immunologic skin lesions which have very similar clinical presentation: oral mucosal lesions, skin lesions, rupture bullae and susceptible surface left to infection.

Answer B is incorrect. IgG autoantibodies are present against epidermal intercellular cement substance in both.

Answer C is incorrect. Immunofluorescence can be diagnostic in both diseases, with encircling epidermal cells (pemphigus vulgaris) and linear bands (bullous pemphigoid) shown in each.

Answer E is incorrect. Histologically, one would expect to find intraepidermal bullae with pemphigus vulgaris and subepidermal bullae with bullous pemphigoid.

26. **The correct answer is B.** *S. pyogenes* is a group A beta hemolytic, gram positive. Streptolysin O and S as its major virulence factors. It is implicated in many cases of glomerulonephritis, pharyngitis, pyogenic infections, meningitis, scarlet and rheumatic fever.

    Answer A is incorrect. *B. pertussis* infection causes whooping cough.

    Answer C is incorrect. *H. influenzae* infection causes meningitis (in children).

    Answer D is incorrect. *H. pylori* infection is implicated in peptic ulcers and gastritis.

    Answer E is incorrect. *F. tularensis* infection causes tularemia (transmitted via tick bite).

27. **The correct answer is B.** Obligate anaerobes typically grow well in nonoxygenated environments. Oxygen requirements can categorize bacteria, also: obligate aerobes require oxygen for growth, obligate anaerobes lack superoxide dismutase and/or catalase, thus cannot live in oxygen-containing environments, and facultative anaerobes can grow in the presence or lack of oxygen (using fermentation for energy when necessary).

    Answer A is incorrect. Gram-positive microorganisms contain LTA in their cell walls. Gram stain differentiates based on cell-wall composition: gram positive contain LTA and have a thick peptidoglycan wall with no endotoxin; gram negative are the opposite with LPS in their walls.

    Answer C is incorrect. Spores are produced by gram-positive rods only. Thus, spore production can also differentiate bacteria.

    Answer D is incorrect. Only one bacterium is differentiated by the acid-fast stain. This bacterium is *Mycoplasma pneumonia*.

    Answer E is incorrect. Bacteria designated as cocci are microscopically round. Another bacteria is classified is by shape, such as cocci (round), bacilli (rods), spirochetes (spiral), and pleomorphic (multiple shapes).

28. **The correct answer is A.** Rheumatic fever is an acute inflammatory disease which presents with the above symptoms: polyarthritis, erythema marginatum, chorea, carditis, subcutaneous nodules, and fever. The disease develops weeks after an untreated streptococcal infection. The most common age for rheumatic fever is 5-15 years old. Patients are normally asymptomatic in the latent period between streptococcus infection and rheumatic fever onset. Mild cases last from 3-4 weeks, whereas more severe illnesses can take up to 3 months to clear.

    Answer B is incorrect. Measles is a disease characterized by Koplik spots (characteristic rash) as well as a fever, cough, and conjunctivitis.

    Answer C is incorrect. Pneumonia is a disease which involves inflammation of the lungs. It is of viral or bacterial origin.

    Answer D is incorrect. Mumps is a viral disease which is characterized by swelling of the salivary glands. Rashes may also be seen.

    Answer E is incorrect. Parvovirus rarely affects humans, but can cause a rash and arthritis. Blood cells can also be affected.

29. **The correct answer is C.** Type III hypersensitivity reactions occur with rheumatic fever. This inflammatory disease is not actually an infection, but rather an inflammatory reaction to an infection. As with this type of hypersensitivity reaction, antigen/antibody complexes are formed to the bacterial infection which eventually attacks the endocardium and valves. From this, permanent damage to the heart and its valves often occurs. This "phase" is referred to as rheumatic heart disease. The mitral, aortic, and tricuspid valves are most commonly affected; the pulmonic valve is rarely damaged.

    Answer A is incorrect. Type I hypersensitivity reactions are allergic in nature and seen with anaphylaxis and asthma.

Answer B is incorrect. Type II hypersensitivity reactions are cytotoxic and are seen in such diseases as Goodpasture and erythroblastosis fetalis.

Answer D is incorrect. Type IV hypersensitivity reactions are cell mediated and are seen in cases of contact dermatitis.

Answer E is incorrect. A hypersensitivity reaction does occur.

30. **The correct answer is E.** Lines of Zahn are found to be associated with arterial thrombi; they are seen morphologically as red and white laminations within the thrombus.

Answer A is incorrect. Anitschkow cells are large, unusual cells included in the grouping of Aschoff bodies.

Answer B is incorrect. Multinucleated giant cells (Aschoff myocytes) are included in the grouping of Aschoff bodies.

Answer C is incorrect. Aschoff myocytes are a form of multinucleated giant cells. They are included in the grouping of Aschoff bodies.

Answer D is incorrect. Focal interstitial myocardial inflammation with fragmented collagen and fibrinoid material is included in the grouping of Aschoff bodies.
   Note that Aschoff bodies are a grouping of pathological findings seen in association with rheumatic fever.

31. **The correct answer is A.** Group A beta-hemolytic streptococcal strain are known to cause rheumatic fever if left untreated for long periods of time. This bacterium, also known as *Streptococcus pyogenes*, contains hyaluronidase, streptokinase, erythrogenic toxin, and streptolysin O and S as its major virulence factors. It is implicated in pyogenic infections, pharyngitis, glomerulonephritis, meningitis, and scarlet fever, as well as rheumatic fever.

Answer B is incorrect. Group C streptococci are very rarely found in humans.

Answer C is incorrect. Group B beta-hemolytic streptococci include S. *agalactiae*

and cause neonatal illnesses (meningitis and sepsis).

Answer D is incorrect. Alpha-hemolytic streptococci are found in dental caries and endocarditis, and is of the Viridans group.

Answer E is incorrect. Group D streptococci include Enterococci and S. *bovis*, and cause UTIs and endocarditis, respectively.

32. **The correct answer is C.** The Jones criteria are used to diagnose rheumatic fever. The diagnosis can be made based on clinical findings of at least 2 major or 1 major and 1 minor criterion. The major criteria include carditis, arthritis, chorea, erythema marginatum, and subcutaneous nodules. The minor criteria include fever, arthralgias, history of rheumatic fever, and ECG changes. Also involved in the diagnosis of rheumatic fever are pathological changes such as Aschoff bodies and laboratory findings including an increase in ASO titers and increase in erythrocyte sedimentation rate.

Answers A, B, D, and E are incorrect. These are not the proper number of major and minor Jones criteria.

33. **The correct answer is C.** Myocardial infarcts are an example of coagulative necrosis. This type of necrosis is characterized by ischemia, protein denaturation, preservation of tissue architecture, and a triangular-shaped area of infarction.

Answer A is incorrect. Ischemia is seen with coagulative necrosis. Gangrenous necrosis, a subgroup seen here, is ischemic with putrefaction and an example is gangrene.

Answer B is incorrect. Fatty acids are released with liquefactive necrosis. Liquefactive necrosis shows enzymatic digestion, suppuration, and loss of tissue architecture. An example is focal bacterial infections. Acute pancreatitis, an example of fat necrosis (a subgroup of liquefactive), has areas of adipose liquefaction and fatty acid release.

Answer D is incorrect. Caseous necrosis is seen in tuberculosis infection. It is characterized by granulomatous inflammation and a clumped, cheesy material.

Answer E is incorrect. Granulomas are considered as being characteristic of caseous necrosis.

34. **The correct answer is D.** TGF-β is secreted by B cells as well as monocytes, macrophages, and T cells. It functions as an anticytokine, inhibits of T cells, B cells, PMNs, monocytes, macrophages, and NK cells, and stimulation of collagen formation and wound healing. Interleukin function is vast and is secreted by different cells.

Answer A is incorrect. IL-4 is in interleukin which is secreted from TH-2 cells and stimulates B cells and IgE.

Answer B is incorrect. INF-γ is secreted by TH-1 cells and stimulates monocyte, macrophage, NK cell, and PMN activation.

Answer C is incorrect. IL-2 is secreted by TH-1 cells and stimulates other TH and TC cells.

Answer E is incorrect. TNF-α is secreted by monocytes and stimulates adhesion molecules.

35. **The correct answer is B.** Cyanide poisoning causes inhibition of cellular oxidation.

Answer A is incorrect. Methanol poisoning can lead to blindness.

Answer C is incorrect. Lead poisoning can lead to basophilic stippling of red blood cells.

Answer D is incorrect. Mercury poisoning can lead to pneumonitis.

Answer E is incorrect. Carbon tetrachloride poisoning can lead to fatty liver.
    Not listed above is carbon monoxide, which causes systemic hypoxia if overexposure occurs.

36. **The correct answer is A.** The epitactic concept of calculus formation states that protein and carbohydrate complexes and/or bacteria induce focal mineralization on teeth which eventually forms a calcified mass.

Answer B is incorrect. Materia alba is composed of desquamated cells, food, and plaque which is easily washed off the teeth.

Answer C is incorrect. Subgingival plaque is gram-negative anaerobic bacilli and spirochetes.

Answer D is incorrect. Chlorhexidine gluconate is the most effective antiplaque mouthrinse.

Answer E is incorrect. Supragingival plaque is largely composed of gram-positive facultative cocci.

37. **The correct answer is D.** Necrotizing ulcerative gingivitis is characterized by punched-out interproximal papillae, plaque, fetid odor of the mouth, gingival bleeding, marginal gingival pseudomembrane formation, and pain. It is commonly associated with emotional stress, malnutrition, smoking, and/or immunocompromise. Spirochetes are a common finding in the microbial flora.

Answer A is incorrect. Chronic periodontitis is characterized by peridontal attachment loss. The amount of periodontal destruction is often consistent with the presence of subgingival plaque and calculus accumulation.

Answer B is incorrect. Aggressive periodontitis is characterized by attachment loss that is often not consistent with the amount of subgingival microbial deposits detected. It typically affects people less than 30 years old.

Answer C is incorrect. Plaque-induced gingivitis is characterized by gingival inflammation in the absence of peridontal attachment loss.

Answer E is incorrect. Candidiasis is a fungal infection and does not have a direct effect on the periodontium.

38. **The correct answer is B.** Addison disease is an adrenal hypofunction or insufficiency that is either caused by pathological changes in the adrenal cortex or hypofunction of the adrenal cortex. Both of the diseases present with the same clinical findings of lethargy, depression, and hypotension. There is also a

decrease in cortisol, increased serum sodium, and increased serum potassium.

Answer A is incorrect. Cushing disease would show an increase in cortisol levels.

Answer C is incorrect. Primary hyperparathyroidism leads to increased PTH in the blood.

Answer D is incorrect. Cushing syndrome would show an increase in cortisol levels.

Answer E is incorrect. Plummer disease would have an increase in thyroid hormone and nearly opposite clinical symptoms of Addison disease.

39. **The correct answer is D.** The ACTH stimulation test is used to differentiate between primary and secondary Addison disease. Primary Addison is due to autoimmune, infectious, neoplastic, or hemorrhagic damage to the adrenal cortex. Secondary Addison is caused by a decrease in ACTH from the pituitary gland, thus hypofunction of the adrenal cortex. Thus, the stimulation test is accomplished by administering ACTH exogenously to a suspect patient. If cortisol increases, then primary Addison is suspected (adrenal cortex still functioning). If cortisol levels stay the same, then secondary Addison is suspected. This is due to inability of the adrenal cortex to respond to the ACTH.

Answer A is incorrect. Primary and secondary hyperparathyroidism would be differentiated by disease of the parathyroid glands or another separate source, respectively.

Answer B is incorrect. Hyper- and hypothyroidism would be differentiated by determining thyroid function. This could be done by evaluating T3 and T4 values, as well as TSH levels.

Answer C is incorrect. Cushing disease and syndrome would be differentiated by looking at levels of ACTH. When elevated, Cushing disease is evident (ie, caused by a pituitary tumor).

Answer E is incorrect. Acromegaly and dwarfism would be differentiated by levels

of excessive or deficient growth hormone, respectively.

40. **The correct answer is A.** In Addison disease, primary or secondary, there is a lack of cortisol. This is due to ill-response of the adrenal cortex to stimulation by ACTH. Thus, exogenous cortisol would overcome this decreased function and help to reverse symptoms of the disease.

Answer B is incorrect. Aldosterone administration would affect the kidneys. It would not be an adequate treatment for Addison disease.

Answer C is incorrect. Androgen administration would affect the HPA axis. It would not be an adequate treatment for Addison disease.

Answer D is incorrect. Growth hormone administration would affect the thyroid gland. It would not be an adequate treatment for Addison disease.

Answer E is incorrect. PTH administration would affect calcium and phosphate balance. It would not be an adequate treatment for Addison disease.

41. **The correct answer is A.** Hyperparathyroidism is a condition characterized by an increase in PTH. There are two forms: primary and secondary. Both primary and secondary hyperparathyroidism share the same clinical characteristics: cystic bone lesions (eg, osteitis fibrosa cystica, von Recklinghausen disease), nephrocalcinosis (renal calculi), and metastatic calcifications. The difference between the two is the causative factor of the symptoms: with primary, there is typically a secreting adenoma of the parathyroid gland which causes an increase in PTH; with secondary, this is usually due to hypocalcemia (secondary to chronic renal disease) which causes a subsequent increase in parathyroid gland function. The labs seen with primary hyperparathyroidism include increased calcium and phosphorus, and a decrease in alkaline phosphatase; secondary hyperparathyroidism has a decrease in calcium and increase in phosphorus. The main cause of damage with hyperparathyroidism is

due to PTH-activation of osteoclasts. The actions of osteoclasts lead to bone lesions, kidney stones, pain, and peptic ulcers.

Answer B is incorrect. Grave disease presents with exophthalmos and hyperthyroidism.

Answer C is incorrect. Hyperthyroidism presents with fatigue, weight loss, anxiety, and sweating. Other symptoms may be evident.

Answer D is incorrect. Hypoparathyroidism presents with cramping, pain, and paresthesias.

Answer E is incorrect. Addison disease presents with weight loss, fatigue, diarrhea, sweating, and vomiting.

42. **The correct answer is C.** These two tests will confirm the suspected lack of calcium in a patient. Briefly, hypocalcemia can be caused by numerous mechanisms (eg, renal disease) and can lead to many systemic problems (bone loss, tetany, etc). In the example of tetany (due to hypoparathyroidism or decreased vitamin D), when blood calcium falls to 6 mg% (from normal 10 mg%), the CNS and PNS are disturbed. Thus, muscle twitching, cramping, carpopedal spasm, and if severe, laryngospasm and seizures occur. If tetany is suspected, one may attempt two tests: Chvostek sign is viewed by tapping the facial nerve near the earlobe/mandibular angle—if tetany is present, the upper lip twitches; Trousseau sign is seen by applying a blood pressure cuff to arm and inflating-carpopedal spasm (thumb adduction and phalangeal extension) confirms tetany.

Answer A is incorrect. Chronic hypocalcemia would show symptoms of paresthesia, tetany, and possibly arrhythmias.

Answer B is incorrect. Acute hypercalcemia would show symptoms of depression, confusion, fatigue, nausea, and vomiting.

Answer D is incorrect. Acute hypocalcemia would show symptoms of tetany and paresthesia.

Answer E is incorrect. Hyperphosphatemia would show symptoms of calcifications throughout the body.

43. **The correct answer is B.** Neurofibromatosis and von Hippel-Lindau disease (as well as multiple endocrine neoplasia) are often associated with pheochromocytoma, not neuroblastoma.

Answer A is incorrect. Pheochromocytoma causes an increase in catecholamine release. It is a chronic chromaffin cell tumor (benign) which is uncommon and affects men and women of any age (usually 30-60).

Answer C is incorrect. The N-myc gene is found mutated in neuroblastoma.

Answer D is incorrect. Metastatic spread to the liver is a sequela of neuroblastoma. Other complications include local invasion and direct spread.

Answer E is incorrect. The symptoms of pheochromocytoma include paroxysmal HTN and hyperglycemia. Other symptoms include hypermetabolic rate and abdominal distension.

Pheochromocytoma and neuroblastoma are tumors of the adrenal medulla. Neuroblastoma is the most common malignant tumor of childhood and infancy.

44. **The correct answer is A.** Ceroid is an endogenous pigment formed via autooxidation, which accumulates in Kupffer cells, and is indicative of hepatocellular injury.

Answer B is incorrect. Lipofuscin is a yellow-brown pigment, which is known as a wear-and-tear pigment. It's derived from lipid peroxidation, accumulates in the heart, liver, and brain, and is indicative of brown atrophy and increased age.

Answer C is incorrect. Hemosiderin is a pigment that is golden brown in color, derived from heme, and is actually aggregates of ferritin micelles. It can be identified by Prussian blue stain and accumulates in phagocytes of the bone marrow, liver, and spleen. It's indicative of hemosiderosis and hemochromatosis.

Answer D is incorrect. Melanin is a brown-black pigment derived from tyrosine which accumulates in skin, eyes, and hair. If increased, it indicates normal physiology, suntan, and

Addison disease; if decreased, it shows albinism and vitiligo.

Answer E is incorrect. Bilirubin is a yellowish pigment of the bile which is derived from heme. When it accumulates in the skin, it causes jaundice and is indicative of biliary tree obstruction, hepatocellular injury, and hemolytic anemias.

45. **The correct answer is B.** Innate immunity does NOT exhibit immunological memory; this is a function of acquired immunity.

Answer A is incorrect. Acquired immunity includes cell- and antibody-mediated defense. There are two types of immune defense: innate (natural) and acquired (adaptive). There are two types of acquired immunity: cell mediated (T cells) and antibody mediated (B cells, immunoglobulins).

Answer C is incorrect. Active and passive defense are different ways to classify acquired immunity. Acquired immunity is also classified as either active (after exposure to foreign antigen) or passive (after exposure to preformed antibody from another host).

Answer D is incorrect. Lysozymes are an example of innate immunity. Innate immunity functions immediately after microbial infiltration. It is nonspecific and has no memory. Examples include NK cell, PMNs, and complement.

Answer E is incorrect. B-lymphocytes are an example of acquired immunity. Acquired immunity takes days after microbial insult to function. This type of defense is specific for certain antigen, exhibits diversity, and has immunologic memory.

46. **The correct answer is E.** Interferon is a cytokine which is produced by monocytes, macrophages, and lymphocytes. Its function is to interfere with virus replication.

Answer A is incorrect. Neuraminidase functions to cleave salicylic acid residues. It is a primary cytoplasmic granule found in PMNs.

Answer B is incorrect. Hydrolase will hydrolyze chemical bonds. It is a primary cytoplasmic granule found in PMNs.

Answer C is incorrect. Myeloperoxidase causes the respiratory burst by producing hypochlorous acid. It is a primary cytoplasmic granule found in PMN.

Answer D is incorrect. Lactoferrin has a high affinity for iron which helps its antimicrobial potency. It is a secondary cytoplasmic granule found in PMN.

47. **The correct answer is B.** This patient presents with symptoms consistent with measles/rubeola. This disease is caused by the measles virus, under the family paramyxovirus. It is single, linear, with no treatment, but a vaccine is available.

Answer A is incorrect. The rhabdovirus family contains the rabies virus.

Answer C is incorrect. The papovirus family contains the human papilloma virus.

Answer D is incorrect. The reovirus family has both the rotavirus and orbivirus.

Answer E is incorrect. The calicivirus family contains hepatitis E and Norwalk virus.

48. **The correct answer is A.** The polio virus, of the family picornavirus, is an RNA nonenveloped virus.

Answer B is incorrect. Rubella virus is an RNA enveloped virus.

Answer C is incorrect. Human T-cell leukemia virus is an RNA enveloped virus.

Answer D is incorrect. HIV is an RNA enveloped virus.

Answer E is incorrect. Hepatitis C virus is an RNA enveloped virus.
Note the following with RNA enveloped viruses: the viral envelope, in general, is an outer membrane. It is composed of plasma membrane lipoproteins and glycoproteins. These are obtained from the host cell upon budding.

49. **The correct answer is C.** For adults allergic to penicillins, the correct dose for clindamycin is 600 mg PO 1 hour prior to dental procedures.

Microbiology and Pathology

Answer A is incorrect. For adults unable to take oral medication: ampicillin 2 g IM or IV 30 minutes prior to procedure.

Answer B is incorrect. For children allergic to penicillins: cephalexin 50 mg/kg PO 1 hour prior to procedure.

Answer D is incorrect. For adult standard prophylaxis: penicillin 2 g PO 1 hour prior to procedure.

Answer E is incorrect. For children allergic to penicillin: clindamycin 20 mg/kg PO 1 hour prior to procedure.

Note that for some adult patients who are allergic to penicillins and unable to take oral medicines, clindamycin may be given IV at a dose of 600-mg IV 30 minutes prior to procedure, or cefazolin 1-g IM or IV within 30 minutes of dental procedure.

50. **The correct answer is A.** Antitoxin vaccine is a form of passive immunity. There are two forms of immunity when developing bacterial vaccines: active and passive. Both types of immunity are meant to present some form of bacteria, which elicits an immune response that confers protection from bacterial offense in the future.

Answer B is incorrect. Immunity from cholera is provided via killed vaccine.

Answer C is incorrect. Active immunity includes whole bacteria, capsular polysaccharides, or toxoids. It includes live attenuated (TB, tularemia), killed (cholera, typhoid fever, pertussis), toxoid (tetanus, diphtheria), capsular polysaccharide (pneumonia, meningitis—both of the bacterial form).

Answer D is incorrect. Antitoxin vaccine contains antibodies to bacterial exotoxins.

Answer E is incorrect. Passive immunity includes preformed antibody preparations which elicit immunity. It includes antitoxin (tetanus, diphtheria, botulism).

51. **The correct answer is B.** Cellular dysplasia involves atypical cells that do not invade the basement membrane.

Answer A is incorrect. Dysplasia is a nonmalignant cellular growth that can become malignant.

Answer C is incorrect. It is characterized by disorganized, structureless maturation and spatial arrangement of cells that are atypical and without invasion.

Answer D is incorrect. It is reversible, and is caused by such things as chronic irritation, chemicals, cigarette smoke, and chronic inflammatory irritation, to name a few.

Answer E is incorrect. The cells display pleomorphism and an increased in mitosis. Involving the epithelial layer, acanthosis is noted, which is an abnormal thickening of the prickle cell layer.

52. **The correct answer is C.** AFP is the tumor marker for hepatoma and yolk sac tumors, and enolase is the marker for neuroblastoma.

Answer A is incorrect. CEA is the tumor marker for adenocarcinoma.

Answer B is incorrect. LSA is the tumor marker for lymphoma.

Answer D is incorrect. hCG is the tumor marker for choriocarcinoma.

Answer E is incorrect. Desmin is the tumor marker for rhabdomyosarcoma.

These common tumor markers can often be analyzed in blood draws, thus leading the doctor to suspect certain regions of pathology to further investigate.

53. **The correct answer is A.** Peptic ulcer disease is an erosion of the stomach (or duodenal) lining. It most often occurs in men 20-50 years old, and duodenal (80%) or gastric (20%) ulceration is the complication. It is caused by either bacterial infection (*Helicobacter pylori*) or due to an imbalance between acid and mucosal protection. For example, NSAIDs cause a decrease in mucosal protection which leads to a decrease in prostaglandin production. Also, acid hypersecretion can cause ulceration. The main symptom is pain, with bleeding complication (erosion into blood vessels or ulcer bleeding), and perforation

(transmural ulceration → acute peritonitis; often duodenal ulcers). Malignant change is uncommon. Treatment is based on the causative factor, so antibiotics, antacid medications, or proton pump inhibitors are used to treat.

Answer B is incorrect. Duodenal ulcers present with the same symptoms as peptic ulcer disease. If left untreated, perforation is common with this type of ulcer.

Answer C is incorrect. Gastroesophageal reflux disease presents with heartburn, regurgitation of food, hoarse voice, wheezing, and coughing.

Answer D is incorrect. Hiatal hernia presents with heartburn, dysphagia, and belching.

Answer E is incorrect. Inflammatory bowel disease presents with abdominal pain and obstruction. Bloody diarrhea is also possible (occult/microscopic or gross).

54. **The correct answer is E.** GERD is a chronic condition caused by acid reflux due to backflow from the stomach into the esophagus. The most often complication is a weak lower esophageal sphincter and risk factors include scleroderma and hiatal hernia. Symptoms would be heartburn, food regurgitation, hoarse voice, wheezing, and coughing. This condition is treated by antacids and proton pump inhibitors. Left untreated, this chronic irritation of esophageal lining leads to Barrett esophagus (which is premalignant).

Answer A is incorrect. Achalasia is caused by nerve dysfunction. It is characterized by a decrease in propulsion of food down the esophagus. Hence, there is a decrease in peristalsis.

Answer B is incorrect. Mallory-Weiss syndrome is also caused by a weak LES, but is not due to acid reflux (it is due to mucosal lacerations from chronic vomiting).

Answer C is incorrect. Hiatal hernia is caused by the protrusion of part of the stomach through the diaphragm into the thoracic cavity.

Answer D is incorrect. Intestinal lymphangiectasia is caused by enlargement of the lymph nodes lining the small intestine. It results in fluid retention.

55. **The correct answer is B.** Basal cell carcinoma is a benign condition.

Answer A is incorrect. Basal cell carcinoma is locally aggressive. It is also destructive and tends to ulcerate and bleed.

Answer C is incorrect. Basal cell carcinoma is the most common form of skin cancer.

Answer D is incorrect. Clinically, basal cell carcinoma presents as a pearly papule. More than 90% occur on regions of the body most exposed to sun (head and neck, upper face) as a pearly papule with telangiectatic vessels.

Answer E is incorrect. It is the most common form of skin cancer in the United States and is derived from the basal cells of the epidermis.

56. **The correct answer is B.** Basal cell carcinoma rarely metastasizes due to its benign nature.

Answer A is incorrect. The stage of treatment is vital with basal cell carcinoma. The prognosis is very good when found and treated early.

Answer C is incorrect. Basal cell carcinoma can be quite disfiguring, disabling, and destructive when left untreated.

Answer D is incorrect. Histologically, there are clusters of darkly staining basaloid cells with a palisading arrangement of nuclei at the periphery of the tumor cells.

Answer E is incorrect. Surgical excision is the best treatment with radiation in lesions which may have questionable margins after excision.

57. **The correct answer is C.** From the given options and based on the clinical situation, one would suspect the patient is suffering from an asthma attack. Asthma is a chronic reactive airway disorder which is caused by airway obstruction. Very few adults (3.5% over 30) are affected by asthma. On the other hand, nearly 50% of asthma cases occur in children less

Microbiology and Pathology

than 10 years old with a 2:1 male predilection. The symptoms are dyspnea, expiratory wheezes, chest tightness, and cough. There are two types of asthma (generally speaking): extrinsic (allergic/atopic/immune) and intrinsic (nonimmune, idiosyncratic).

Answer A is incorrect. Chronic bronchitis is seen in patients with a history of smoking, in most cases.

Answer B is incorrect. Emphysema is seen in patients with a history of smoking, in many cases.

Answer D is incorrect. Asbestosis is seen in patients with a positive history of asbestos exposure.

Answer E is incorrect. Anthracosis presents in patients who have had years of exposure to carbon dust.

Chronic bronchitis, emphysema, asbestosis, and anthracosis affect older adults and not children. This is due to the fact that years and years of pathological changes are necessary to cause illness to occur.

58. **The correct answer is C.** There is an increased Reid index seen in patients afflicted with chronic bronchitis. The Reid index measures the ratio of mucous gland thickness to bronchial wall thickness.

Answer A is incorrect. Chronic bronchitis sufferers have mucous hypersecretion in the bronchi and smaller airways. This illness is caused by a long history of cigarette smoking. It is defined as at least 3 months of the year, for 2 years, of having a chronic productive cough.

Answer B is incorrect. Clinically, there is also wheezing and rhonchi/noisy chest on auscultation along with a productive, sputum-filled cough.

Answer D is incorrect. Patient stricken with chronic bronchitis have an increased PO_2. Complications include pulmonary hypertension and increased risk of lung cancer.

Answer E is incorrect. "Blue bloaters" is the term used to describe patients with chronic

bronchitis. This is due to their barrel-chested, cyanotic appearance.

59. **The correct answer is E.** The aortic valve is most often distorted in cases of aortic dissection.

Answer A is incorrect. Rupture can cause pericardial tamponade. Rupture can also lead to hemomediastinum/hemothorax and distortion of the aortic valve.

Answer B is incorrect. The carotid artery may become occluded, leading to stroke. Occlusion of branches of the aorta and their effects include carotid—stroke, coronary—myocardial infarct, splanchnic—organ infarction, renal—acute renal failure.

Answer C is incorrect. It can be life threatening. This life-threatening condition is caused by blood dissecting the adventitial layer of the aorta from the intima.

Answer D is incorrect. Blood "dissects" between the intima and adventitia of the aorta. Symptoms include a tearing chest pain as well as blood pressure measurements which differ on one arm from the other.

60. **The correct answer is D.** Preeclampsia is a form of secondary hypertension which is pregnant women of at least 20 weeks gestation. It is characterized by hypertension (> 140 systolic and > 90 diastolic), proteinuria, and edema. Predisposing conditions for it include hypertension, diabetes, autoimmune diseases, hyperuricemia, and thrombocytopenia. This can lead to eclampsia, which includes episodes of seizures.

Answer A is incorrect. Malignant hypertension is characterized by a sudden rapid increase in blood pressure without a precipitating event (usually). It can be life threatening. It's most common in African Americans.

Answer B is incorrect. Aortic aneurysm is characterized by abnormal, localized dilation of the aorta. It is caused by atherosclerosis, cystic medial necrosis, infection aortitis, and vasculitis. Rupture is a major risk.

Answer C is incorrect. Primary hypertension is characterized by an increase in blood pressure. There is no identifiable cause. It is, though, related to increase in cardiac output and total peripheral resistance.

Answer E is incorrect. Cardiac tamponade is characterized by an extrinsic compression of the heart, typically from fluid. Cardiac compression ensures with decreased venous return, decreased cardiac output, and death.

61. The correct answer is D. Hypoaldosteronism does not lead to secondary hypertension. Secondary hypertension is hypertension of known causes (5%-10% of all hypertensive cases). It is often correctable. It is caused by, most commonly, renal disease (RAS system—leads to renal parenchymal diseases or renal artery stenosis).

Answer A is incorrect. Cushing syndrome can contribute to secondary hypertension. This is due to increased sensitivity to catecholamines, increased angiotensinogen, and increased aldosterone receptors.

Answer B is incorrect. Diabetes may contribute to secondary hypertension. This is due to vascular insult from not controlling the disease.

Answer C is incorrect. Pheochromocytoma may contribute to secondary hypertension. This is due to increased catecholamine production.

Answer E is incorrect. Hyperthyroidism may contribute to secondary hypertension. This is due to an increase in the body's metabolic rate.

62. The correct answer is A. *Streptococcus viridans* is known to cause subacute bacterial endocarditis in more than 50% of all cases. It is seen in patients with preexisting cardiac valvular damage and is caused by an oral source.

Answer B is incorrect. *Staphylococcus epidermidis* is not greatly implicated in endocarditis.

Answer C is incorrect. *Staphylococcus aureus* infections cause approximately 50% of acute endocarditis cases. However, it is usually secondary to systemic infection or intravenous drug use.

Answer D is incorrect. *Streptococcus sanguis* is not greatly implicated in endocarditis.

Answer E is incorrect. *Streptococcus mutans* is not greatly implicated in endocarditis.

63. The correct answer is A. The Libman-Sacks form of endocarditis occurs in systemic lupus erythematous. The mitral valve is most often implicated, and small vegetation form on the leaflet.

Answer B is incorrect. Dental seeding and intravenous drug use cause the infective form.
Typically, infective form is usually caused by an intrinsic bacteremia from the oral cavity, upper respiratory tract, urologic tract, lower gastrointestinal tract, and also intravenous drug use and introduced/extrinsic bacteria.

Answer C is incorrect. The mitral valve is most often affected in the Libman-Sacks form. The tricuspid valve is also often affected with this form of endocarditis, especially in intravenous drug users.

Answer D is incorrect. The rheumatic form occurs in areas of greatest hemodynamic stress. The mitral valve is often involved and calcification (stenosis, insufficiency, or both) occurs.

Answer E is incorrect. The mitral valve is most often affected in rheumatic form.

64. The correct answer is D. Hydropericardium is the accumulation of serous fluid within the pericardial space. Pleural effusion is the general term for any fluid accumulation in the pericardial space and can lead to cardiac tamponade (which can be fatal).

Answer A is incorrect. Hemopericardium is the accumulation of blood in the pericardium.

Answer B is incorrect. Acute pericarditis is the inflammation of the pericardium.

Answer C is incorrect. Constrictive pericarditis is a chronic pathology involving thickening and scarring of the pericardium.

Answer E is incorrect. Myocarditis is the inflammation of cardiac tissue.

65. **The correct answer is B.** Splinter hemorrhaging is seen in patients afflicted with endocarditis. This illness is an inflammation of the endocardium and/or heart valves which can develop quickly (acute) or slowly (subacute). The symptoms include fever, nonspecific constitutional symptoms, malaise, headache, and night sweats. Upon further exam, you would expect to find heart murmur, which is secondary to vegetations, splenomegaly, and splinter hemorrhages.

    Answer A is incorrect. Cardiac tamponade shows symptoms of distended neck veins, hypotension, decreased heart sounds, tachypnea, and weak or absent peripheral pulse.

    Answer C is incorrect. Primary hypertension typically does not have any clinically identifiable symptoms.

    Answer D is incorrect. Coronary artery disease shows symptoms of angina. This is the classical symptom.

    Answer E is incorrect. Angina shows symptoms of squeezing substernal chest discomfort. It may radiate to the left arm, jaw, shoulder blade, and neck.

66. **The correct answer is B.** Haptens are antigens that must bind to a carrier protein to elicit an immune response.

    Answer A is incorrect. Most antigens are proteins. Antigens are considered molecules that react with antibody to induce an immune response.

    Answer C is incorrect. Adjuvants, related to antigenicity, are molecules that enhance the immune response to an antigen.

    Answer D is incorrect. The binding site for on antigen is an epitope.

    Answer E is incorrect. Antigens induce an immune response by binding to antibody.

They are comprised of proteins, polysaccharides, lipoproteins, and nucleoproteins.

67. **The correct answer is C.** Macrophages present antigen via class II MHC.

    Answer A is incorrect. Macrophages are derived from bone marrow histiocytes, exist in plasma as monocytes and in tissue as macrophages.

    Answer B is incorrect. Other than phagocytose, macrophages also present antigen via class II MHC and produce cytokines.

    Answer D is incorrect. Macrophages are a form of agranular leukocytes which function to phagocytose materials.

    Answer E is incorrect. Macrophages can be activated by numerous components, including bacterial lipopolysaccharide, peptidoglycan, DNA, and interferon gamma.

68. **The correct answer is A.** Eosinophils are granular leukocytes which defend against parasitic infection. Other functions include phagocytosis and binding of IgG or IgE (when antigen-bound), thus mediating hypersensitivity reactions. They do not present antigen to T cells.

    Answer B is incorrect. Basophils mediate hypersensitivity reactions.

    Answer C is incorrect. Mast cells mediate hypersensitivity reactions.

    Answer D is incorrect. PMNs produce cytokines and function in phagocytosis.

    Answer E is incorrect. Dendritic cells present antigen to other cells.

69. **The correct answer is E.** PMNs do not present antigen; their main function is phagocytosis of materials, as well as to produce cytokine.

    Answer A is incorrect. Monocytes function as antigen presenting cells.

    Answer B is incorrect. B cells function as antigen presenting cells.

    Answer C is incorrect. Macrophages can function as antigen presenting cells.

Answer D is incorrect. Langerhans cells function as antigen presenting cells. They are the major dendritic cells of the oral gingival epithelium,

These cells present antigen throughout the body via their MHC II proteins. The presentation is made to CD4 T cells.

70. **The correct answer is E.** DiGeorge syndrome is due to defective development of the 3rd and 4th pharyngeal arches. Thus, patients will present with deformity of the ear and lip, as well as cardiac malformation (more specifically, that of the aortic arch). Also, patients will have defective immune defense due to thymic hypoplasia. Their parathyroids are also impaired.

Answer A is incorrect. Common variable immunodeficiency affects B-cell maturation into plasma cells.

Answer B is incorrect. Wiskott-Aldrich syndrome is a combined B- and T-cell pathology which is caused by defective IgM response to bacterial LPS.

Answer C is incorrect. SCID (severe combined immunodeficiency) is a defect in stem-cell differentiation that causes a lack of lymphoid tissue.

Answer D is incorrect. Bruton is caused by pre-B cells not differentiating into mature B cells.

71. **The correct answer is D.** Job syndrome is a disease characterized by pathological T cells. In this syndrome, T-helper cells are not producing interferon-gamma. Thus, there are increased bacterial infections due to poor PMN chemotaxis. There is also an increase in IgE levels. *Staphylococcus aureus* is a common infection seen with this disease.

Answer A is incorrect. Bruton X-linked agammaglobulinemia is seen in patients with defective B cell function.

Answer B is incorrect. Wiskott-Aldrich syndrome has a combined B- and T-cell pathology.

Answer C is incorrect. Isolated IgA deficiency is seen in patients with defective B-cell function.

Answer E is incorrect. Ataxia telangiectasia is seen in patients with defective B-cell function.

72. **The correct answer is A.** DiGeorge syndrome causes a decrease in blood calcium levels. The parathyroid gland is also pathological, thus decreased PTH which causes this hypocalcemia.

Answer B is incorrect. Thymic hypoplasia is seen with these patients. This causes a T-cell defect.

Answer C is incorrect. Microdeletion of chromosome 22 causes this syndrome.

Answer D is incorrect. Palatal clefting is a clinical presentation with these patients leading to hypocalcemia. These patients are more susceptible to viral and fungal infections, as well as a decrease in type IV hypersensitivity reactions.

Note that cardiac abnormalities and abnormal facies are also common clinical symptoms with these patients.

73. **The correct answer is C.** A type IV hypersensitivity reaction involves the binding of a class II MHC to a TCR. It also involves the presentation of antigen by macrophage to T cells, thus producing tissue destruction. This damage to tissue is mediated by lymphokines. Malfunction of T cells will alter the effectiveness of this hypersensitivity reaction.

Answer A is incorrect. This type of reaction (type IV) is mediated by T cells.

Answer B is incorrect. A type IV hypersensitivity reaction is not immediate. This is due to the fact that it is cell mediated.

Answer D is incorrect. Hemolytic anemia is an example of a type II hypersensitivity reaction.

Answer E is incorrect. Atopic allergy is an example of a type I hypersensitivity reaction.

Examples of diseases associated with this reaction include contact dermatitis, tuberculin testing (PPD), tuberculosis, sarcoidosis, and leprosy.

74. **The correct answer is B.** An allograft involves the transplantation of tissue between two genetically different individuals within

the same species. Transplantation is a complicated process by which means immunosuppression is often necessary to suppress and allow the immune system to accept a graft.

Answer A is incorrect. A xenograft is transplantation of tissue between two different species.

Answer C is incorrect. An autograft is grafting between different sites within the same individual.

Answer D is incorrect. An isograft is transplantation of tissue between two genetically identical individuals of the same species.

75. **The correct answer is B.** IgG can readily cross the placental barrier and function in passive immunity. IgG is the most abundant antibody in humans and is located within the plasma. It is the main antimicrobial defense of the secondary response, and it opsonizes bacteria, activates complement, and neutralizes bacterial toxins and viruses. It also has four subclasses.

Answer A is incorrect. IgA cannot cross the placental barrier.

Answer C is incorrect. IgD cannot cross the placental barrier.

Answer D is incorrect. IgE cannot cross the placental barrier. It functions to mediate type I hypersensitivity reactions.

Answer E is incorrect. IgM cannot cross the placental barrier.

76. **The correct answer is E.** IgA acts to prevent mucosal membrane attachment of microbes.

Answer A is incorrect. IgA does not mediate type I hypersensitivity reactions. It does not have a major function in any hypersensitivity reactions.

Answer B is incorrect. IgA does not activate complement.

Answer C is incorrect. Its response is not uncertain. IgA is secreted in an exocrine manner from glands.

Answer D is incorrect. IgA is not the main antimicrobial defense in the primary immunological response.

IgA is the 2nd most abundant antibody in humans (1st is IgG) and is comprised of two subunits. The other antibodies are secreted by either B cells (IgM-monomer, IgD), mast cells, basophils and eosinophils (IgE), or plasma (IgM-pentamer, IgG).

77. **The correct answer is A.** Antibody can activate complement via the classical pathway, not alternate. It is a Y-shaped glycoprotein that is secreted by plasma cells. It is comprised of two identical light chains and two identical heavy chains held together by disulfide bonds.

Answer B is incorrect. The Fab regions of the heavy and light chains are considered variable, specific for binding antigen, and determine idiotype.

Answer C is incorrect. The Fc regions of the heavy chains are considered constant and determine the isotype.

Answer D is incorrect. The constant regions of antibody bind APC (antigen presenting cells) or C3b (of the complement cascade).

Answer E is incorrect. The variable regions of antibody bind specific antigen.

78. **The correct answer is E.** Trisomy 18 is seen in Edward syndrome. This syndrome is characterized by mental retardation, small head, micrognathia, pinched facial appearance, and malformed ears (amongst other systemic findings). The prognosis for these patients is grim, surviving only months.

Answer A is incorrect. Patau syndrome is defined as trisomy 13 and is characterized by mental retardation, microcephaly, microphthalmia, cleft lip and palate, and brain abnormalities with a life expectancy of less than 1 year.

Answer B is incorrect. Klinefelter syndrome is defined as having XXY chromosomal abnormality.

Answer C is incorrect. Down syndrome is trisomy 21 with the characteristics of retardation, epicanthal folds, large protruding tongue, small head with low-set ears, simian crease, and a broad flat fact.

Answer D is incorrect. Turner syndrome patients have a XO chromosomal arrangement.

79. **The correct answer is E.** Influenza is not found to be teratogenic.

Answers A, B, C, and D are incorrect. Cytomegalovirus, rubella, toxoplasmosis and herpes simplex virus are known teratogens. These agents can all be passed on from the mother to the fetus during pregnancy. This is known as the TORCH complex. The acronym stands for toxoplasmosis, other agents, rubella, Cytomegalovirus, herpes simplex virus. Teratogens can cause death, growth retardation, malformation, and functional impairment to the fetus. The mechanism of such is specific to each teratogen, and susceptibility of the fetus to the offending agent depends on such factors as the developmental stage and dose.

80. **The correct answer is C.** Impetigo is caused by *Staphylococcus aureus* or *Streptococcus pyogenes* infection.

Answer A is incorrect. Impetigo is a highly contagious disease. It is the ooze which is contagious.

Answer B is incorrect. This is a common skin infection in preschool age children, typically in warm weather.

Answer D is incorrect. This infection is very superficial. Clinically, it presents as a sore, which progresses to a blister that breaks and oozes. Acute glomerulonephritis can occur occasionally in *Streptococcus* infection if left untreated.

Answer E is incorrect. The cure rate is extremely high with little scarring. Treatment is topical antimicrobial or oral antibiotic.

81. **The correct answer is C.** Cystic fibrosis patients have an error with chromosome 7q. This chromosome encodes the cystic fibrosis transmem-

brane regulator which controls Cl^- and Na^+ transport across epithelial membranes. CF is the most common fatal genetic disease in Caucasian children. The life expectancy is 28 years.

Answer A is incorrect. Chloride transporters malfunction due to an error with chromosome 7q. Sodium channels are affected, especially mucous and sweat glands.

Answer B is incorrect. Meconium ileus is a common clinical symptom with these patients. It is characterized by intestinal obstruction.

Answer D is incorrect. Pancreatic exocrine insufficiency is a common clinical symptom with these patients.

Answer E is incorrect. Bronchiectasis is a common clinical symptom with these patients. This is due to thick mucous obstruction and leads to lung infection.

82. **The correct answer is E.** Vitiligo is characterized by hypopigmentation due to an acquired loss of melanocytes. The other diseases are all of the hyperpigmentation variety.

Answer A is incorrect. Neurofibromatosis (type 1) is the most frequent neurocutaneous syndrome.

Answer B is incorrect. Tuberous sclerosis presents clinically with café au lait spots.

Answer C is incorrect. Fanconi anemia presents clinically with café au lait spots.

Answer D is incorrect. McCune-Albright syndrome presents clinically with café au lait spots.
Café au lait spots are due to an increase in melanin content with giant melanosomes.

83. **The correct answer is A.** A mural thrombus typically forms after an MI or atrial fibrillation. This type of thrombus is from the endocardial surface and protrudes into the lumen of the heart or large vessel. It is caused by MI, a-fib, or aortic atherosclerosis.

Answer B is incorrect. Agonal thrombi are intracardiac and caused by prolonged heart failure.

Answer C is incorrect. Red thrombi are mostly composed of RBCs and caused by their accumulation.

Answer D is incorrect. White thrombi are mostly comprised of platelets and caused by their accumulation.

Answer E is incorrect. Fibrin thrombi are mostly composed of fibrin and caused by their accumulation.

84. **The correct answer is D.** Metabolic acidosis is a characteristic of the progressive stage of shock.

    Answer A is incorrect. The nonprogressive/early stage of shock is considered to be compensated. This means that the body can overcome the changes it incurs.

    Answer B is incorrect. The body is still maintaining perfusion to vital organs in the nonprogressive/early stage of shock.

    Answer C is incorrect. There is increased total peripheral resistance to organs in the nonprogressive/early stage of shock.

    Answer E is incorrect. There is an increase in sympathetic nervous output in the nonprogressive/early stage of shock.
    The other two stages of shock are progressive (decreased cardiac perfusion, cardiac depression, decreased cardiac output, metabolic acidosis, no longer compensated), and irreversible (organ damage, decrease in high-energy phosphate reserves, death).

85. **The correct answer is A.** Septic shock can cause systemic vasodilation.

    Answer B is incorrect. This form of shock occurs due to bacteria with subsequent endotoxin release.

    Answer C is incorrect. Septic shock is caused by infection of gram-negative bacteria.

    Answer D is incorrect. Neurogenic shock is caused by CNS injury.

    Answer E is incorrect. Anaphylactic shock is caused by type I hypersensitivity, histamine release, and vasodilation (eg, allergy).

Note that Hypovolemic shock is caused due to decreased blood volume (eg, hemorrhage), cardiogenic shock is caused by pump failure and sudden decrease in cardiac output (eg, massive MI).

86. **The correct answer is C.** Caisson disease is caused by air gaining entry into the circulatory system. The result of this is an air embolism.

    Answer A is incorrect. A solid mass occluding a vessel would not be seen here. This could be caused by a thromboemboli or tumor embolism.

    Answer B is incorrect. Fatty emboli are not seen in Caisson disease. Fat embolism is commonly seen with long bone fractures.

    Answer D is incorrect. Blood clots are not seen in this disease. This could be caused by a thromboemboli (most common type; because of blood clot).

    Answer E is incorrect. Emboli caused by amniotic fluid are not seen in Caisson disease. This amniotic fluid embolism is seen at time of delivery and can activate DIC.
    Emboli are some type of intravascular mass such as solid, liquid, and gas. They travel within a blood vessel and may lodge at a distant site, thus occluding flow and possibly leading to infarction.

87. **The correct answer is B.** Chronic passive congestion of the liver is caused more directly by right-sided heart failure. The passive form can further be broken down into acute (shock or right-sided heart failure) and chronic (lung congestion).

    Answer A is incorrect. Active hyperemia is caused by increased arteriolar dilation. It leads to inflammation.

    Answer C is incorrect. Passive hyperemia is caused by decreased venous return. It leads to obstruction.

    Answer D is incorrect. Inflammation and blushing is a clinical finding of active hyperemia.

Answer E is incorrect. Obstruction and increased back pressure is a clinical finding of chronic hyperemia.

Hyperemia, which is another term for congestion, is due to an increased volume of blood in local capillaries and small vessels.

88. **The correct answer is C.** A deficiency of vitamin B_{12} will cause pernicious anemia. This is an autoimmune disorder in which intrinsic factor fails to form. There are anti-intrinsic factor and anti–parietal cell antibodies. Thus, without intrinsic factor, no B_{12} may be absorbed. Achlorhydria is also seen with this illness. Pernicious anemia is also characterized by macrocytic red blood cells, and abnormal Schilling test, hypersegmented neutrophils, lemon-yellow skin, stomatitis, glossitis, and subacute degeneration of the spinal cord.

Answer A is incorrect. Aplastic anemia is due to decreased production of RBCs.

Answer B is incorrect. Sickle cell anemia is from abnormal Hb-S.

Answer D is incorrect. Plummer-Vinson syndrome is anemia due to iron deficiency (with esophageal webbing).

Answer E is incorrect. Folate deficiency anemia is caused by a lack of dietary folate.

89. **The correct answer is C.** Polycythemia is a general term for an increase in RBCs. Relative polycythemia is decreased plasma volume causing increased concentration of RBCs. It is known as Gaisböck syndrome.

Answer A is incorrect. True polycythemia is increased RBC mass and increased total blood volume.

Answer B is incorrect. Primary polycythemia, known as polycythemia vera, is a genetic, myeloproliferative disease. It is characterized by decreased sensitivity of myeloid precursors to erythropoietin.

Answer D is incorrect. Secondary polycythemia is increased RBCs due to conditions other than polycythemia vera. These include renal disease, chronic hypoxia, tumors, androgen therapy, and Bartter syndrome.

Answer E is incorrect. In primary polycythemia, erythropoietin levels are decreased.

90. **The correct answer is B.** This patient most likely has type II diabetes mellitus. The symptoms of this disease include polyuria, polydipsia, polyphagia, blurred vision, paresthesias, and weakness. It is typically a disease associated with increased age/adulthood in obese peoples. Insulin production may or may not be normal, rather there is insulin resistance with receptors. The genetic predisposition is strong. Treatment includes diet, weight loss, and oral hypoglycemic drugs.

Answer A is incorrect. Hyperthyroidism presents clinically with symptoms of irritability, weight loss, tremor, diarrhea, and sweating.

Answer C is incorrect. Hypothyroidism presents clinically with symptoms of mental slowing, cold intolerance, weight gain, constipation, and dry skin.

Answer D is incorrect. Addison disease presents clinically with symptoms of weakness, fatigue, depression, hypotension, and skin bronzing.

Answer E is incorrect. Type I diabetes presents clinically with symptoms of polyuria, polydipsia, polyphagia, paresthesias, weakness, and blurred vision.

91. **The correct answer is A.** Kidney tubules are not sensitized to ADH in patients with nephrogenic diabetes insipidus.

Answer B is incorrect. It has a genetic component, as it is sex linked and it affects men.

Answer C is incorrect. In nephrogenic diabetes insipidus, ADH production and secretion is normal, but there is resistance of ADH receptors.

Answer D is incorrect. The result of desensitization to ADH receptors is a large volume of dilute urine.

Answer E is incorrect. Nephrogenic diabetes insipidus can be caused by patients taking Lithium, as well as other medications.

92. **The correct answer is A.** The symptoms experienced with both type I and II diabetes

mellitus are the same. In each case, patients experience the 3 Ps (polyuria, polyphagia, polydipsia), as well as blurred vision, paresthesias, weakness, and fatigue.

Answer B is incorrect. The cause is different in type I and II diabetes. Type I diabetes is due to a lack of insulin production, whereas in type II diabetes there is a desensitization of insulin receptors.

Answer C is incorrect. There is a genetic predisposition in both type I and II diabetes. There is a much stronger genetic component to type II diabetes.

Answer D is incorrect. The treatment differs between the two types of diabetes. Type I diabetes is treated with mainly insulin injections, whereas type II diabetes is mainly diet controlled.

Answer E is incorrect. The age of onset for type I and II diabetes is not the same. Type I diabetes is a disease which has an early age of onset. Type II diabetes occurs in the later stages of life.

The incidence of type I diabetes is far less (only 15% of diabetics have this form) than type II. Insulin production is nearly nonexistent, and it is caused by either a viral or immune destruction of B cells. It has a weak genetic predisposition. Ketoacidosis is a real concern with this type of diabetes (unlike type II). The treatment is insulin injection and diet control.

93. **The correct answer is C.** Hyperglycemia is characterized by a blood glucose level greater than 125 mg/dL. Other values of importance include hypoglycemia (blood glucose level less than 50 mg/dL), glycosuria (blood glucose levels greater than 160-180 mg/dL), and normal range (blood glucose in range of 70-110 mg/dL). These values can be ascertained by evaluating plasma glucose levels with either overnight fasting, 72-hour fasting, or oral glucose tolerance tests.

Answers A, B, D, and E are incorrect. These values are too low to be characterized as hyperglycemia.

94. **The correct answer is B.** Ketoacidosis is rare in type II diabetes, but a very common concern in type I diabetics.

Answer A is incorrect. This reaction occurs in cases of severe insulin deficiency or starvation.

Answer C is incorrect. Ketoacidosis is caused by an accumulation of ketone bodies which are synthesized from free fatty acids.

Answer D is incorrect. Blood ketones consist of acetoacetic acid and beta-hydroxybutyric acid.

Answer E is incorrect. In advanced cases of type II diabetes, ketoacidosis may become a concern. It can be life threatening when left untreated.

95. **The correct answer is D.** The normal range of glycosylated hemoglobin is from 4%-7%.

Answer A is incorrect. HbA1c is used to assess long-term control of diabetics, not the short term.

Answer B is incorrect. Glycosylated hemoglobin, also known as HbA1c, is formed from the irreversible glycosylation of hemoglobin.

Answer C is incorrect. This value reflects glucose levels over the past 2-3 months.

Answer E is incorrect. The reaction is a nonenzymatic glycosylation.

Note that HbA1c is a form of an advanced glycosylated end product (other products formed from glycosylation are Schiff bases and Amadori products → both are reversible). Levels greater than 7% would lead one to believe that a patient is poorly controlling their diabetes.

96. **The correct answer is C.** Bence-Jones proteins are found in patients with multiple myeloma. This finding is sensitive, but not specific. Therefore, it can confirm the diagnosis of multiple myeloma, but the absence of the protein cannot rule it out. Multiple myeloma is a cancer of plasma cells, and it arises in the bone marrow. There is an increase in plasma cells which interferes with other bone marrow cell lineages. Also, patients tend to have osteolytic lesions due to the plasma cell proliferation and expansion in the bone marrow.

Answer A is incorrect. Non-Hodgkin lymphoma would have symptoms similar to Hodgkin, but an absence of Reed-Sternberg cells.

Answer B is incorrect. Burkitt lymphoma has a chromosomal change located at t(8;14).

Answer D is incorrect. Patients with CML (chronic myelogenous leukemia) have the Philadelphia chromosome, which can be seen in genetic testing.

Answer E is incorrect. Patients with AML (acute myelogenous leukemia) have a rapid increase in myelocytes. This can be noted on laboratory exam.

97. The correct answer is A. One would find a decrease in the platelet count in cases of multiple myeloma. This causes difficulty with blood clotting.

Answer B is incorrect. Patients with multiple myeloma have a decreased white blood cell count. Thus, they are susceptible to increased infections.

Answer C is incorrect. Patients with multiple myeloma have a decreased red blood cell count. Thus, they typically have anemia.

Answer D is incorrect. Patients with multiple myeloma have an increased plasma cell count. Thus, plasma cells are functioning abnormally which leads to increased infection rate.

Answer E is incorrect. Patients with multiple myeloma have an increase in osteolytic lesions. This is due to increased osteoclastic function.

98. The correct answer is A. Amyloidosis can lead to development of type II diabetes mellitus. This is a rare chronic disease affecting middle-aged and older people. It is due to accumulation of amyloid (which is abnormal fibrillar scleroprotein). These deposit in various organs and tissues of the body, and eventually compromise such normal function. These disease states may be inflammatory, hereditary, or neoplastic. The deposition of amyloid may be local, generalized, or systemic. If the amyloid deposits in islet cells, it can cause type II diabetes mellitus by damaging receptors. Amyloid can be seen with Congo red stain.

Answers B, C, D and E are incorrect. Pheochromocytoma, small cell carcinoma, neuroblastoma, and rheumatoid arthritis do not lead to development of diabetes.

99. The correct answer is B. The mandible, not the maxilla, is the most commonly affected region from an eosinophilic granuloma.

Answer A is incorrect. This condition is mostly benign and affects males in the early 3rd decade of life.

Answer C is incorrect. Intraorally, mobile teeth and periodontal inflammation is present.

Answer D is incorrect. Clinically, one would find an asymptomatic patient with possibly some localized pain. There would be swelling of the mouth, with the mandible being most affected.

Answer E is incorrect. It is a histiocytosis X disease. Therefore, it involves increased abnormal histiocytes.

100. The correct answer is C. Haberman disease is not one of the Histiocytosis X diseases. Rather, it is a skin condition characterized by eruption of polymorphous skin macules, papules, and hemorrhaging vesicles. It does not involve histiocytes. The diseases of histiocytosis X all include an increase in abnormal histiocytes.

Answer A is incorrect. Letterer-Siwe disease presents clinically with a rash, fever, anemia, hemorrhage, splenomegaly, and lymphadenopathy.

Answer B is incorrect. Hand-Schüller-Christian disease has the clinical presentation of exophthalmos, diabetes insipidus, bone destruction, and some intraoral pathology.

Answer D is incorrect. Eosinophilic granuloma causes clinical symptoms consistent with asymptomatic swelling of mandible and intraoral regions.

Microbiology and Pathology

Note that the treatment for Histiocytosis X is radiation and/or chemotherapy, and typically the prognosis is poor.

101. **The correct answer is B.** The hyperacute phase of tissue graft rejection is most directly mediated by preformed antibody to graft antigen. This occurs within minutes after transplantation.

Answer A is incorrect. T cells attacking foreign class I MHC occurs during the acute phase of graft rejection. This occurs over weeks after transplantation.

Answer C is incorrect. The chronic phase occurs months to years after transplantation, and is characterized by antibody-mediated necrosis of graft vasculature.

Answer D is incorrect. T cells attacking foreign class II MHC occurs during the acute phase of graft rejection.

Answer E is incorrect. PMN attack of graft antigen does not occur during the acute phase of graft rejection.

102. **The correct answer is E.** Patients with blood type AB are considered the universal recipients.

Answer A is incorrect. Anti-B antibody is found in patients which are blood type A.

Answer B is incorrect. Blood type O has neither A nor B antigens on red blood cells.

Answer C is incorrect. Patients with erythrocyte antigen A have anti-B plasma antibody.

Answer D is incorrect. Both plasma antibody A and B are seen in patients with blood type O.

Note that ABO blood typing deals with the alloantigens located on all erythrocytes. There are only two genes involved in this (A and B), with four possible antigenic combinations of blood types: A (contain erythrocyte A antigen, patients have anti-B plasma antibody), B (B antigen, anti-A plasma antibody), AB (both A and B antigen, no plasma antibody, "universal recipient"), O (no erythrocyte antigens, have anti-A and -B plasma

antibody, "universal donor"). If blood types are mismatched, hemagglutination occurs.

103. **The correct answer is B.** Hemagglutination would occur when blood type AB is given to a patient with anti-A plasma antibody. This concept deals with a reaction which occurs between a mismatch of donor and recipient blood.

Answer A is incorrect. Blood type A can be given to a patient with anti-B plasma antibodies. This recipient cannot receive blood type B.

Answer C is incorrect. Blood type B can be given to a patient with anti-A plasma antibodies. This recipient cannot receive blood type A.

Answer D is incorrect. Blood with erythrocyte antigen A can be given to a patient with anti-B plasma antibodies. This recipient cannot receive blood type B.

Answer E is incorrect. Blood with erythrocyte antigen B can be given to a patient with anti-A plasma antibodies. This recipient cannot receive blood type A.

Note that if a patient whose plasma contains antibodies to, for example, erythrocyte antigen A (patient would be blood type B), they cannot be transfused with blood type A (which has erythrocytes containing antigen A). If this occurs, hemagglutination, which is a clumping of blood cells because of an antibody-antigen reaction, will cause rejection of the transfusion.

104. **The correct answer is C.** Cyanide poisoning causes malfunction of oxidative phosphorylation. Thus, patients suffering from cyanide intoxication cannot optimally produce ATP within mitochondrion. Death will ensue because of this.

Answer A is incorrect. Lead poisoning causes stippling of RBCs. This causes a decrease in oxygen-carrying capacity.

Answer B is incorrect. Carbon monoxide poisoning will cause hypoxia due to decreased oxygen binding.

Answer D is incorrect. Mercury poisoning causes renal tubular necrosis as well as pneumonitis, GI ulceration, and gingival lesions.

105. **The correct answer is E.** Alkaline phosphatase is elevated in the body of patients who are suffering from bone, liver, and skeletal abnormalities, to name a few.

Answer A is incorrect. CK-MB is a cardiac enzyme. It is found elevated in a patient which just experienced a myocardial infarction.

Answer B is incorrect. Troponin T is a cardiac enzyme. It is found elevated in a patient who just experienced a myocardial infarction.

Answer C is incorrect. Myoglobin is a cardiac enzyme. It is found elevated in a patient who just experienced a myocardial infarction.

Answer D is incorrect. Creatine phosphokinase is a cardiac enzyme. It is also found in the brain and skeletal muscle. It is found elevated in a patient who just experienced a myocardial infarction.

106. **The correct answer is E.** All of the answer choices listed in the question can lead to tissue hypoxia. Tissue hypoxia results from decreased oxygen being delivered to tissue.

Answer A is incorrect. Carbon monoxide poisoning can lead to tissue hypoxia. This is due to hemoglobin's increased affinity for CO compared to O_2.

Answer B is incorrect. Decreased tissue perfusion can lead to tissue hypoxia. An example of this is seen in shock and cardiac failure.

Answer C is incorrect. Decreased blood oxygenation can lead to tissue hypoxia. An example of this is seen in anemia, and pulmonary disease.

Answer D is incorrect. Vascular ischemia can lead to tissue hypoxia. This is due to a decrease in blood flow, thus decreased oxygenation of tissue.

Note that tissue hypoxia affects the heart, brain, and lungs most severely.

107. **The correct answer is A.** Karyorrhexis is a type of cell injury which is irreversible. There

are two types of cellular injury, irreversible and reversible. These changes occur to cells based mainly on the severity and duration of insult. It also depends on the cells' own adaptive mechanism to the offending agent.

Answer B is incorrect. Ribosomal detachment from endoplasmic reticulum is an example of reversible cell injury.

Answer C is incorrect. Chromatin clumping is an example of reversible cell injury.

Answer D is incorrect. Cellular and organelle swelling is an example of reversible cell injury. This is due to a Ca^{2+} influx which ultimately reverses itself.

Answer E is incorrect. Bleb formation is an example of reversible cell injury.

Note that another example of reversible cell injury includes increased lipid deposition. Irreversible cell injury includes: extensive plasma membrane damage, massive Ca^{2+} influx, diminished oxidative phosphorylation within mitochondrion, lysosomal enzyme release into cytoplasm, nuclear fragmentation (karyorrhexis), and cell death.

108. **The correct answer is B.** Hypertrophy is a term describing an increase in cell mass, not in number of cells.

Answer A is incorrect. Aplasia describes the complete lack of cells.

Answer C is incorrect. Metaplasia is a term which describes cellular change from one type to another cell type. It is a morphological change.

Answer D is incorrect. Atrophy describes a decrease in cellular mass.

Answer E is incorrect. Hypoplasia is a term which describes the decrease in the number of cells.

Note that these changes can occur in specific tissue and organs and can be caused by such conditions as decreased neurovascular supply, nutrition, endocrine dysfunction, and stress.

109. **The correct answer is B.** *Taenia solium* is a helminth which is transmitted by ingestion of

undercooked pork. It causes cysticercosis. Helminths (also known as metazoans) are associated with numerous forms of human infection.

Answer A is incorrect. *Taenia saginata* causes tapeworm infection. It can be transmitted from undercooked beef. It does not cause cysticercosis.

Answer C is incorrect. *Trichinella spiralis* causes trichinosis. It can be transmitted from ingestion of undercooked meat. It causes muscle pain, periorbital edema, fever, and eosinophilia.

Answer D is incorrect. *Enterobius vermicularis* causes pinworm infection. It is transmitted from ingestion of worm eggs. It causes perianal pruritus.

Answer E is incorrect. *Giardia lamblia* causes giardiasis, a parasitic infection of the intestine. It causes severe diarrhea and stomach upset. Giardia infection is one of the most common waterborne diseases in the United States.

110. **The correct answer is C.** Nemathelminthes are a type of Metazoa, not Protozoa. Parasites are unicellular eukaryotes which infect blood cells, intestinal and urogenital tissue, and meninges.

Answer A is incorrect. Sporozoans are a type of Protozoa. Protozoa are subdivided into Sarcodina (amebas), Sporozoa (aporozoans), Mastigophora (flagellates), and Ciliata (ciliates).

Answer B is incorrect. There are two groups of parasites: Protozoa and Metazoa.

Answer D is incorrect. "Flatworms" is another name for Platyhelminthes. They further subdivide into Trematoda (Flukes), Cestoda (Tapeworms), and Nemathelminthes (Roundworms).

Answer E is incorrect. Trematoda and Cestoda are subgroups of Platyhelminthes. Platyhelminthes are a subgroup of Metazoa.

111. **The correct answer is B.** *Pneumocystis* is transmitted through inhalation. This protozoa causes pneumonia in immunocompro-

mised patients. The other protozoa listed in the question have other routes of transfer.

Answer A is incorrect. *Cryptosporidium parvum* is transmitted via fecal-oral route and causes giardiasis.

Answer C is incorrect. *Entamoeba histolytica* causes amebiasis and dysentery by the fecal-oral route.

Answer D is incorrect. *Toxoplasma gondii* is transmitted not only via fecal-oral route, but also transplacental, and causes toxoplasmosis which is a CNS infection.

Answer E is incorrect. *Trichomonas vaginalis* is transmitted sexually and causes trichomoniasis, vaginitis, and urethritis.

112. **The correct answer is A.** Clotrimazole is an antifungal agent, which inhibits ergosterol synthesis via troche form. Antifungal agents are typically used to treat such problems as candidiasis, amongst other types of fungal infection.

Answer B is incorrect. Ketoconazole is an antifungal (in tablet form), which functions by blocking fungal cytochrome p450.

Answer C is incorrect. Fluconazole is an antifungal (in table form), which functions by blocking fungal cytochrome p450.

Answer D is incorrect. Nystatin is an antifungal (in topical and oral suspension form), which functions by binding ergosterol.

Answer E is incorrect. Amphotericin B is an antifungal (in topical, oral suspension, and intravenous form), which functions by binding ergosterol.
  Note that Clotrimazole is an antifungal (in troche form), which inhibits ergosterol synthesis. Ergosterol is a component of fungal cell membranes which alters their permeability.

113. **The correct answer is D.** Dermatophytosis is a disease caused by molds which includes tinea corporis, tinea capitis, tinea cruris, tinea pedis, and tinea unguium.

Answer A is incorrect. Histoplasmosis is a dimorphic fungus which is found in bird and bat droppings in the Ohio and Mississippi Valleys and causes damage within host macrophages.

Answer B is incorrect. Coccidioidomycosis is also dimorphic, endemic in the southwest USA and Latin America, and causes respiratory infection when inhaled from arthrospores.

Answer C is incorrect. Blastomycosis, also dimorphic, is endemic in North America and causes respiratory infection after inhalation of microconidia.

Answer E is incorrect. Mucormycosis is caused by a mold and inhalation of it causes respiratory, skin, paranasal sinus, and brain infection.

114. **The correct answer is C.** Trimethoprim is a bacteriostatic antibiotic. It would not be effective in this situation.

Answer A is incorrect. Miconazole would be effective in this situation. It is an antifungal, which affects fungal membrane permeability by inhibition of ergosterol.

Answer B is incorrect. Clotrimazole would be effective in this situation. It is an antifungal, which affects fungal membrane permeability by inhibition of ergosterol.

Answer D is incorrect. Tolnaftate would be effective in this situation. It is an antifungal, which affects fungal membrane permeability by inhibition of ergosterol.

Answer E is incorrect. Griseofulvin would be effective in this situation. It is an antifungal, which affects fungal membrane permeability by inhibition of ergosterol.

115. **The correct answer is A.** Fungi are gram positive.

Answer B is incorrect. Their cell walls are composed primarily of chitin, and their membranes formed from ergosterol.

Answer C is incorrect. These microorganisms are either obligate or facultative aerobes.

Answer D is incorrect. Fungi are eukaryotic microorganisms.

Answer E is incorrect. Fungi reproduce either sexually (via spores) or asexually (via conidia). Examples of fungal spores include zygospores, ascospores, and basidiospores, and examples of conidia include arthrospores, chlamydospores, blastospores, and sporangiospores.

116. **The correct answer is C.** Hepatitis C is the disease described in this patient. Hepatitis C is a viral disease characterized by increased incidence of chronic liver disease, cirrhosis, and hepatocellular carcinoma. Symptoms include fever, loss of appetite, nausea, and jaundice.

Answer A is incorrect. Symptoms of HIV are similar, with constitutional symptoms being present. No jaundice would be expected, though.

Answer B is incorrect. Syphilis presents clinically with varying forms and symptoms. There is a primary, secondary, latent, and tertiary form of the disease. Each one has a differing presentation.

Answer D is incorrect. Gonorrhea presents clinically with dysuria in males and females, as well as a discharge which could be present.

Answer E is incorrect. Chlamydia presents clinically with symptoms of the genital, ocular, or joint regions. Each region presents a different clinical symptom.

117. **The correct answer is C.** Acute hepatitis B infection would have a lab finding of the HBs Ag. This antigen designated chronicity of disease with hepatitis B, as well as acute infection of the virus.

Answer A is incorrect. Acute hepatitis C infection would have anti-HCV markers seen in lab results during this phase.

Answer B is incorrect. Acute hepatitis A infection has IgM anti-HAV markers in this stage. There is no particular marker in chronic disease.

Answer D is incorrect. Chronic hepatitis E infection would have no markers in this stage. Although, one would expect to find

IgM anti-HEV markers on lab studies with acute hepatitis E infection.

Answer E is incorrect. Chronic hepatitis B infection is evidenced by a lab finding of HBsAg. It is the same marker found in the acute stage.

Note that Hepatitis D has IgM anti-HDV markers in lab studies.

118. **The correct answer is B.** Hepatitis B is the form of hepatitis infection in which a vaccine is commonly administered to healthcare workers. Hepatitis B is very easily transmissible through blood contact with an infected patient.

Answer A is incorrect. Hepatitis A does not have a vaccine which is commonly given to healthcare workers. A vaccine does exist for it, though.

Answer C is incorrect. Hepatitis C does not have a vaccine which is commonly given to healthcare workers. No vaccine exists for this virus.

Answer D is incorrect. Hepatitis D does not have a vaccine which is commonly given to healthcare workers. No vaccine exists for this virus.

Answer E is incorrect. Hepatitis E does not have a vaccine which is commonly given to healthcare workers. No vaccine exists for this virus.

Note that only hepatitis B and hepatitis A have vaccines (hepatitis A → killed vaccine; hepatitis B → immune globulin vaccine/passive immunity and subunit vaccine/active immunity).

119. **The correct answer is A.** Picornavirus is responsible for hepatitis A infection. It is a single-stranded RNA virus, which lacks an envelope.

Answer B is incorrect. Hepadnavirus is a double-stranded DNA virus, which causes hepatitis B infection.

Answer C is incorrect. Flavivirus is a single-stranded RNA virus responsible for hepatitis C infection.

Answer D is incorrect. Hepatitis D infection is caused by Deltavirus, a single-stranded RNA virus.

Answer E is incorrect. Hepatitis E is caused by infection of the single-stranded RNA virus, Calicivirus.

120. **The correct answer is A.** Autoclaving is the only way to be sure that hepatitis B virus is effectively destroyed. This form of sterilization uses moist heat to denature proteins at 121°C/205°F in 15-20 minutes. It is the most common form of sterilization and can corrode or dull carbon-steel instruments.

Answer B is incorrect. Ethylene oxide gas is used mostly in hospitals for heat-sensitive materials and is very slow (8-10 hours).

Answer C is incorrect. Chemical vapor uses a combination of alcohol and formaldehyde and does not corrode or dull instruments.

Answer D is incorrect. Formaldehyde is a less efficacious form of sterilization which uses a 37% solution in water, formalin, to sterilize.

Answer E is incorrect. Glutaraldehyde is used for heat-sensitive materials and is very slow, taking up to 10 hours.

121. **The correct answer is C.** Glutaraldehyde 2% is a sterilization technique which alkylates nucleic acids and proteins to achieve sterile conditions.

Answer A is incorrect. It is a slow process, though, taking up to 10 hours.

Answer B is incorrect. Glutaraldehyde 2% is associated with hypersensitivity reaction.

Answer D is incorrect. It does not denature proteins. It is used mostly for heat-sensitive materials.

Answer E is incorrect. The preferred method of sterilizing liquid solutions is filtration, which physically and electrostatically traps microorganism larger than its pore size.

122. **The correct answer is D.** An endemic infection is one that occurs at a minimal level within a population.

Answer A is incorrect. An infection occurring more frequently than normal within a population is called an epidemic.

Answer B is incorrect. An infection occurring at a worldwide level is called a pandemic.

Answer C is incorrect. An infection which occurs within different countries does not have a specific classification.

123. **The correct answer is D.** Ludwig angina does not involve the parapharyngeal fascial space.

     Answer A is incorrect. The sublingual fascial space is involved in Ludwig angina.

     Answer B is incorrect. The submandibular fascial space is involved in Ludwig angina.

     Answer C is incorrect. The submental fascial space is involved in Ludwig angina.

     Note that Ludwig angina is a cellulitis which rapidly progresses to involve the submandibular, sublingual, and submental fascial spaces. The key to this infection is that it occurs bilaterally and treatment is emergent in that it can quickly obstruct the airway, thus compromising oxygenation.

124. **The correct answer is D.** A cyst is a fluid-filled sac lined by true epithelium. The other terms listed in the question have definitions which are similar, yet correct usage and differentiation of them is vital when describing pathology.

     Answer A is incorrect. A granuloma is a chronic inflammatory lesion consisting of granulation tissue (fibrosis, angiogenesis, inflammatory cells).

     Answer B is incorrect. An abscess is an acute inflammatory lesion with pus being surrounded by a fibrous wall.

     Answer C is incorrect. Cellulitis is an acute, diffuse swelling along fascial planes that separate muscle bundles.

125. **The correct answer is E.** The carrier stage is the infectious state characterized as having active growth of microorganisms with or without symptoms.

Answer A is incorrect. The chronic stage is the infectious state in which there is long-term active growth of microorganisms. There are symptoms present.

Answer B is incorrect. The acute stage is the infectious state in which there is short-term active growth of microorganism. There are symptoms present.

Answer C is incorrect. The latent stage is the infectious state with no active growth of microorganisms. Reactivation is possible, though.

Answer D is incorrect. The subclinical stage is the infectious state that is only detectable via serology. The patient is clinically asymptomatic.

126. **The correct answer is A.** Autoclaving (moist heat sterilization) is a process which must be done with heat at 121°C/250°F for 15-20 minutes. Other forms of sterilization are carried out at differing levels of heat and at variable time intervals.

     Answer B is incorrect. Dry heat sterilization is completed at 160°C/320°F for 2 hours.

     Answer C is incorrect. Dry heat sterilization is completed at 170°C(340°F) for 1 hour.

     Answer D is incorrect. There is no sterilization method which uses these parameters for treatment.

     Answer E is incorrect. Chemical vapor sterilization is completed at 132°C/270°F for 20-30 minutes.

     Note that the sterilization method of using ethylene oxide gas is for 8-10 hours, and glutaraldehyde 2% for 10 hours. Glutaraldehyde 2% and filtration have no specific time interval.

127. **The correct answer is A.** Hepatitis B infection presents the greatest risk of bloodborne infection amongst healthcare workers. Because of the high risk of bloodborne infection with this and other diseases, universal precautions have been implicated in the dental office (as well as in hospital settings). It says that all human blood, as well as other body fluids which contain blood, should be

Microbiology and Pathology

treated as infectious for HIV, hepatitis B, and other bloodborne pathogens.

Answer B is incorrect. HSV (herpes simplex virus) poses a risk.

Answer C is incorrect. HIV (human immunodeficiency virus) poses a bloodborne risk to healthcare workers. This risk is not greater than hepatitis B, though.

Answer D is incorrect. HPV (human papilloma virus) poses a risk to healthcare workers. This virus is contractible via touching of the lesion.

Answer E is incorrect. HCV (hepatitis C virus) poses a bloodborne risk to healthcare workers. This risk is not greater than hepatitis B, though.

128. **The correct answer is B.** Regarding tuberculosis infection, Ghon complex is characteristic of the primary and secondary form of TB. In the primary form, the bacterium is between the upper and middle lobes of lung. Ghon complex consists of parenchymal lesion and hilar lymphadenopathy.

Answer A is incorrect. The miliary form is widely disseminated. The lesions found look like "millet seed" with multiple extrapulmonary sites. In the secondary form, the lung apices are involved due to high oxygen tension, and Ghon complex reactivated.

Answer C is incorrect. Tuberculosis is caused by a bacterium. The offending agent is *Mycobacterium tuberculosis*, an acid fast, strict anaerobe. Because of this, it lives viably within the lungs.

Answer D is incorrect. This disease is contracted by aerosolized droplets which are inhaled.

Answer E is incorrect. Tuberculosis does involve the lymph nodes. Hilar lymphadenopathy is part of the Ghon complex.

129. **The correct answer is C.** Hemoptysis is not a clinical symptom of emphysema. Hemoptysis is the coughing up of blood and/or blood-streaked sputum. It is seen in the following diseases: respiratory infection, bronchitis, tuberculosis, pneumonia, bronchogenic carcinoma, and idiopathic pulmonary hemosiderosis.

Answer A is incorrect. Patients with pneumonia typically have bouts of hemoptysis.

Answer B is incorrect. Patients with tuberculosis typically have bouts of hemoptysis.

Answer D is incorrect. Patients with bronchitis pneumonia typically have bouts of hemoptysis.

Answer E is incorrect. Patients with idiopathic pulmonary hemosiderosis typically have bouts of hemoptysis.

130. **The correct answer is B.** Ascites is not a characteristic of pneumonia. It occurs when excess fluid accumulates in the space between the membranes lining the abdomen and abdominal organs. It can be free serous or protein-laden fluid. Disorders associated with this include cirrhosis, hepatitis, portal vein thrombosis, constrictive pericarditis, congestive heart failure, liver cancer, nephrotic syndrome, and pancreatitis.

Answer A is incorrect. Patients with pancreatitis may have symptoms of ascites.

Answer C is incorrect. Patients with congestive heart failure may have symptoms of ascites.

Answer D is incorrect. Patients with constrictive pericarditis may have symptoms of ascites.

Answer E is incorrect. Patients with nephrotic syndrome may have symptoms of ascites.

131. **The correct answer is A.** Steatorrhea is a result of certain malabsorptive disorders. This symptom is soft, bulky, foul-smelling, light-colored stool. It occurs when fat is not absorbed. This can be seen in such cases as pancreatic disease (decrease in digestive enzymes) and bile obstruction (decrease bile for emulsification).

Answer B is incorrect. Celiac disease is caused by gluten sensitivity, not infection.

Answer C is incorrect. There is no correlation between increased length of breastfeeding and Whipple disease.

Answer D is incorrect. Malabsorption is due to nutrients not being absorbed by the small intestine. It can cause growth retardation, failure to thrive, and in adults, weight loss.

Answer E is incorrect. Sore tongue is not a clinical complication of Whipple disease.

Note that other forms of malabsorption include tropical sprue (etiology unknown; probably an infection) and Whipple disease (caused by *Tropheryma whippelii* infection).

132. **The correct answer is C.** The most detrimental effect on salivary pH is the frequency of carbohydrate intake.

Answer A is incorrect. Dental caries is caused by bacteria which synthesize glucans (dextrans) and fructans (levans) from metabolism of dietary sucrose. These contribute to bacterial adherence to tooth surfaces and plaque formation.

Answer B is incorrect. Lactic acid is a byproduct of this metabolism and it reduces salivary pH. This creates sites of enamel demineralization and cavitation.

Answer D is incorrect. The reverse is true. Glucans (and fructans) are the by-products of sucrose metabolism.

Answer E is incorrect. Also detrimental to salivary pH is the quantity of carbohydrate intake.

133. **The correct answer is E.** By-products of viral replication are not typically a major component of dental calculus.

Answer A is incorrect. Calcium is a component of dental calculus. This is an inorganic component of it, which makes up roughly 70%-90% of calculus.

Answer B is incorrect. Hydroxyapatite is a component of dental calculus. It is made up of calcium and phosphorus.

Answer C is incorrect. Carbohydrate is a component of dental calculus. This is an organic component, which makes up roughly 10%-30% of calculus.

Answer D is incorrect. Desquamated cells are a component of dental calculus. This is an organic component, which makes up roughly 10%-30% of calculus.

134. **The correct answer is D.** Catalase is an antioxidant, thus rids the body of free radical injury.

Answer A is incorrect. Free radicals can cause various forms of cellular injury. These include membrane lipid peroxidation, nucleic acid denaturation, and cross-linking of proteins.

Answer B is incorrect. They are generated from redox reactions. Also, radiation, drugs and chemicals, and reperfusion injury can cause free radical formation.

Answer C is incorrect. They initiate autocatalytic reactions which cause cellular damage.

Answer E is incorrect. Free radicals are induced by activated oxygen species.

Examples of antioxidants include superoxide dismutase, catalase, vitamin E, and ceruloplasmin.

135. **The correct answer is C.** Serum calcium is normal in dystrophic calcification. There are two types of pathologic calcification—dystrophic and metastatic.

Answer A is incorrect. Metastatic calcification does not occur in damaged heart valves. This calcification occurs at such locations as the stomach, lungs, and kidneys. Metastatic calcification is defined as calcification of normal tissue.

Answer B is incorrect. There are abnormal serum calcium levels. Pathogenesis involves the precipitation caused by tissue acidity and increased calcium concentration. It is associated with hyperparathyroidism, vitamin D intoxication, and bone destruction.

Answer D is incorrect. Dystrophic calcification is the calcification of degenerate or necrotic tissue. The serum calcium levels remain normal. The pathogenesis is enhanced by collagen and acidic phosphoproteins, and it is commonly seen in hyalinized scars, degenerated leiomyoma foci, caseous nodules, damaged heart valves, and atherosclerotic plaques.

Microbiology and Pathology

Answer E is incorrect. Eggshell calcification can be seen on chest x-ray.

136. **The correct answer is A.** The calor sign of acute inflammation is due to increased tissue perfusion. It is seen clinically as a localized heat.

   Answer B is incorrect. Tumor is a swelling. It is due to tissue edema.

   Answer C is incorrect. Rubor is a clinical redness. It is due to vasodilation and increased vascular permeability.

   Answer D is incorrect. Function laesa is the loss of function. It is due to swelling and pain.

   Answer E is incorrect. Dolor is pain. It is due to inflammatory mediators and pressure due to edema.
   Note that these classical signs of inflammation comprise the initial responses to tissue injury.

137. **The correct answer is B.** It is not granuloma, but abscess formation which includes pus from neutrophils, necrotic cells, and exudates. Acute inflammation is the initial response to tissue injury. It is largely leukocyte infiltration with rids of the offending factor and degrades necrotic tissue from the damage.

   Answer A is incorrect. PMNs are the first leukocyte to respond.

   Answer C is incorrect. Regeneration is the first stage of wound repair following inflammation. It involves the resolution of affected tissues. Also, repair (fibrosis of affected tissues), abscess formation, and chronic inflammation are the other stages of wound repair.

   Answer D is incorrect. Chronic inflammation differs from acute in that monocytes and macrophages are present in this chronic phase.

   Answer E is incorrect. Elimination of infectious agents and ridding of necrotic tissue occur in the initial response to tissue injury.

138. **The correct answer is D.** Down syndrome is the most frequent autosomal chromosomal

disorder. This syndrome occurs at a frequency of 1 in 700 births.

   Answer A is incorrect. Next most common autosomal chromosomal abnormality is Edward syndrome at 1 in 3000 births.

   Answer B is incorrect. Patau syndrome is the third most common autosomal chromosomal abnormality. It occurs at a frequency of 1 in 5000 births.

   Answer C is incorrect. Klinefelter syndrome is not autosomal, rather it is sex related. It occurs at a frequency of 1 in 500 male births.

   Answer E is incorrect. Turner syndrome is not autosomal. It is a sex-related chromosomal abnormality that occurs 1 in 3000 female births.

139. **The correct answer is E.** There is decreased cross-sectional area of capillaries and arterioles in cases of primary hypertension. Primary hypertension accounts for 90%-95% of all hypertensive cases, and there is no identifiable cause. Although, it is related to increased cardiac output and increased total peripheral resistance.

   Answer A is incorrect. In primary hypertension, there is hypertrophy of arteries and arterioles and not the capillaries (because there is no smooth muscle in capillaries).

   Answer B is incorrect. There is also increased wall-to-lumen ratio of arteries and arterioles (due to increased smooth muscle cell growth) seen in primary hypertension.

   Answer C is incorrect. Patients have decreased arteriolar and capillary density with primary hypertension.

   Answer D is incorrect. There is increased smooth muscle growth in patients with primary hypertension.

140. **The correct answer is C.** Being a premenopausal woman is not a risk factor for atherosclerosis. The risk factors for atherosclerosis include smoking, hypertension, nephrosclerosis, and diabetes. This is a disease in which degenerative changes occur in artery walls. Plaques

(fatty material) accumulate under the walls of vessels (commonly arteries). This disease is the most important contributor to arterial thrombosis and the most susceptible arteries are the aorta and coronary arteries.

Answer A is incorrect. Smoking is a risk factor for atherosclerosis.

Answer B is incorrect. Hypertension is a risk factor for atherosclerosis.

Answer D is incorrect. Nephrosclerosis is a risk factor for atherosclerosis.

Answer E is incorrect. Diabetes is a risk factor for atherosclerosis.

141. **The correct answer is C.** Right-sided heart failure can be caused by cor pulmonale. This is defined as increased pulmonary vascular resistance causing right heart strain.

Answer A is incorrect. Isolated right heart failure is uncommon. These pathological changes to the right side of the heart are typically caused by left heart failure.

Answer B is incorrect. Right heart failure usually occurs due to left heart failure. Thus, it is not independent of it.

Answer D is incorrect. The symptoms of right heart failure include elevated venous pressure, hepatomegaly, and dependent edema, as well as systemic venous congestion and peripheral edema (ie, swollen ankles).

Answer E is incorrect. A gallop rhythm is not typically heard when right heart failure is present.

142. **The correct answer is C.** A decrease in alpha-1 antitrypsin is seen in emphysema. Emphysema is typically a disease of smokers. It is either centrilobular (due to cigarette smoking) or panlobular (due to familial antiproteinase deficiency, a decrease in alpha-1 antitrypsin). This allows the destruction of elastic fibers in alveolar walls distal to respiratory bronchioles. Thus, there is a decrease in elastic recoil, decrease in radial traction, and decrease in functioning parenchyma.

Answer A is incorrect. Asthma is a hypersensitivity reaction due to overreactive airways.

Answer B is incorrect. Chronic bronchitis is due to chronic inflammation of the bronchial tree. It is often from years of offending cigarette smoke.

Answer D is incorrect. Pneumonia is due to either bacterial or viral infection.

Answer E is incorrect. Tuberculosis is caused by bacterial infection. It is not due to a decrease in alpha-1 antitrypsin.

143. **The correct answer is A.** *Klebsiella* infection can often cause lung abscess in alcoholic patients. Lung abscesses are localized collections of pus in the lung caused by aspiration, bronchial obstruction, or septic emboli. The most commonly found organisms include *Pseudomonas, Klebsiella, Proteus,* and anaerobes. Clinically, one would expect to find a productive cough with large amounts of foul-smelling sputum, fever, dyspnea, chest pain, cyanosis, and a fluid-filled cavity seen on chest x-ray.

Answer B is incorrect. *Staphylococcus* infection does not present with lung abscesses. The clinical presentation of infection with this bacterium varies based upon the species.

Answer C is incorrect. *Streptococcus* infection does not present with lung abscesses. The clinical presentation of infection with this bacterium varies based upon the species.

Answer D is incorrect. Bacillus infection does not present with lung abscesses. The clinical presentation of infection with this bacterium varies based upon the species.

Answer E is incorrect. *Clostridium* infection does not present with lung abscesses. The clinical presentation of infection with this bacterium varies based upon the species.

144. **The correct answer is C.** When viewed histologically, sulfur granules will appear in samples taken from patients infected with *Actinomyces israelii. A israelii* is an anaerobic bacterium which contains no virulence factors.

Microbiology and Pathology

It causes actinomycosis. This disease is characterized by not only sulfur granules but also slow-growing, lumpy abscesses. The other above bacteria listed do not have characteristic histological findings as listed above with *A israelii.*

Answer A is incorrect. *L monocytogenes* can be identified microscopically with its long actin tails. It can also be detected by molecular biology techniques.

Answer B is incorrect. *S aureus* can be identified microscopically by its characteristic grapelike clusters. It can also be grown on blood-rich agar places.

Answer D is incorrect. *C botulinum* can be identified microscopically with special staining—gentian violet. It also can be identified using monoclonal antibodies.

Answer E is incorrect. *C tetani* can be identified microscopically with its tennis racket appearance.

145. **The correct answer is E.** *Pseudomembranous colitis* is not caused by *Neisseria*; it is due to antibiotic-induced overgrowth of *Clostridium difficile*. *Neisseria* genus is a gram-negative cocci which has two species: *N meningitides* (aerobic; contains LPS, IgA protease, and polysaccharide capsule), and *N gonorrhoeae* (aerobic; contains LOS, fimbriae, and IgA protease).

Answer A is incorrect. Septic arthritis is caused by *N gonorrhoeae.*

Answer B is incorrect. Waterhouse-Friderichsen syndrome is caused by *N meningitides.*

Answer C is incorrect. Meningitis is caused by *N meningitides.*

Answer D is incorrect. Gonorrhea is caused by *N gonorrhoeae.*

146. **The correct answer is B.** *Clostridium perfringens* causes the symptoms of necrotizing fascitis and myonecrosis after becoming inoculated from ingestion of reheated meats. It is anaerobic, and its virulence factor is alpha toxin, which causes gas gangrene. *Clostridium* genus is a gram-positive bacilli.

Answer A is incorrect. *C difficile* is an anaerobic bacterium. Its virulence factors are exotoxin A and B and it can cause pseudomembranous colitis.

Answer C is incorrect. *C tetani* is an anaerobic bacterium. Its virulence factor is tetanus toxin, and it causes tetanus.

Answer D is incorrect. *C botulinum* is an anaerobic bacterium. Its virulence factor is botulinum toxin, and it causes botulism.

147. **The correct answer is A.** *Shigella* species causes dysentery. This bacterium is facultative and has virulence factors including enterotoxin and endotoxin.

Answer B is incorrect. *Excherichia coli* is a facultative bacterium. Its virulence factors are enterotoxin and endotoxin, and infection causes urinary tract infections, traveler's diarrhea, and neonatal meningitis.

Answer C is incorrect. *Klebsiella pneumoniae* is a facultative bacterium. Its virulence factor includes endotoxin infection, and it causes pneumonia and urinary tract infections.

Answer D is incorrect. *Vibrio cholerae* is a facultative bacterium. Its virulence factors are endotoxin and enterotoxin, and infection causes cholera.

Answer E is incorrect. *Helicobacter pylori* is a facultative bacterium. Its virulence factor is endotoxin, and infection causes gastritis, peptic ulcers, and gastric carcinoma.

148. **The correct answer is B.** Syphilis infection is treated with penicillin.

Answer A is incorrect. The tertiary form is characterized by gumma formation. This gumma can be found on the palate and the tongue.

Answer C is incorrect. Syphilis is a disease caused by the spirochete *Treponema pallidum.*

Answer D is incorrect. The secondary form includes a highly infectious maculopapular rash. Also, condyloma lata is present on the skin and mucosa.

Answer E is incorrect. The primary form is characterized by a painless ulcer/chancre at the site of local contact.

149. **The correct answer is C.** *Mycoplasma pneumonia* is the smallest bacterium. It is a wallless bacteria with a cell membrane that contains cholesterol. It causes atypical pneumonia. These bacteria are classified in a group by themselves.

Answer A is incorrect. *C trachomatis* is a bacterium which causes infection of the lower genitourinary tract in both men and women. It cannot be Gram stained. Microscopically, one can view small inclusion bodies.

Answer B is incorrect. *M tuberculosis* is diagnosed microscopically using an acid-fast stain. It causes tuberculosis infection.

Answer D is incorrect. *R rickettsii* is a bacterium which causes Rocky Mountain spotted fever. It is transmitted via tick bites.

Answer E is incorrect. *B burgdorferi* is a bacterium which causes Lyme disease. It is transmitted via tick bite.

150. **The correct answer is D.** Hepatitis B is caused by infection of hepadnavirus. Hepadnavirus is a double-stranded, circular DNA virus which is also associated with hepatocellular carcinoma.

Answer A is incorrect. Aseptic meningitis is caused by Coxsackie A and B viruses. This virus is a subgroup of Picornavirus. Picornavirus is the smallest family of RNA viruses.

Answer B is incorrect. Herpangina is caused by Coxsackie A virus. This virus is a subgroup of Picornavirus.

Answer C is incorrect. Polio is caused by poliovirus. This virus is a subgroup of Picornavirus.

Answer E is incorrect. Common cold is caused by Rhinovirus. This virus is a subgroup of Picornavirus.

Note that acute lymphonodular pharyngitis is caused by Coxsackie A virus. Coxsackie B

virus also causes pleurodynia, myocarditis, and pericarditis. Hepatitis A virus causes hepatitis A infection.

151. **The correct answer is D.** The classic symptom of coronary artery disease is angina.

Answer A is incorrect. Coronary artery disease is characterized by atherosclerotic plaques and decreased blood supply to the myocardium.

Answer B is incorrect. The result of decreased blood supply to the myocardium is ischemia and infarction of the heart. This is due to decreased oxygen and nutrients to the myocardium.

Answer C is incorrect. Risks include hypertension, hyperlipidemia, smoking, obesity, inactivity, diabetes, and being male.

Answer E is incorrect. Ischemia is a common consequence of coronary artery disease.

Note that myocardial infarction can be noted with ECG changes and cardiac enzymes in the blood in patients with coronary artery disease.

152. **The correct answer is A.** A patient experiencing a myocardial infarct would not have pain radiating to the right arm, but rather to the left arm.

Answer B is incorrect. Symptoms seen in patients suffering from an MI include angina, sweating, and nausea.

Answer C is incorrect. ECG changes can also be seen in these patients. This is because of disruption in electrical conductivity in the heart.

Answer D is incorrect. Angina is a common, early symptom experienced by patients having an MI. The pain is said to be crushing.

Answer E is incorrect. Lab values would show an increase in cardiac enzymes in the circulation.

Note that myocardial infarction is due to prolonged interruption of coronary blood flow to the myocardium, thus, coagulative necrosis eventually ensues after the lack of blood flow to the heart. There are two types of cardiac occlusion: complete (transmural infarct-ST elevation on ECG) and partial (subendocardial infarct—non-ST elevation). The prognosis is good if patients are treated quickly.

153. **The correct answer is E.** Stable angina is precipitated by exertion. Angina is characterized as squeezing substernal chest discomfort. This pain may also radiate to the left arm, neck, jaw, and shoulder blades. Angina is caused by ischemia of the myocardium, atherosclerotic narrowing, and vasospasm.

    Answer A is incorrect. Stable angina is the most common type of angina. It is seen with coronary artery disease and atherosclerotic narrowing, and it is precipitated by exertion.

    Answer B is incorrect. Prinzmetal angina is seen clinically as intermittent chest pain at rest. It is due to vasospasm.

    Answer C is incorrect. The most common type of angina is stable angina, not Prinzmetal.

    Answer D is incorrect. Unstable angina will occur even at rest. It is the most severe coronary artery disease, and could be a sign of oncoming myocardial infarct.

154. **The correct answer is C.** This patient is suffering from emphysema. This disease is due to destruction of elastic fibers in alveolar walls. It is most often caused by a history of cigarette smoking, but also has a genetic predilection. Symptoms include dyspnea, labored breathing, and a nonproductive cough. Pulmonary function tests would show increased total lung capacity, increased residual volume, and decreased ratio of forced expiratory volume 1 to forced vital capacity.

    Answer A is incorrect. Chronic bronchitis patients suffer from a productive cough and wheezing. They also have a positive chest auscultation.

    Answer B is incorrect. Dyspnea has clinical symptoms of expiratory wheezes, cough, and chest tightness.

Answer D is incorrect. Patients with pneumonia have constitutional symptoms, productive cough, blood-tinged sputum, dyspnea, and chest pain.

Answer E is incorrect. Tuberculosis patients show hemoptysis, weight loss, night sweats, malaise, and weakness.

155. **The correct answer is A.** Asthma is not precipitated by increased sympathetic stimulation. Asthma is a chronic reactive airway disorder caused by episodic airway obstruction.

    Answer B is incorrect. Cox inhibitors precipitate asthma by leading to an increase in leukotrienes and bronchoconstrictors.

    Answer C is incorrect. Direct bronchoconstrictor release is caused by chemical inhalation or medications.

    Answer D is incorrect. Increased vagal stimulation is due to viral infection and upper respiratory tract infection. This leads to a lowering of the respiratory threshold.

    Answer E is incorrect. Type I hypersensitivity causes mast-cell degranulation which leads to bronchospasm and increased inflammatory-cell recruitment.

    Note that asthma can occur at any age, but greater than half of the cases occur in children under age 10. The mechanism of asthma is broken up into two categories, allergic (immune: type I hypersensitivity) and intrinsic (nonimmune: direct bronchoconstrictor release, increased vagal stimulation, cox inhibitors).

156. **The correct answer is C.** A blue bloater is someone who has chronic bronchitis. Chronic bronchitis is a disease in people with a history of cigarette smoking. By definition, it is someone who has a chronic, productive cough for at least 3 months of the year for two years. These patients are blue due to cyanosis caused by increased partial pressure oxygen.

    Answer A is incorrect. Patients with emphysema are considered "pink puffers." This is because they purse their lips to overcome airway collapse.

Answer B is incorrect. Patients with asthma have clinical symptoms of shortness of breath and chest tightness.

Answer D is incorrect. Patients with pneumonia typically present with a cough, fever, increased respiratory rate, and possibly rales (when auscultating).

Answer E is incorrect. Patients with bronchiectasis typically present with frequent respiratory infections and the symptoms which accompany them.

157. **The correct answer is D.** Noncaseating granulomas are not a possible complication of chronic bronchitis. Chronic bronchitis is a disease which causes a productive cough, wheezing, and positive chest auscultation (noisy chest, rhonchi).

Answer A is incorrect. Peripheral edema is a complication of chronic bronchitis. This is due to pulmonary hypertension (which causes right ventricular overload and cor pulmonale/right heart failure).

Answer B is incorrect. Chronic productive cough is a complication of chronic bronchitis. This is due to volume overload.

Answer C is incorrect. Right ventricular overload is a complication of chronic bronchitis. This occurs secondary to pulmonary hypertension, and leads to cor pulmonale and peripheral edema.

Answer E is incorrect. Bronchogenic carcinoma is a complication of chronic bronchitis. This increased lung cancer risk is due to squamous metaplasia from chronic lung inflammation.

158. **The correct answer is D.** Increased elastic recoil is not a mechanism of airway obstruction. Airway obstruction can be caused by many mechanisms.

Answer A is incorrect. Decreased elastic recoil causes airways to collapse and, thus, airway obstruction. An example of this is seen with patients that have emphysema.

Answer B is incorrect. Increased mucous can cause airway obstruction. An example of this is seen in chronic bronchitis.

Answer C is incorrect. Airway hyperreactivity, for example bronchospasm, can cause airway obstruction. An example of this occurs in patients with asthma.

159. **The correct answer is E.** An ELISA test is a substrate-activated enzyme reaction labeling antigen-antibody complexes. If the reaction is positive, there will be a visible color reaction. This type of testing is used to detect antigen or antibody in patient specimens.

Answer A is incorrect. Precipitation reactions are characterized by antibody cross-linking with a soluble antigen. This test detects serum antigen or antibody.

Answer B is incorrect. Radioimmunoassay reactions are characterized by radio-labeled antibody cross-linking with unlabeled antigen. This test is used to detect serum antigen or hapten.

Answer C is incorrect. Immunofluorescence reactions are characterized by fluorescent-labeled antibody bind to unlabeled antigen. This test is used to detect antigen in histologic sections or tissue specimen.

Answer D is incorrect. Agglutination reactions are characterized by antibody cross-linking with particulate antigen. This test is used in ABO blood typing.

160. **The correct answer is D.** TH-2 cells signal B cells to differentiate into plasma cells. T cells are lymphocytes which differentiate in the thymus. They have a long life span which ranges from months to years.

Answer A is incorrect. TH-2 cells function to signal B cells. They secrete the cytokines IL-4 and IL-5.

Answer B is incorrect. CD8 cells (also called TC cells) function to kill virus-infected, tumor, and allograft cells. They respond to MHC I receptors. TH-1 cells signal CD8 and macrophages. They also secrete IL-2 and INF-γ.

Microbiology and Pathology

Answer C is incorrect. Memory T cells function by responding to reexposure of antigen.

Answer E is incorrect. CD4 cells (also called TH cells) function by responding to antigen associated with MHC II.

Note that T cells also have a CD3-associated T-cell receptors which recognize antigen only in conjunction with MHC proteins.

161. **The correct answer is C.** Skeletal muscle does not exhibit tissue regeneration. Tissue regeneration is a concept in which a tissue or organ may restore itself by way of an adaptive mechanism. This can occur at many tissue levels: liver, bone, cartilage, intestinal mucosa, and surface epithelium are all capable of regeneration. There are also some tissues that cannot regenerate, including: skeletal muscle, cardiac muscle, and neurons. For example, the regenerative capacity of the liver makes it a very uncommon site for infarction.

Answers A, B, D, and E are incorrect. Tissue regeneration occurs with liver, cartilage, bone, and intestinal mucosa tissues.

162. **The correct answer is A.** One function of histamine is to cause vasodilation. Histamine is a molecule which functions generally as an inflammatory mediator.

Answer B is incorrect. The bronchial response to histamine causes broncho-constriction.

Answer C is incorrect. Histamine also activates a type I hypersensitivity response (involving in anaphylaxis).

Answer D is incorrect. Histamine is secreted by mast cells and basophils.

Answer E is incorrect. Histamine does not activate complement. It binds to receptors to cause its cell-specific reaction.

Note that histamine is derived from the amino acid histidine.

163. **The correct answer is C.** Nitric oxide is not derived from histidine. Rather, it is derived from arginine. The major inflammatory mediators of the body have numerous specific responses, but in general they cause changes in vascular permeability, pain, inflammatory mediation, immunological mediation, and tissue damage.

Answer A is incorrect. Serotonin is derived from the amino acid, tryptophan.

Answer B is incorrect. Complement protein is derived from hepatocytes.

Answer D is incorrect. Bradykinin is derived from its proform, kininogen.

Answer E is incorrect. Leukotrienes are derived from the cell-membrane molecule, arachidonic acid.

164. **The correct answer is B.** Fibroblasts do not secrete TGF-β. TGF-β is an important inflammatory cytokine. Cytokines are small peptides secreted by many cell types and are involved in host defense and immunity. It is secreted by many cells, including monocytes, macrophages, T cells, and B cells. Its function is to inhibit T cells, B cells, PMNs, monocytes, macrophages, and NK cells. TGF-β also stimulates collagen formation and wound healing.

Answer A is incorrect. Monocytes secrete TGF-β. TGF-β is known as the anticytokine.

Answer C is incorrect. T cells secrete TGF-β.

Answer D is incorrect. B cells secrete TGF-β.

Answer E is incorrect. Macrophages secrete TGF-β.

165. **The correct answer is D.** vasodilation is not part of the cellular stage of acute inflammation. Acute inflammation is the initial response to tissue injury and it consists largely of leukocyte infiltration ridding of bacteria and necrotic tissue. There are two main stages: vascular and cellular. The vascular stage is mediated by histamine-producing cells (including mast cells, basophils, and platelets).

An exudative edem (straw-colored, protein-rich exudates of extravascular fluid) is clinically evident.

Answer A is incorrect. Diapedesis is part of the cellular stage of acute inflammation. It is a part of the cellular stage.

Answer B is incorrect. Margination is part of the cellular stage of acute inflammation. It is a part of the cellular stage. Phagocytosis and leukocyte degranulation lead to microbial cell lysis as well as host tissue damage.

Answer C is incorrect. Chemotaxis is part of the cellular stage of acute inflammation. It is a part of the cellular stage. Mostly PMNs are activated toward the site of injury.

Answer E is incorrect. Adhesion is part of the cellular stage of acute inflammation. It is a part of the cellular stage.

166. **The correct answer is B.** Subgingival plaque is not affected by diet and saliva.

Answer A is incorrect. Supragingival plague is located at or coronal to the gingival margin. Subgingival plaque is located apical to the gingival margin.

Answer C is incorrect. Supragingival is comprised mostly of gram-positive facultative cocci. Subgingival plaque is largely comprised of gram-negative anaerobic bacilli and spirochetes.

Answer D is incorrect. Supragingival plaque is affected by diet and saliva. Subgingival plaque is not affected by diet and saliva.

Answer E is incorrect. Supragingival plaque is found attached to gingival epithelial and tooth surfaces, as well as loosely adherent to intraoral structures.

167. **The correct answer is C.** The host cell is not destroyed in the lysogenic cycle of bacteriophage activity.

Answer A is incorrect. There are two pathways of bacteriophage replication: the lytic and lysogenic cycles.

Answer B is incorrect. The lysogenic cycle includes a prophage. It does this by incorporation of their DNA into the host-cell chromosome. The host cell is kept vital.

Answer D is incorrect. Bacteriophages are viruses. They infect bacterial cells.

Answer E is incorrect. Viral DNA is incorporated into the host-cell chromosome in the lysogenic cycle. This integrated DNA is termed a prophage and it is replicated when host DNA is damaged.

Note that the lytic cycle of virus replication states that the process by which a phage replicates within the host cell is via production of hundreds of new progeny phage. The host cell is eventually destroyed.

168. **The correct answer is A.** Infectious mononucleosis cannot be prevented with a vaccine. This disease is self-limiting, typically lasting anywhere from 2 to 3 weeks.

Answer B is incorrect. Primary varicella (varicella zoster virus) has a vaccine for its prevention. This virus can cause the following: chickenpox, macular lesions, and is sometimes associated with Reye syndrome.

Answer C is incorrect. Smallpox (variola virus) has a vaccine for its prevention.

Answer D is incorrect. Hepatitis B (hepadnavirus) has a vaccine for its prevention.

Answer E is incorrect. Hepatocellular carcinoma (hepadnavirus) has a vaccine for its prevention.

169. **The correct answer is A.** Human immunodeficiency virus does not contain only one strand of RNA; rather, it contains two strands. HIV is of the retrovirus family. It is a single, linear RNA virus. There are two viruses associated with this family, HTLV (adult T-cell leukemia, chronic progressive myelopathy) and HIV (AIDS).

Answer B is incorrect. gp120 protein mediates attachment to CD4 molecules.

Answer C is incorrect. gp41 protein mediates fusion to the host cell.

Answer D is incorrect. p24 and p7 proteins combine to form the nucleocapsid.

Answer E is incorrect. HIV contains reverse transcriptase. It uses this to replicate within the nucleus of a host cell.

Microbiology and Pathology

170. **The correct answer is B.** Cephalosporins contain beta lactam rings.

    Answer A is incorrect. Cephalosporins function by inhibition of peptidoglycan cross-linking via blockage of transpeptidase during the last stage of cell-wall synthesis.

    Answer C is incorrect. These antibiotics are bacteriocidal.

    Answer D is incorrect. There are currently four generations of this drug: first (narrow spectrum: gram-positive cocci and some gram-negative bacilli), second (broader spectrum: fewer gram-positive cocci and more gram-negative bacilli), third (broader spectrum: fewer gram-positive cocci and more gram-negative bacilli, anaerobes), and fourth (broader spectrum: fewer gram-positive cocci and more gram-negative bacilli, anaerobes).

    Answer E is incorrect. They contain beta lactam rings in their formulation. Thus, cephalosporins have a 10% cross-hypersensitivity with penicillins.

171. **The correct answer is E.** Infection by *H. influenzae* does not cause enterocolitis. This disease is caused by such bacteria as *Salmonella*, *Shigella*, and *Campylobacter* (all referred to as enteric bacilli). *Haemophilus influenzae* is a gram-negative, "respiratory" bacilli. It is a facultative anaerobe and it produces endotoxin as its major virulence factor.

    Answer A is incorrect. Otitis media is a disease caused by *H. influenzae*. It is an infection of the middle ear.

    Answer B is incorrect. Epiglottitis media is a disease caused by *H. influenzae*. It is an infection of the throat.

    Answer C is incorrect. Meningitis in children. Otitis media is a disease caused by *H. influenzae*. This is an infection of the meninges of the brain.

    Answer D is incorrect. Upper respiratory tract infection, Otitis media is a disease caused by *H. influenzae*.

172. **The correct answer is A.** This patient is most likely afflicted with osteomalacia. Osteomalacia is a disease of the bones which is due to bone softening secondary to decreased vitamin D. Thus, the osteoid matrix does not calcify without vitamin D. Radiologic findings include diffuse radiolucency which mimics osteoporosis. In order to diagnose, lab values are important as it is difficult to distinguish osteoporosis from osteomalacia on bone biopsy. There is a predilection for females with this disease.

    Answer B is incorrect. Paget disease is seen clinically with odd-shaped, abnormal, enlarged bones.

    Answer C is incorrect. Fibrous dysplasia is seen clinically only in certain instances. If bone of the head and neck region is involved, one may see bone which is enlarging due to tumor growth within the medullary spaces.

    Answer D is incorrect. Osteoporosis is seen clinically with weakened, brittle bones causing weakness and an increased predilection for fracture.

    Answer E is incorrect. Osteitis fibrosa cystica is seen clinically with painful bones and possible pathologic fractures.

173. **The correct answer is C.** Increased phosphate intake is not a cause of vitamin D deficiency. The opposite is true. Vitamin D deficiency can lead to numerous diseases of the bone including osteoporosis and osteomalacia.

    Answer A is incorrect. Vitamin D deficiency can be caused by decreased dietary intake of the vitamin.

    Answer B is incorrect. Vitamin D deficiency can be caused by decreased absorption of the vitamin.

    Answer D is incorrect. Vitamin D deficiency can be caused by decreased sunlight exposure.

    Answer E is incorrect. Vitamin D deficiency can be caused by kidney failure.

    Note that there are other reasons for vitamin D deficiency: hereditary or acquired disorders of vitamin D metabolism, acidosis, and medication side effects.

174. **The correct answer is A.** The laboratory findings of anemia, increased alkaline phosphatase, and increased urinary hydroxyproline indicate that Paget disease is present. Paget disease is a metabolic bone disease (referred to as osteitis deformans) which occurs mostly in the elderly. The etiology of this disease is unknown, although it is believed to be associated with viral infection such as mumps, measles, and paramyxovirus. There is also a genetic component. It is characterized by cycles of bone destruction and regrowth of abnormal bone (which is enlarged and weakened). Its presentation is widespread and it will localize to one or two areas of the skeleton. Dealing with the head and neck, there is increased skull size, cranial nerve foramina constriction, and teeth displacement. Lab findings show anemia, increased alkaline phosphatase (marker of osteoblastic activity), and increased urinary hydroxyproline (marker of osteoclastic activity). These patients have an increased risk of osteosarcomas.

Answer B is incorrect. Fibrous dysplasia has lab values showing a decrease in phosphorus levels, and increased calcium and alkaline phosphate. These alone are not diagnostic.

Answer C is incorrect. Osteoporosis may have lab values showing low calcium levels, although these alone are not diagnostic.

Answer D is incorrect. Osteochondrosis has lab values which are not of diagnostic value. This disease is caused by a decrease in blood supply to bone. Thus, a cycle of necrosis, regeneration, and reossification occurs.

Answer E is incorrect. Osteopetrosis has lab values of increased acid and alkaline phosphatase levels. This alone is not diagnostic, though. One must also view imaging studies to search for osteosclerosis.

175. **The correct answer is D.** Complete fractures occur when a bone is broken into two distinct segments. In general, a fracture is a break in bone. It is the most common bone lesion and occurs when force exerted overcomes bone strength.

Answer A is incorrect. A greenstick fracture is when bone is broken only on one side. It is not through and through.

Answer B is incorrect. A comminuted fracture is when bone is crushed into two or more pieces.

Answer C is incorrect. An open fracture is when bone breaks and pierces the skin.

Answer E is incorrect. A single fracture is when bone is broken in one place.

Note that there is another term to define fracture classification: bending (no break). Bone then heals in three phases after fracture: inflammatory (formation of blood clot), reparative (formation of cartilage callus → replaced by bony callus), and remodeling (cortex is revitalized). A nonunion is a fracture which fails to heal, whereas a malunion is a bone which heals in an abnormal position.

176. **The correct answer is C.** This patient has Alzheimer disease. Alzheimer is a disease characterized as being neurodegenerative due to amyloid plaques and neurofibrillary tangles. Common symptoms include dementia seen in the elderly.

Answer A is incorrect. Multiple sclerosis, a demyelinating disease, is due to damage of white matter and symptoms of visual changes, hemisensory findings, and loss of bladder control.

Answer B is incorrect. Myasthenia gravis is a neuromuscular disease characterized by weakness of voluntary muscles due to an autoimmune attack of postsynaptic receptors in neuromuscular junctions.

Answer D is incorrect. Parkinson disease is a neurodegenerative disease caused by Lewy bodies and depigmentation of the substantia nigra.

Answer E is incorrect. Eaton-Lambert syndrome has the same symptoms as myasthenia gravis but it is not autoimmune (rather, it is caused by a decrease in acetylcholine).

Microbiology and Pathology

177. **The correct answer is B.** Dementia is not part of the triad of symptoms seen with multiple sclerosis. Multiple sclerosis is a demyelinating disease of autoimmune etiology.

Answer A is incorrect. Scanning speech is part of the clinical triad seen clinically with multiple sclerosis.

Answer C is incorrect. Intention tremor is part of the clinical triad seen clinically with multiple sclerosis.

Answer D is incorrect. Nystagmus is part of the clinical triad seen clinically with multiple sclerosis.

Note that these symptoms are due to a decrease or block in nerve transmission and it usually begins at age 20-40 and has a predilection for females. Lab findings include an increase in IgG in cerebrospinal fluid. Intravenous interferon can decrease the frequency of relapses.

178. **The correct answer is D.** Sudden paralysis and numbness of the body on the ipsilateral side of the stroke is not common: these symptoms are seen on the contralateral side of the stroke.

Answer A is incorrect. A stroke is due to an infarction of the cerebrum or another part of the brain.

Answer B is incorrect. It is caused by arterial occlusion to and/or in the brain. This occlusion is caused by thrombus or embolism and hemorrhage/brain bleed.

Answer C is incorrect. Symptoms depend on the area of the brain affected. They often include hemiparesis and numbness on the side of the body opposite the stroke.

Answer E is incorrect. Hemorrhage of the brain can cause a stroke. This is due to ischemia secondary to blood loss.

179. **The correct answer is A.** Alzheimer disease is not characterized by the presence of Lewy bodies. Patients stricken with Alzheimer disease show the presence of amyloid plaques and neurofibrillary tangles.

Answer B is incorrect. Lewy bodies are seen with Parkinson disease.

Answer C is incorrect. Werdnig-Hoffman disease is neurodegenerative disease seen with floppy babies (clinically, one would find a patient with tongue fasciculations, as well).

Answer D is incorrect. Poliomyelitis is a lower motor neuron disease.

Answer E is incorrect. Huntingdon disease is an autosomal dominant disease with symptoms of chorea and dementia.

180. **The correct answer is B.** A myxoma is not a malignant tumor derived from connective tissue. It is, in fact, derived from connective tissue but is a benign disease. The other tumors listed in the question are all benign.

Answer A is incorrect. The choristoma is a small benign nonneoplastic mass of normal tissue misplaced within another organ (ie, pancreatic tissue in the stomach wall).

Answer C is incorrect. A teratoma is a neoplasm comprised of all three embryonic germ cell layers (it MAY become malignant, though).

Answer D is incorrect. Adenomas are benign neoplasm of glandular epithelium of several variants: papillary cystadenoma (adenomatous papillary processes extending into cystic spaces) and fibroadenoma (proliferating connective tissue surrounding neoplastic glandular epithelium).

Answer E is incorrect. A papilloma is a benign tumor of surface epithelium.

181. **The correct answer is A.** Ultraviolet light does not produce free radicals that can attack DNA bases. This is actually the definition of ionizing radiation (form gamma and x-rays). Ultraviolet light causes cross-linking of adjacent pyrimidine bases, and viruses cause frameshift mutations of deletions.

Answer B is incorrect. Dimers (eg, thymine dimers) interfere with DNA replication.

Answer C is incorrect. Chemicals (nitrous oxide, alkylating agents, benzpyrene) alter existing bases and bind existing DNA bases to cause frameshifts.

Answer D is incorrect. Viruses cause frameshift deletions.

182. **The correct answer is D.** Breast cancer is characterized clinically by peau d'orange (swollen, pitted surface on breast) and enlarged axillary lymph nodes. This neoplasm is the most common cancer in women. It usually does not affect women until they have reached menopause. There is a strong genetic component of the disease and it is due to mutation of the BRCA-1 and BRCA-2 genes. Other clinical symptoms include a painless mass in the breast and skin/nipple retraction. The left breast is more often affected. Metastasis and spread goes to the chest wall, axillary nodes, and other distant sites (other breast, liver, bone, brain). Histologically, the appearance is that of adenocarcinoma and the prognosis is made based on the nodal involvement.

Answer A is incorrect. The clinical signs of squamous cell carcinoma are totally dependent on the area of concern. For example, sites on the skin may have unusual, nonhealing areas which are growing and/or changing appearance.

Answer B is incorrect. The clinical signs of lung cancer are coughing, dyspnea, hemoptysis, chest pain, and wheezing.

Answer C is incorrect. The clinical signs of colorectal cancer are changes in stool appearance and/or consistency, as well as anorexia and malaise.

Answer E is incorrect. The clinical signs of uterine cancer are unusual bleeding and pain in the pelvic region.

183. **The correct answer is C.** Nerve cells have the lowest radiosensitivity. This concept is based on a cell's rate of proliferation: the higher the rate of proliferation, the more sensitive the cell is to radiation. Thus, with an increased rate of mutagenesis comes an increase in the response to radiation therapy.

Answer A is incorrect. Lymphocytes have a high cell turnover. Thus, they have an increased radiosensitivity.

Answer B is incorrect. Reproductive cells have a high turnover. Thus, they have an increased radiosensitivity.

Answer D is incorrect. Epithelial cells have a high turnover. Thus, they have an increased radiosensitivity.

Answer E is incorrect. Bone marrow cells have high turnover. Thus, they have an increased radiosensitivity.

Note that cells with low turnover and thus low radiosensitivity include: nerve cells, mature bone cells, and muscle cells.

184. **The correct answer is B.** A medulloblastoma is a highly malignant cerebellar tumor that is also of primitive neuroectodermal origin. This type of tumor occurs in children.

Answer A is incorrect. Glioblastoma multiforme occurs in adults. It is the most common primary brain tumor in humans.

Answer C is incorrect. A low-grade astrocytoma occurs in children. It occurs in the posterior cranial fossa.

Answer D is incorrect. A craniopharyngioma occurs in children. It is a benign tumor, and can cause bitemporal hemianopia. It is derived from Rathke pouch.

Answer E is incorrect. An ependymoma is a tumor which occurs in children. This happens, often, in the 4th ventricle, can cause hydrocephalus.

Note these other tumors which occur in humans: meningioma (adults: 2nd most common primary brain tumor, arises from arachnoid) and pituitary adenoma (adults: usually secrete prolactin, can present as bitemporal hemianopia).

185. **The correct answer is C.** The cancer with the highest incidence in men is prostate

cancer. It is the 2nd highest cause of cancer death in men.

Answer A is incorrect. Colorectal cancer has the 2nd highest incidence of cancer in men. It also has the 3rd highest cause of cancer death in men.

Answer B is incorrect. Urinary tract cancer has the 4th highest incidence of cancer in men.

Answer D is incorrect. Lung cancer has the 2nd highest incidence of cancer in men. It is the highest cause of cancer death in men.

Answer E is incorrect. Leukemia has the 4th highest cause of cancer death in men.

Note: The cause of prostate cancer is unknown, although it is possibly due to an increase in testosterone (increase in dietary fat leads to increased testosterone). Laboratory findings include an increase in prostate-specific antigen (PSA) and increased acid phosphatase. Histologically, it mimics adenocarcinoma and its common sites of metastasis include bones and lungs.

186. **The correct answer is B.** This patient most likely has basal cell carcinoma. This type of neoplasm is the most common skin cancer (75% of all skin cancers) and is the most common form of all cancers in the United States. It is derived from basal cells of the epidermis. Clinically, most occur on sun-exposed areas of the head and neck. It appears as a pearly papule with overlying telangiectatic vessels. Basal cell carcinoma is locally aggressive, invasive, and destructive. It ulcerates, bleeds, and appears nonhealing. The histology shows darkly staining basaloid cells with a typical palisade arrangement of nuclei at the periphery of tumor cell clusters. The prognosis is good when treated early.

Answer A is incorrect. Dermatofibroma presents clinically with benign skin lumps on the body. There is a predilection for the legs.

Answer C is incorrect. Squamous cell carcinoma presents with many different clinical presentations, depending on the part of the body affected.

Answer D is incorrect. Actinic keratosis presents clinically with scaly, crust-ridden, thicker than normal skin. It is premalignant.

Answer E is incorrect. Melanoma presents clinically with lesion that is asymmetric, has ragged borders, an odd color, and a larger diameter.

187. **The correct answer is A.** Of the listed neoplasms, pigmented nevus is the only one that is benign. The other cancers are all malignant. Pigmented nevus is a benign neoplasm, which presents in four forms: nevocellular (common mole: hamartoma, cluster of nevus cells derived from melanocytes), junctional (confined to epidermal-dermal junction), compound (occurs at epidermal-dermal junction and in the dermis), and intradermal (within the dermis and often not pigmented).

Answer B is incorrect. Squamous cell carcinoma presents with symptoms that are totally dependent on the area affected.

Answer C is incorrect. Melanoma presents with a lesion that has atypical shape, irregular borders, multiple colors, and a large diameter.

Answer D is incorrect. Keratocanthoma presents with a lesion which is usually solitary, firm, round, skin-colored, and it rapidly progresses to a dome-shaped nodule.

188. **The correct answer is C.** Squamous cell carcinoma of the skin is not normally treated with chemotherapy. Treatment is excision and sometimes radiation therapy. This type of cancer is malignant and of epithelial origin. It is more aggressive than basal cell carcinoma and the mean age is 50 years old.

Answer A is incorrect. Histologically, there are sheets and islands of neoplastic epidermal cells in the middle of the epidermis, as well as keratin pearls.

Answer B is incorrect. These malignant cells have increased laminin receptors.

Answer D is incorrect. Causes include the sun, radiation, x-ray exposure, and chemical carcinogens.

Answer E is incorrect. Clinically, it may appear as normal skin, damaged skin (burn, scar, chronic inflammation), or sun-damaged skin (face, dorsal hands). The lesion is scaling, indurated, ulcerated, and painless initially. Squamous cell carcinoma is locally invasive and metastasizes to nodes and organs.

189. **The correct answer is E.** Regarding melanoma of the skin, the initial phase of growth is not vertical. The histology shows growth phases that begin in a radial phase (no metastasis, lateral spread, characteristic of the "spreading" types of melanoma) and subsequent vertical phase (into reticular dermis or deeper, metastasis possible, depth of growth determines prognosis, and this type is characteristic of nodular melanoma).

Answer A is incorrect. It is a malignant tumor of melanocytes or nevus cells and has a high incidence. Causes are sunlight (specifically, sunburns at an early age).

Answer B is incorrect. The most common form of melanoma of the skin is the superficial spreading type.

Answer C is incorrect. Melanoma is the most deadly form of skin cancer. It is most common in fair-skinned persons or those with blue/green eyes and red/blonde hair.

Answer D is incorrect. The clinical course may include very rapid spread. Melanoma of the skin occurs in many forms. It may appear on what were normal skin, a mole, and other skin area that has changed appearance.

190. **The correct answer is A.** Ewing sarcoma is a disease in which histology alone is not specific for diagnostic purposes.

Answer B is incorrect. Ewing sarcoma is highly radiosensitive.

Answer C is incorrect. This form of cancer typically afflicts children aged 10-20 years old.

Answer D is incorrect. This cancer originates in the bone marrow and invades long and flat bones such as the femur, tibia, fibula, and humerus, as well as the pelvis, ribs, skull, vertebra, and facial bones. Symptoms are few,

sometimes with increasing pain with time. One-third of children have metastasis at time of diagnosis.

Answer E is incorrect. Ewing sarcoma is a nonosseous malignant bone tumor.

191. **The correct answer is E.** Type I hypersensitivity reaction is not a possible cause of disseminated intravascular coagulation. This condition is life threatening and involves uncontrolled, cyclic bleeding and clotting throughout the body. There is extensive microclot formation and the bleeding accompanies fibrinolysis (thus increased fibrin split products/D-dimers → important indicators of DIC). Lab findings include decreased platelet count, increased PT and PTT, hypofibrinogenemia, and decreased levels of all clotting factors and fibrinolytic proteins.

Answer A is incorrect. Major trauma is a possible cause of disseminated intravascular coagulation.

Answer B is incorrect. Malignancy is a possible cause of disseminated intravascular coagulation.

Answer C is incorrect. Gram-negative sepsis is a possible cause of disseminated intravascular coagulation.

Answer D is incorrect. Amniotic fluid embolism is a possible cause of disseminated intravascular coagulation.

192. **The correct answer is C.** Iron deficiency does not result in macrocytic anemia. Iron deficiency leads to a form of anemia called hypochromic microcytic (pale, small RBCs).

Answer A is incorrect. Chronic blood loss can cause iron deficiency, thus leading to a form of anemia.

Answer B is incorrect. Clinical findings of iron deficiency include pallor, fatigue, shortness of breath, glossitis, and koilonychias.

Answer D is incorrect. Iron deficiency can lead to Plummer-Vinson syndrome. This is iron-deficiency anemia due to upper esophageal webbing.

Answer E is incorrect. Iron deficiency can be caused by a poor diet.

193. **The correct answer is B.** Duodenal resection would not cause vitamin B_{12} deficiency.

    Answer A is incorrect. Pernicious anemia is caused by decreased intrinsic factor. This is due to autoimmune gastritis.

    Answer C is incorrect. Gastric resection is the removal of cells producing intrinsic factor, thus, parietal cells.

    Answer D is incorrect. Dietary deficiency of B_{12} is commonly seen in strict vegetarians.
    Note that ileal resection (removal of intestinal cells that absorb B_{12}) can cause anemia. This type of deficiency results in megaloblastic anemia. Patients would have an abnormal Schilling test, fatigue, shortness of breath, tingling sensations, difficulty walking, and diarrhea.

194. **The correct answer is E.** Proteinuria would be seen with nephrotic syndrome. This type of kidney disorder is due to inflammation affecting the glomeruli. This inflammation leads to numerous types of glomerulonephropathies (rapidly progressive nephritic syndrome, nephrotic syndrome, chronic nephritic syndrome). Nephrotic syndrome can occur at any age and is characterized by proteinuria, hypoalbuminemia, hyperlipidemia, and edema. The specific cause of these symptoms is increased glomerular capillary permeability, thus leading to decreased blood protein and increased protein in the urine. This syndrome is associated with many diseases and the clinical symptoms are vast, including loss of appetite, malaise, puffy eyelids, abdominal pain, frothy urine, muscle wasting, and tissue edema.

    Answer A is incorrect. Hypoalbuminemia is a common lab finding seen with nephrotic syndrome. It is characterized by a decrease of the protein-carrier albumin in the blood.

    Answer B is incorrect. Hyperlipidemia is a common lab finding seen with nephrotic syndrome. It is characterized by an increase of lipids in the blood.

    Answer C is incorrect. Hypercholesterolemia is a common lab finding seen with nephrotic syndrome. It is characterized by an increase of cholesterol in the blood.

    Answer D is incorrect. The renal glomeruli are not function properly with nephrotic syndrome. Thus, filtration is malfunctioning.

195. **The correct answer is B.** Rubella infections are largely associated with lymphocytosis.

    Answer A is incorrect. Giardia is a parasite. Thus, they would be associated with eosinophilia.

    Answer C is incorrect. Fever is a common systemic response to infection.

    Answer D is incorrect. Leukocytosis is a common result of bacterial, parasitic, and viral infection. The systemic effects of inflammation can be generalized by three types of leukocytosis: neutrophilia, eosinophilia, and lymphocytosis.

    Answer E is incorrect. Clostridium is a bacterium. Thus, it is largely associated with neutrophilia.
    Note that these responses are based on the type of offending organism within the body. Bacterial infections are associated with neutrophilia, parasitic infections are associated with eosinophilia, and viral infections are associated with lymphocytosis. Fever also occurs with most of these types of leukocytosis.

196. **The correct answer is B.** Regarding edema, there is an increase in interstitial fluid colloid osmotic pressure. Edema is an abnormal accumulation of fluid in interstitial spaces of body cavities.

    Answer A is incorrect. There is an increase in capillary permeability seen with tissue edema.

    Answer C is incorrect. There is an increase in plasma colloid osmotic pressure seen with tissue edema.

    Answer D is incorrect. There is an increase in capillary hydrostatic pressure seen with tissue edema.

Answer E is incorrect. Fluid tends to move out of the intravascular space in instances of tissue edema.

Note that there are two main types of edema: transudative (more watery/serious, noninflammatory, due to altered intravascular hydrostatic or osmotic pressure) and exudative (more protein-rich, inflammatory, due to increased vascular permeability with inflammation).

197. The correct answer is A. There is a decrease in urinary output in patients suffering from systemic shock. Shock is a condition due to decreased tissue perfusion.

Answer B is incorrect. Patients experiencing shock become hypotensive. This is typically due to a loss of blood.

Answer C is incorrect. There is a decrease in blood flow in patients that are undergoing shock.

Answer D is incorrect. There is a decrease in cardiac output in patients experiencing shock. This is primarily due to a decrease in stroke volume, and secondarily due to hypovolemia.

Answer E is incorrect. There is a decrease in stroke volume in patients experiencing shock. This is due to hypovolemia.

Note: There are hemodynamic changes which result in decreased blood flow and thus decreased oxygen and metabolic supply to tissues. The end outcome is multiple organ damage or failure. Symptoms include fatigue and confusion. Signs are pallor, thready pulse, hypotension, and decreased urine output. Immediate medical treatment is necessary.

198. The correct answer is E. Portal hypertension does not lead to cirrhosis. It is a result of cirrhosis, though. Cirrhosis is the most common chronic liver disease characterized by scarring/fibrosis, loss of architecture, and formation of regenerative nodules.

Answer A is incorrect. Hemochromatosis can lead to cirrhosis of the liver.

Answer B is incorrect. Biliary obstruction can lead to cirrhosis of the liver.

Answer C is incorrect. Wilson disease can lead to cirrhosis of the liver.

Answer D is incorrect. Viral hepatitis can lead to cirrhosis of the liver.

Note that alcoholism (most common → 75%) and inborn errors of metabolism can also lead to cirrhosis of the liver. Clinically, the patient would be suffering from ascites, splenomegaly, jaundice, coagulopathy, confusion/hepatic encephalopathy, portal hypertension, and esophageal varices.

199. The correct answer is C. There is not a decrease in unconjugated bilirubin in the blood in patients with hemolytic anemia. Hemolytic anemia is a blood disorder characterized by decrease in red blood cell life span and thus increased red blood cell destruction. There is hyperbilirubinemia and hemoglobinemia.

Answer A is incorrect. Bilirubin, the breakdown product of hemoglobin, is increased in its unconjugated form (which is water insoluble) leading to jaundice. This leads to yellow under the tongue and yellow sclera, the first clinical sign of the disease.

Answer B is incorrect. Hyperbilirubinemia is a common laboratory finding in patients with hemolytic anemia. This is due to increased red blood cell breakdown.

Answer D is incorrect. Conjugated bilirubin forms from albumin and unconjugated bilirubin.

Answer E is incorrect. The pathophysiology includes broken down red blood cells in which hemoglobin is liberated and found in the urine and blood. Thus, hemoglobinuria is a common laboratory finding.

Note that the autoimmune form of this anemia is due to IgG antibodies combining with red blood cell surface antigen. This is diagnosed with a positive direct Coombs test.

200. The correct answer is E. Patients with sickle-cell trait are heterozygotic for the disease. Sickle-cell anemia is a disease of primarily African Americans. It is inherited autosomal recessive (Hb-S from both parents) resulting

Microbiology and Pathology

in an abnormal type of hemoglobin. The globin portion has a valine substituted for glutamic acid in the sixth position.

Answer A is incorrect. The heterozygotic form is termed sickle cell trait, and is less severe. The homozygotic version is sickle cell disease, and is more severe.

Answer B is incorrect. The spleen is often affected. This is due to sickled red blood cells becoming entrapped within the spleen.

Answer C is incorrect. African Americans are most commonly affected by sickle cell anemia.

Answer D is incorrect. It is an inherited autosomal recessive disease.

Note: This form of anemia deals with sickled red blood cells, thus, hemoglobin instability when exposed to stress. This results in hypoxic conditions (decreased oxygen). There are four types of crises which can occur because of this: sickle-cell pain crisis (formation of small blood clots), hemolytic crisis (life-threatening breakdown of damaged RBCs), splenic sequestration crisis (enlarged spleen due to trapping of sickled RBCs), and aplastic crisis (infection causes bone marrow to stop producing RBCs). Repeated bouts of sickle cell crises can damage the kidneys, lungs, bones, eyes, and the CNS.

CHAPTER 4

Dental Anatomy and Occlusion

1. Which feature allows one to distinguish between the permanent mandibular lateral incisor and the permanent mandibular central incisor from an occlusal view?

   A. A decreased mesiodistal length of the lateral incisor.
   B. The cingulum location is slightly distal of center on the central incisor.
   C. The distolingual twist of the lateral incisor's incisal edge.
   D. The incisal edge of central incisor is lingual to the root axis line.

2. How many cusp tips can be seen on a mandibular 1st molar when viewed directly from the buccal?

   A. 2
   B. 3
   C. 4
   D. 5

3. All of the following are true regarding the curve of Spee EXCEPT

   A. the curve in the lower arch is concave.
   B. the curve in the upper arch is convex.
   C. the curve is formed by the lingual inclination of the mandibular molars.
   D. the curve is directed anteroposteriorly.

4. Which tooth has the most prominent lingual ridge with mesial and distal fossae?

   A. Maxillary central incisor
   B. Mandibular lateral incisor
   C. Maxillary lateral incisor
   D. Mandibular canine
   E. Maxillary canine

5. On a maxillary molar the palatal root is the longest of the three roots. Among all maxillary teeth, the palatal root of the maxillary 1st molar is the 3rd longest root.

   A. Both statements are true.
   B. Both statements are false.

C. The first statement is true; the second is false.
D. The first statement is false; the second is true.

6. All of the following muscles involved in mastication are innervated by the mandibular branch of trigeminal nerve EXCEPT

   A. temporalis.
   B. masseter.
   C. buccinator.
   D. medial pterygoid.
   E. lateral pterygoid.

7. The horizontal distance between the labioincisal surfaces of mandibular incisors and the linguoincisal surfaces of maxillary teeth is referred to as

   A. overjet.
   B. overbite.
   C. openbite.
   D. crossbite.

8. The primary mandibular 2nd molar most closely resembles which permanent tooth?

   A. Mandibular 1st molar
   B. Mandibular 2nd molar
   C. Maxillary 1st molar
   D. Maxillary 2nd molar

9. The primary teeth erupt in which of the following sequences?

   A. ABCDE
   B. BACDE
   C. ABDCE
   D. ACBDE

10. A triangular outline form is present on which of the following teeth when viewed from the proximal aspect?

   A. Mandibular 1st premolar
   B. Maxillary 1st molar
   C. Mandibular central incisor
   D. Mandibular 1st molar

11. A patient presents to your office with what appears to be five mandibular incisors. However, upon radiographic examination, you count four roots. The most likely explanation for this finding is

    A. concrescence.
    B. hypercementosis.
    C. fusion.
    D. gemination.
    E. fibrous dysplasia.

12. Angle classification of occlusion is based primarily on

    A. the relationship between the maxillary and mandibular anterior teeth.
    B. the position of the maxillary canines.
    C. the relationship between the maxillary and mandibular 1st molars.
    D. the amount of anterior overjet.

13. Primary teeth are more constricted at the cervical 3rd than their permanent counterparts. Pulp chambers are comparatively smaller in primary teeth.

    A. Both statements are true.
    B. Both statements are false.
    C. The first statement is true; the second is false.
    D. The first statement is false; the second is true.

14. Which of the following premolars does not have a transverse ridge?

    A. Maxillary 1st premolar
    B. Maxillary 2nd premolar
    C. Mandibular 1st premolar
    D. Mandibular 2nd premolar (2-cusp type)
    E. Mandibular 2nd premolar (3-cusp type)

15. When the mandible shifts to the left, the right condylar head moves in which direction relative to articular eminence?

    A. Anteriorly, downward, laterally
    B. Anteriorly, downward, medially
    C. Anteriorly, upward, laterally
    D. Anteriorly, upward, medially
    E. Posteriorly, upward, laterally

16. Which tooth has a mesial marginal ridge that is more cervically located than the distal marginal ridge?

    A. Maxillary 1st premolar
    B. Maxillary 2nd premolar
    C. Mandibular 1st premolar
    D. Mandibular 2nd premolar

17. In an ideal occlusion, the lingual cusp of the permanent maxillary 1st premolar occludes where?

    A. Mesial triangular fossa of the mandibular 1st premolar
    B. Distal triangular fossa of the mandibular 1st premolar
    C. Distal marginal ridge of the mandibular 1st premolar
    D. Mesial marginal ridge of the mandibular 2nd premolar
    E. Mesial triangular fossa of the mandibular 2nd premolar

18. Of the mandibular premolars, the 1st premolar has the longest and sharpest buccal cusp. Among maxillary premolars, the 2nd premolar has the longest and sharpest buccal cusp.

    A. Both statements are true.
    B. Both statements are false.
    C. The first statement is true; the second is false.
    D. The first statement is false; the second is true.

19. All of the following are true regarding primary molars in comparison to permanent molars EXCEPT

    A. primary teeth have roots that are longer, more slender, and highly divergent.
    B. primary molars have a much more pronounced buccal cervical ridge.
    C. deciduous enamel is thinner, and has a more consistent depth throughout the crown.
    D. primary molars have shorter root trunks.
    E. primary molars have well-defined occlusal anatomy with pronounced ridges and deep fossae.

20. How many premolars are found in each quadrant of a normal deciduous dentition?

    A. 0
    B. 1
    C. 2
    D. 3
    E. 4

21. Which of the following are supporting cusps?

    A. Distobuccal cusp of maxillary 1st molars
    B. Lingual cusp of mandibular 2nd premolars
    C. Mesiolingual cusp of maxillary 1st molars
    D. Distolingual cusp of mandibular 1st molars

22. Which of the following is TRUE of individuals with anodontia?

    A. They have additional or supernumerary teeth.
    B. They have congenitally missing teeth.
    C. They have additional maxillary and mandibular incisors.
    D. They have all teeth shaped as incisors.
    E. None of the above.

23. The *primary* sensory innervation of the TMJ arises from what cranial nerve?

    A. CN V
    B. CN VII
    C. CN VIII
    D. CN IX
    E. CN XI

24. Which posterior tooth is most symmetrical from an occlusal view?

    A. Maxillary 1st premolar
    B. Maxillary 2nd premolar
    C. Maxillary 1st molar
    D. Mandibular 1st premolar
    E. Mandibular 1st molar

25. In an ideal occlusion, the _____ cusp of the mandibular _____ contacts the central fossa of the maxillary 1st molar.

    A. Buccal; 2nd premolar
    B. Mesiobuccal; 1st molar
    C. Distobuccal; 1st molar

    D. Distal; 1st molar
    E. Distobuccal; 2nd molar

26. Which of the following teeth have a functional lingual surface?

    I. Maxillary incisors
    II. Maxillary canines
    III. Mandibular incisors
    IV. Mandibular canines

    A. I only
    B. I and IV
    C. III and IV
    D. I and II
    E. None of the above

27. How many point angles are found on tooth No. 12?

    A. 1
    B. 2
    C. 3
    D. 4
    E. 5

28. All of the following cusp tips occlude in the central fossa of an opposing tooth during ideal intercuspation EXCEPT

    A. mesiobuccal of mandibular 1st molar.
    B. distobuccal of mandibular 1st molar.
    C. mesiolingual of maxillary 2nd molar.
    D. distobuccal of mandibular 2nd molar.

29. Using the Universal Numbering System, which of the following represents the four permanent adult canines?

    A. 13, 23, 33, 43
    B. 6, 11, 22, 27
    C. C, H, R, M
    D. 6, 12, 22, 27
    E. 53, 63, 73, 83

30. Which tooth is most likely to have two canals in a single root?

    A. Mandibular lateral incisor
    B. Mandibular canine
    C. Mandibular 2nd premolar
    D. Maxillary central incisor
    E. Maxillary canine

31. The mandibular condyle and its associated disc slide against which surface in normal mandibular opening?

    A. Posterior one-fourth of mandibular fossa
    B. Anterior portion of articular eminence
    C. Posterior portion of articular eminence
    D. Articular (glenoid) fossa

32. The crown of the primary maxillary central incisor

    A. has a longer length incisocervically and is smaller mesiodistally than the permanent maxillary central incisor.
    B. has a longer length incisocervically and is larger mesiodistally than the permanent maxillary central incisor.
    C. has a shorter length incisocervically and is smaller mesiodistally than the permanent maxillary central incisor.
    D. has a shorter length incisocervically and is larger mesiodistally than the permanent maxillary central incisor.

33. In a maxillary 1st molar, a depression associated with a furcation might be detectable on all of the following surfaces EXCEPT

    A. buccal.
    B. palatal.
    C. mesial.
    D. distal.

34. Which of these surfaces is a proximal surface?

    A. Facial
    B. Lingual
    C. Incisal
    D. Buccal
    E. Mesial

35. In an ideal occlusion, the mesiobuccal cusp of the permanent maxillary 2nd molar opposes which of the following?

    A. The buccal groove of the mandibular 2nd molar
    B. The distobuccal groove of the mandibular 1st molar
    C. The mesiobuccal groove of the mandibular 2nd molar
    D. The buccal embrasure between the mandibular 1st and 2nd molars

36. Which one of the following normally single-rooted teeth is most likely to have a bifurcated root?

    A. Maxillary central incisor
    B. Maxillary lateral incisor
    C. Maxillary canine
    D. Mandibular canine
    E. Maxillary 1st premolar

37. Which tooth is likely to have root depressions on both the mesial and distal root surfaces?

    A. Maxillary central incisor
    B. Maxillary lateral incisor
    C. Maxillary 2nd premolar
    D. Mandibular 2nd premolar

38. The mandible functions as what type of lever?

    A. Class I
    B. Class II
    C. Class III
    D. Class IV

39. At what age is a child expected to have 12 primary teeth and 12 permanent teeth?

    A. $6^1/_2$ years
    B. $7^1/_2$ years
    C. $8^1/_2$ years
    D. $10^1/_2$ years
    E. $12^1/_2$ years

40. All of the following are true of the functional outer aspect (FOA) in ideal occlusions EXCEPT

    A. it is located on the outer aspect of supporting cusps.
    B. it may contact the inner incline of supporting cusps.
    C. in the mandibular arch, it is a continuous ribbon which runs from the buccal of one 3rd molar to the other, covering the incisal edges of the lower anterior teeth.
    D. it does not exist on maxillary anterior teeth.
    E. it is no more than 1 mm wide.

41. When viewed from the occlusal, the proximal contact between mandibular 1st and 2nd molars is located

    A. slightly lingual to the middle 3rd.
    B. in the middle 3rd.
    C. slightly buccal to the middle 3rd.
    D. in the cervical 3rd.

42. How many teeth in the primary dentition normally have a cingulum?

    A. 6
    B. 8
    C. 10
    D. 12
    E. 14

43. The maxillary buccal and mandibular lingual cusps function as supporting cusps in which of the following occlusal schemes?

    A. Ideal intercuspal relationship
    B. Nonworking side movement
    C. Working-side movement
    D. Posterior crossbite

44. A 25-year-old patient presents with mamelons on the incisors. Which of the following is the most likely explanation for this finding?

    A. Posterior crossbite
    B. Anterior crossbite
    C. Variation of normal
    D. Anterior open bite
    E. Nocturnal bruxism

45. Which muscle inserts in the articular disc and condylar neck?

    A. Masseter
    B. Medial pterygoid
    C. Lateral pterygoid
    D. Temporalis

46. Which of the following has both mesial and distal contact areas located at the same height in the incisal 3rd?

    A. Maxillary central incisor
    B. Maxillary lateral incisor
    C. Mandibular central incisor

D. Mandibular lateral incisor
E. Mandibular canine

47. All posterior teeth have a height-of-contour located in which segment of the crown?

    A. Occlusal 3rd of the lingual surface
    B. Middle 3rd of the buccal surface
    C. Middle 3rd of the lingual surface
    D. Cervical 3rd of the lingual surface

48. The maxillary 1st premolar typically has a pulp chamber of what shape (at the level of the CEJ)?

    A. Round
    B. Egg shaped
    C. Oval (flattened mesiodistally)
    D. Oval (flattened buccolingually)
    E. Rectangular

49. During mandibular movement, which aspect of a mandibular molar will never contact its maxillary antagonist, assuming all occlusal relationships are ideal?

    A. Outer aspect of the buccal cusps
    B. Inner aspect of the buccal cusps
    C. Inner aspect of the lingual cusps
    D. Outer aspect of the lingual cusps

50. Which succedaneous tooth erupts beneath tooth J?

    A. 1
    B. 10
    C. 13
    D. 20
    E. 21

51. The greatest contour of the cervical line (CEJ) can be found on the

    A. mesial aspect of anterior teeth.
    B. mesial aspect of posterior teeth.
    C. distal aspect of anterior teeth.
    D. distal aspect of posterior teeth.

52. Which cusp on permanent maxillary molars generally gets progressively smaller from the 1st to the 3rd molar?

A. Mesiolingual
B. Distolingual
C. Mesiobuccal
D. Distobuccal

53. A working interference is a premature contact of the posterior teeth on the same side as the direction of the mandibular movement. A protrusive interference is a premature contact between the mesial aspects of maxillary posterior teeth and the distal aspects of mandibular posterior teeth.

A. Both statements are true.
B. Both statements are false.
C. The first statement is true; the second statement is false.
D. The first statement is false; the second statement is true.

54. Which of the following teeth contacts only one other tooth in the opposing arch in an ideal occlusion?

A. Maxillary central incisor
B. Maxillary lateral incisor
C. Mandibular central incisor
D. Maxillary 3rd molar
E. Both C and D

55. Which of the following has the highest frequency of impaction?

A. Maxillary lateral incisor
B. Maxillary canine
C. Maxillary 1st molar
D. Mandibular canine
E. Mandibular 2nd premolar

56. A cervical ridge is found on the facial surface of how many primary teeth?

A. 4
B. 8
C. 12
D. 16
E. 20

57. Which cusp has two triangular ridges on the maxillary 1st molar?

A. Mesiolingual
B. Distolingual

C. Cusp of Carabelli
D. Mesiobuccal
E. Distobuccal

58. The incisal edge or cusp tip of which tooth ideally lies in the facial embrasure between the mandibular canine and mandibular 1st premolar?

A. Maxillary lateral incisor
B. Maxillary canine
C. Maxillary 1st premolar
D. Maxillary 2nd premolar

59. Which cusp is most likely to be absent on a maxillary 2nd molar?

A. Mesiolingual
B. Distolingual
C. Cusp of Carabelli
D. Mesiobuccal
E. Distobuccal

60. The bud stage of tooth development starts at about

A. 6 weeks in utero.
B. 8 weeks in utero.
C. 9 weeks in utero.
D. 11 weeks in utero.
E. 18 weeks in utero.

61. As a dentist, how many determinants of occlusion can you directly control?

A. 0
B. 1
C. 2
D. 3
E. 4

62. Molar crowns typically taper from buccal to lingual when viewed from the occlusal. Which tooth, as an exception, is most likely to taper from lingual to buccal?

A. Mandibular 1st molar
B. Mandibular 2nd molar
C. Maxillary 1st molar
D. Maxillary 2nd molar

63. How many teeth contact both anterior and posterior segments of the opposing arch in ideal intercuspation?

    A. 0
    B. 2
    C. 4
    D. 6
    E. 8

64. Which cusp is the longest and largest on a maxillary 1st molar?

    A. Mesiolingual
    B. Distolingual
    C. Mesiobuccal
    D. Distal
    E. Distobuccal

65. Unique features of the primary mandibular 1st molar include all of the following EXCEPT

    A. the mesial marginal ridge is overdeveloped and resembles a cusp.
    B. the mesiolingual cusp is the largest.
    C. the occlusal table distal to the transverse ridge is larger than the portion mesial to the transverse ridge.
    D. there is no central fossa.
    E. the crown is much wider mesiodistally than buccolingually.

66. Which tooth is most likely to have a cervical enamel projection?

    A. Maxillary central incisor
    B. Maxillary canine
    C. Mandibular 1st premolar
    D. Mandibular 2nd premolar
    E. Mandibular 2nd molar

67. The mandibular canine is most likely to occlude with the _____.

    A. maxillary canine only
    B. maxillary canine and 1st premolar
    C. maxillary 1st premolar only
    D. maxillary lateral incisor only
    E. maxillary lateral incisor and canine

68. Which of the following teeth has the roundest pulp chamber (at the level of the CEJ)?

    A. Maxillary central incisor
    B. Maxillary lateral incisor
    C. Maxillary canine
    D. Mandibular central incisor
    E. Mandibular lateral incisor

69. Which of the following muscles is/are most active in maintaining centric occlusion?

    I. Masseter
    II. Medial pterygoid
    III. Lateral pterygoid
    IV. Temporalis

    A. I only
    B. I and II
    C. I and IV
    D. II and III
    E. I, II, and IV

70. In total, how many grooves can be found on the buccal and lingual surfaces of both mandibular 1st and 2nd molars?

    A. 2
    B. 3
    C. 4
    D. 5
    E. 6

71. Which of the following is the best description of where primate spaces are located?

    A. Between all the primary anterior teeth
    B. Between the canine and 1st premolar in the mandible
    C. Distal to the primary canines in the maxilla
    D. Between the canine and 1st and 2nd primary molars
    E. Distal to primary canines in the mandible

72. How many transverse ridges exist on a maxillary molar?

    A. 0
    B. 1
    C. 2
    D. 3
    E. 4

73. In an ideal dentition, which of the following teeth occludes with only one other tooth in the opposing arch during the full range of mandibular movements?

    A. Mandibular 1st molar
    B. Mandibular lateral incisor
    C. Mandibular central incisor
    D. Maxillary lateral incisor
    E. Maxillary central incisor

74. A maxillary molar has _____ fossae; and the mandibular molar has _____ fossae on the occlusal surface.

    A. 3; 3
    B. 3; 4
    C. 4; 3
    D. 4; 4

75. Maxillary 1st molars are wider mesiodistally on the buccal than the lingual. Mandibular 1st molars are wider on the lingual than buccal.

    A. Both statements are true.
    B. Both statements are false.
    C. The first statement is true; the second is false.
    D. The first statement is false; the second is true.

76. What TMJ ligament is derived from the 1st branchial arch?

    A. Temporomandibular
    B. Sphenomandibular
    C. Stylomandibular
    D. Lateral

77. Which of the following is the term for a supernumerary tooth in the maxillary anterior region?

    A. Mesiodens
    B. Distodens
    C. Dens-in-dente
    D. Paramolar
    E. Talon cusp

78. Which of the following cusp tips passes through the buccal groove of mandibular 1st molar during a working-side movement?

    A. MB of maxillary 1st molar
    B. DB of maxillary 1st molar
    C. ML of maxillary 1st molar
    D. DL of maxillary 1st molar
    E. Buccal of maxillary 2nd premolar

79. The primary maxillary 1st molar most closely resembles which permanent tooth?

    A. Mandibular 1st molar
    B. Mandibular 2nd molar
    C. Maxillary 1st premolar
    D. Maxillary 1st molar
    E. Maxillary 2nd molar

80. The facial height-of-contour of the maxillary 2nd premolar is in what segment of the crown?

    A. Incisal 3rd
    B. Junction of the incisal and middle 3rds
    C. Middle 3rd
    D. Junction of the middle and cervical 3rds
    E. Cervical 3rd

81. Ordinarily, a 7-year-old child would have what teeth clinically visible in the mouth?

    A. All 20 primary teeth and 4 permanent 1st molars
    B. 18 primary teeth and 2 permanent teeth
    C. 16 primary teeth and 8 permanent teeth
    D. 12 primary teeth and 12 permanent teeth

82. In an Angle class III malocclusion, the cusp tip of the maxillary canine is located

    A. distal to the buccal embrasure created by the mandibular canine and 1st premolar.
    B. centered in the embrasure created by the mandibular canine and 1st premolar.
    C. mesial to the buccal embrasure created by the mandibular canine and 1st premolar.
    D. none of the above.

83. The 2nd largest cusp on a mandibular 2nd molar is the

    A. mesiolingual.
    B. distolingual.
    C. mesiobuccal.
    D. distobuccal.
    E. distal.

84. All of the following are true of the articular disc EXCEPT

    A. it is biconcave, with a central avascular intermediate zone.
    B. it is composed of dense hyaline cartilage.
    C. it consists of thick anterior and posterior bands.
    D. fibers of the lateral pterygoid attach to its most anterior portion.
    E. it divides the area between the glenoid fossa and the condyle into two compartments: superior and inferior.

85. After preparing an ideal endodontic access for tooth No. 3, you notice a 4th canal. In which root is this 4th canal most likely located?

    A. Mesiobuccal
    B. Distobuccal
    C. Palatal
    D. Any of the above

86. Which tooth has the greatest root-to-crown ratio?

    A. Maxillary central incisor
    B. Maxillary canine
    C. Mandibular canine
    D. Mandibular 1st molar

87. Which of the following is correct?

    A. VDR = VDO – FS
    B. VDO = CO – FS
    C. VDR = VDO + FS
    D. VDO = CO + CR
    E. VDR = VDO + CO

88. A 30-year-old patient presents with shallow, cup-shaped depressions on the cervicofacial surface of the maxillary anterior teeth. The posterior teeth also exhibit extensive loss of the occlusal surface, including numerous noncarious class VI lesions. Tooth No. 30 has an amalgam restoration that extends about 1 mm above the level of the tooth structure. Which of the following is the most likely cause of this wear?

    A. Abfraction
    B. Attrition

C. Erosion
D. Abrasion

89. Mandibular molar crowns tilt lingually at the cervix. Maxillary molar crowns are aligned directly over the roots.

    A. Both statements are true.
    B. Both statements are false.
    C. The first statement is true; the second is false.
    D. The first statement is false; the second is true.

90. Which of the following primary teeth has the longest root?

    A. Maxillary central incisor
    B. Maxillary canine
    C. Maxillary 2nd molar
    D. Mandibular canine
    E. Mandibular 2nd molar

91. The crowns of all primary teeth begin to calcify at what time?

    A. 2-4 months in utero
    B. 4-6 months in utero
    C. 6-8 months in utero
    D. At birth
    E. 2-4 months postpartum

92. Which is the principal muscle that protrudes the mandible?

    A. Masseter
    B. Medial pterygoid
    C. Lateral pterygoid
    D. Temporalis

93. Which of the following is the most reproducible mandibular position?

    A. Centric occlusion
    B. Functional occlusion
    C. Postural position
    D. Centric relation

94. Mandibular molars usually have how many roots?

    A. 1
    B. 2

C. 3
D. 4
E. 5

95. A "zig-zag" occlusal pattern can be found on which of the following teeth?

A. Mandibular 2nd molar
B. Mandibular 1st molar
C. Maxillary 2nd molar
D. Maxillary 1st molar
E. Maxillary 2nd premolar

96. Which of the following points in the sagittal view of Posselt envelope of motion below is centric occlusion?

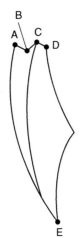

A. A
B. B
C. C
D. D
E. E

97. All anterior teeth develop from how many lobes?

A. 2
B. 3
C. 4
D. 5
E. 6

98. After a difficult extraction of tooth No. 31, you notice that your patient's jaw cannot close. You diagnose the problem as a right-side TMJ

dislocation. What is the initial direction that you should redirect the mandible to treat the problem?

A. Push the ramus superiorly
B. Push the ramus posteriorly
C. Push the ramus downward
D. Slide the ramus mesially
E. Slide the ramus laterally

99. Which of the following teeth is most likely to be congenitally absent?

A. Maxillary lateral incisor
B. Maxillary canine
C. Mandibular canine
D. Mandibular 1st premolar
E. Mandibular 2nd premolar

100. In which age range would one normally expect to see all 20 primary teeth present, but no permanent teeth yet visible?

A. 0.5-1 years
B. 1-1.5 years
C. 1-2 years
D. 2.5-5.5 years
E. 3.5-6.5 years

101. Which of the following is the smallest tooth of both arches?

A. Maxillary central incisor
B. Maxillary lateral incisor
C. Mandibular central incisor
D. Mandibular lateral incisor

102. In an ideal occlusion, the mesiolingual cusp of the mandibular 1st molar articulates with which of the following?

A. The distal marginal ridge of the maxillary 2nd premolar
B. The lingual embrasure between the maxillary 2nd premolar and 1st molar
C. The mesial marginal ridge of the maxillary 1st molar
D. The central fossa of the maxillary 1st molar
E. The lingual embrasure between the maxillary 1st and 2nd molar

103. Which of the following pulp canal configurations has two separate canals exiting the pulp chamber, but merge together to form one canal just short of the apex?

    A. Type I
    B. Type II
    C. Type III
    D. Type IV

104. The primary mandibular 1st molar most closely resembles which permanent tooth?

    A. Mandibular 1st molar
    B. Mandibular 2nd molar
    C. Maxillary 1st molar
    D. Maxillary 2nd molar
    E. None of the above

105. Which of the following has the greatest mesial cervical line (CEJ) curvature?

    A. Maxillary central incisor
    B. Maxillary lateral incisor
    C. Maxillary canine
    D. Maxillary 1st premolar
    E. Maxillary 2nd premolar

106. In an ideal occlusion, the lingual cusp of the maxillary 2nd premolar contacts which of the following?

    A. Mesial marginal ridge of the mandibular 2nd premolar
    B. Distal triangular fossa of the mandibular 2nd premolar
    C. Distal marginal ridge of the mandibular 2nd premolar
    D. Mesial marginal ridge of the mandibular 1st molar
    E. Mesial triangular fossa of the mandibular 1st molar

107. A 12-year-old boy fractures the neck of his right condyle after falling off his bicycle. The mandible will deviate to the right side because the left lateral pterygoid is still functional.

    A. Both the statement and the reason are correct and related.
    B. Both the statement and the reason are correct but not related.

C. The statement is correct, but the reason is not.
D. The statement is not correct, but the reason is correct.
E. Neither the statement nor the reason is correct.

108. The incisal edge (cusp tip) is positioned more to the lingual of the root axis line in which of the following teeth?

    A. Maxillary incisors
    B. Mandibular incisors
    C. Maxillary canine
    D. Mandibular canine
    E. B and D

109. The cingulum is centered mesiodistally on the

    A. maxillary central incisor.
    B. mandibular lateral incisor.
    C. maxillary canine.
    D. all of the above.
    E. none of the above.

110. Humans are classified as having which types of dentition?

    A. Homodont, diphyodont
    B. Heterodont, polyphyodont
    C. Heterodont, diphyodont
    D. Homodont, monophyodont
    E. Homodont, polyphyodont

111. Permanent incisors often erupt _____ to their primary counterparts.

    A. buccal
    B. lingual
    C. directly underneath
    D. lateral

112. In ideal maximum intercuspation, the oblique ridge of the maxillary 1st molar opposes which of the following areas of the mandibular 1st molar?

    A. Buccal groove
    B. Distobuccal groove
    C. Lingual groove
    D. Mesial marginal ridge
    E. Distal marginal ridge

113. Which of the following teeth has a nearly straight crown-root profile on the mesial surface when viewed from the facial?

    A. Maxillary central incisor
    B. Maxillary lateral incisor
    C. Maxillary canine
    D. Mandibular canine
    E. Mandibular 1st premolar

114. How many cusps does the primary mandibular 2nd molar typically have?

    A. 1
    B. 2
    C. 3
    D. 4
    E. 5

115. Which ligament helps retain the condyle within the glenoid fossa?

    A. Sphenomandibular ligament
    B. Temporomandibular ligament
    C. Stylomandibular ligament
    D. Pterygomandibular ligament

116. An individual diagnosed with posterior bite collapse will most likely have a decrease in which of the following?

    A. Freeway space
    B. Postural position
    C. VDR
    D. Maximum opening
    E. VDO

117. The only tooth with three different occlusal schemes is the

    A. mandibular 1st premolar.
    B. mandibular 2nd premolar.
    C. mandibular 1st molar.
    D. mandibular 2nd molar.

118. Which tooth has the longest root in the permanent dentition?

    A. Maxillary central incisor
    B. Maxillary lateral incisor
    C. Maxillary canine
    D. Maxillary 1st molar
    E. Mandibular canine

119. A nonworking side interference would be present on which of the following surfaces?

    A. Inner aspects of a supporting cusp
    B. Outer aspects of a guiding cusp
    C. Inner aspects of a guiding cusp
    D. Outer aspects of a supporting cusp

120. You suspect a 2nd canal on tooth No. 23. In which direction should you look?

    A. Mesial
    B. Distal
    C. Buccal
    D. Lingual
    E. None, there is no possibility of a 2nd canal

121. You are having a hard time mobilizing tooth No. 18 during a routine extraction. After looking at the radiograph again, you cannot see a PDL space all the way around the roots. Which of the following would best describe the reason why you can't elevate the tooth?

    A. It is ankylosed.
    B. It is a taurodont.
    C. It has a dilaceration.
    D. It has hypercementosis.
    E. It has a cervical enamel projection.

122. All of the primary teeth have just completed root formation at what age?

    A. 1-1$\frac{1}{2}$ years
    B. 1$\frac{1}{2}$-2 years
    C. 2-3 years
    D. 3-4 years
    E. 4-5 years

123. Which of the following jaw positions is determined almost exclusively by the behavior of the musculature?

    A. Centric occlusion
    B. Centric relation
    C. Postural position
    D. All of the above

124. In comparison to the maxillary canine, the mandibular canine has a

A. sharper cusp.
B. more pronounced labial ridge.
C. more cervical mesial contact.
D. centered cingulum.
E. more narrow mesiodistal crown width.

125. All primary maxillary molars have three roots. All primary mandibular molars have two roots.

A. Both statements are true.
B. Both statements are false.
C. The first statement is true; the second statement is false.
D. The first statement is false; the second statement is true.

126. Anterior guidance allows only the molars to disarticulate during protrusive movement. Cusp length is generally longest with a deep overbite and minimal overjet.

A. Both statements are true.
B. Both statements are false.
C. The first statement is true; the second statement is false.
D. The first statement is false; the second statement is true.

127. Permanent canine cusps have mesial cusp ridges shorter than distal cusp ridges. Their crowns are wider faciolingually than mesiodistally.

A. Both statements are true.
B. Both statements are false.
C. The first statement is true; the second is false.
D. The first statement is false; the second is true.

128. Aside from the mandibular lateral incisor, a distolingual twist of the incisal edge can be found on which of the following teeth?

A. Mandibular central incisor
B. Maxillary lateral incisor
C. Maxillary canine
D. Mandibular canine

129. The terminal hinge position occurs when the condyles are in the most _____ location within the glenoid fossa.

A. Anterior and superior
B. Anterior and inferior
C. Medial and superior
D. Lateral and superior
E. Posterior and superior

130. Calcification of the permanent dentition typically starts at what time?

A. 4-6 months in utero
B. 6-8 months in utero
C. Birth
D. 1-2 months postpartum
E. 2-4 months postpartum

131. In which Angle classification would you typically find a deep overbite with proclined maxillary lateral incisors?

A. Class I
B. Class II, division I
C. Class II, division II
D. Class III, division I
E. Class III, division II

132. Which incisor exhibits the most variability?

A. Maxillary central
B. Maxillary lateral
C. Mandibular central
D. Mandibular lateral

133. A labial ridge can be found on which tooth type?

A. Incisor
B. Canine
C. Premolar
D. Molar

134. Which of the following is not TRUE of primary teeth compared to permanent teeth?

A. They are generally whiter.
B. Their crowns are more bulbous.
C. Their CEJs are more constricted.
D. Their root trunks are longer.
E. Their pulp chambers are larger.

135. The length of the permanent maxillary arch is about 8 mm longer than the permanent mandibular arch. The permanent arches are generally more circular than the primary arches.

    A. Both statements are true.
    B. Both statements are false.
    C. The first statement is true; the second statement is false.
    D. The first statement is false; the second statement is true.

136. The lingual height-of-contour of all anterior teeth is in what segment of the crown?

    A. Incisal 3rd
    B. Junction of the incisal and middle 3rds
    C. Middle 3rd
    D. Junction of the middle and cervical 3rds
    E. Cervical 3rd

137. Which of the following best describes a Bennett shift?

    A. The lateral movement of the working-side condyle in the opposite direction of the excursive movement
    B. The lateral movement of the working-side condyle in the same direction of the excursive movement
    C. The anterior translation of both condyles during protrusive movement
    D. The anterior translation of the contralateral condyle during lateral excursive movement
    E. The anterior translation of the ipsilateral condyle during lateral excursive movement

138. Two pulp canals are most commonly found in which of the following teeth?

    A. Maxillary 1st premolar
    B. Mandibular 1st premolar
    C. Maxillary 2nd premolar
    D. Mandibular 2nd premolar

139. Which of the following premolars has a shorter buccal cusp than lingual cusp?

    A. Maxillary 1st premolar
    B. Maxillary 2nd premolar

    C. Mandibular 1st premolar
    D. Mandibular 2nd premolar
    E. None of the above

140. Maxillary incisor protrusion, anterior open bite, crowded laterals, and a high palatal vault are most likely caused by which of the following?

    A. Mouth breathing
    B. Thumb sucking
    C. Tongue thrusting
    D. Nocturnal bruxism

141. Which of the following is the 1st succedaneous tooth to erupt?

    A. Maxillary 1st molar
    B. Mandibular 1st molar
    C. Maxillary central incisor
    D. Mandibular central incisor
    E. None of the above

142. Which premolar has the most square occlusal table shape?

    A. Maxillary 1st premolar
    B. Maxillary 2nd premolar
    C. Mandibular 1st premolar
    D. Mandibular 2nd premolar

143. Which of the following is a microdont?

    A. Geminated incisor
    B. Cusp of Carabelli
    C. Peg-shaped lateral
    D. Dens evaginatus
    E. Mulberry molar

144. All of the following are true of primary canines EXCEPT

    A. when viewed from the facial, the crown shapes are pentagonal.
    B. they have cingula.
    C. the mesial cusp ridge of the maxillary canine is longer than the distal cusp ridge.
    D. the distal cusp ridge of the mandibular canine is longer than the mesial cusp ridge.
    E. all of the above.

145. In an ideal occlusion, protrusive contacts can occur on which of the following surfaces?

    A. Maxillary distal inclines and mandibular mesial inclines
    B. Maxillary mesial inclines and mandibular distal inclines
    C. Maxillary distal inclines and mandibular distal inclines
    D. Maxillary mesial inclines and mandibular mesial inclines

146. The principal muscle that protrudes the tongue is innervated by which cranial nerve?

    A. CN V
    B. CN VII
    C. CN IX
    D. CN X
    E. CN XII

147. Which portion of the maxillary 1st molar root typically has the greatest surface area?

    A. Root trunk
    B. MB root
    C. DB root
    D. Palatal root

148. All of the following are features of the permanent mandibular canine EXCEPT

    A. the mesial cusp ridge is shorter than distal cusp ridge.
    B. the mesial cusp ridge is almost horizontal.
    C. the mesial crown outline is in line with the root.
    D. the cusp tip is located labial to the mid—root-axis line.

149. Which of the following points in the horizontal view of Posselt envelope of motion below is the anterior edge-to-edge position?

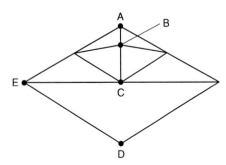

A. A
B. B
C. C
D. D
E. E

150. Which is the only premolar with a longer mesial buccal cusp ridge than distal buccal cusp ridge?

    A. Maxillary 1st premolar
    B. Maxillary 2nd premolar
    C. Mandibular 1st premolar
    D. Mandibular 2nd premolar

151. On average, how much root structure must be formed before a tooth erupts?

    A. 0%-25%
    B. 25%-33%
    C. 33%-50%
    D. 50%-66%
    E. 66%-75%

152. The glenoid fossa is a portion of which bone?

    A. Zygomatic
    B. Temporal
    C. Maxilla
    D. Mandible
    E. Palatine

153. Which of the following is the smallest primary molar?

    A. Maxillary 1st
    B. Maxillary 2nd
    C. Mandibular 1st
    D. Mandibular 2nd

154. A posterior bitewing radiograph reveals a 2 mm × 2 mm radiopaque mass on the distal surface of tooth No. 2, just apical to the CEJ. Which of the following is most likely the finding?

    A. Enamel pearl
    B. Cervical enamel projection
    C. Taurodont
    D. Distodens
    E. Hypercementosis

155. In an unworn dentition, tooth-to-tooth contacts may be characterized as all of the following EXCEPT

   A. point-to-point.
   B. point-to-area.
   C. edge-to-edge.
   D. edge-to-area.
   E. area-to-area.

156. All of the following teeth typically have one root canal EXCEPT

   A. maxillary central incisor.
   B. maxillary lateral incisor.
   C. maxillary canine.
   D. mandibular canine.
   E. all of the above.

157. Which of the following teeth is most likely to have a trifurcation?

   A. Maxillary 1st premolar
   B. Mandibular 1st premolar
   C. Maxillary 1st molar
   D. Mandibular 1st molar

158. Tooth No. 18 has what general crown shape when viewed from the distal?

   A. Square
   B. Rectangular
   C. Rhomboidal
   D. Trapezoidal
   E. Oval

159. Which two muscles form a sling around the mandible?

   A. Masseter and temporalis
   B. Medial pterygoid and lateral pterygoid
   C. Masseter and medial pterygoid
   D. Masseter and lateral pterygoid
   E. None of the above

160. During working-side excursion, the distobuccal cusp of the maxillary 1st molar passes through which of the following?

   A. Lingual groove of the mandibular 1st molar
   B. Lingual embrasure between the mandibular 1st and 2nd molar
   C. Buccal groove of the mandibular 1st molar
   D. Distobuccal groove of the mandibular 1st molar
   E. Buccal embrasure between the mandibular 1st and 2nd molar

161. The proximal contact positions of the maxillary canine are in which areas?

   A. Mesial: Incisal 3rd; Distal: Junction of the incisal and middle 3rds
   B. Mesial: Incisal 3rd; Distal: Middle 3rd
   C. Mesial: Junction of the incisal and middle 3rds; Distal: Junction of the incisal and middle 3rds
   D. Mesial: Junction of the incisal and middle 3rds; Distal: Middle 3rd
   E. Mesial: Middle 3rd; Distal: Junction of the incisal and middle 3rds

162. All of the following are true of eruption EXCEPT

   A. boys' teeth generally erupt before girls' teeth.
   B. mandibular teeth generally erupt before maxillary teeth.
   C. teeth generally erupt in contralateral pairs.
   D. eruption starts after at least 50% of root formation is complete.
   E. all of the above are true.

163. The occlusal surface of the primary maxillary 1st molar is

   A. square.
   B. rectangular.
   C. trapezoidal.
   D. rhomboidal.

164. An individual who never formed 3rd molars has which of the following?

   A. Anodontia
   B. Hypodontia
   C. Oligodontia
   D. Hyperdontia
   E. Metadontia

165. The nonworking pathway of the mesial cusps on mandibular posterior teeth is in which direction?

   A. Distofacial
   B. Distolingual
   C. Mesiofacial
   D. Mesiolingual

166. The mesial proximal contact area of tooth No. 29 is located where?

   A. Incisal 3rd
   B. Junction of the incisal and middle 3rds
   C. Middle 3rd
   D. Junction of the middle and cervical 3rds
   E. Cervical 3rd

167. Which of the following intrinsic muscle fibers flattens and broadens the tongue?

   A. Vertical
   B. Horizontal
   C. Longitudinal
   D. Transverse

168. Anterior teeth have 4 line angles. Posterior teeth have 6 line angles.

   A. Both statements are true.
   B. Both statements are false.
   C. The first statement is true; the second is false.
   D. The first statement is false; the second is true.

169. If not coincidental, the average slide from centric relation to centric occlusion is

   A. 1-2 mm.
   B. 2-4 mm.
   C. 4-6 mm.
   D. 6-8 mm.

170. You are evaluating maxillary and mandibular CT scans for a patient who has recently had facial trauma. Out of curiosity, you notice the natural inclination of roots within the alveolar bone on the sagittal slices. Which tooth root has the greatest horizontal axial inclination?

   A. Maxillary central incisor
   B. Maxillary lateral incisor
   C. Maxillary canine
   D. Mandibular central incisor
   E. Mandibular canine

171. On a 3-cusped mandibular 2nd premolar, how many cusps can be seen from the mesial and distal, respectively?

   A. 2 from the mesial; 2 from the distal
   B. 3 from the mesial; 2 from the distal
   C. 2 from the mesial; 3 from the distal
   D. 3 from the mesial; 3 from the distal

172. Which of the following is typically the last primary tooth to exfoliate?

   A. Maxillary canine
   B. Mandibular canine
   C. Maxillary 2nd molar
   D. Mandibular 2nd molar
   E. Maxillary 1st molar

173. Which of the following cusps on a mandibular 1st molar has the largest pulp horn?

   A. Mesiobuccal
   B. Distobuccal
   C. Mesiolingual
   D. Distolingual
   E. Distal

174. In which of the following mandibular positions would you find the greatest increase in VDO from centric occlusion?

   A. Centric relation
   B. Maximum protrusion
   C. Anterior edge-to-edge position
   D. Postural position
   E. Maximum opening

175. Which of the following chronic conditions may cause tooth abrasion?

   A. GERD
   B. Nocturnal bruxism
   C. Occlusal trauma
   D. Pipe smoking
   E. Cigarette smoking

176. What are the typical positions of the maxillary and mandibular teeth, and the tongue during empty-mouth swallowing?

A. Centric occlusion; the tongue touches the palate.
B. Centric occlusion; the tongue touches the lingual aspects of the anterior teeth.
C. Retruded contact; the tongue touches the palate.
D. Retruded contact; the tongue touches the lingual aspects of the anterior teeth.
E. Rest position; the tongue touches the palate.

177. On which primary tooth can one find an oblique ridge and, occasionally, a fifth cusp of Carabelli?

A. Mandibular 1st molar
B. Mandibular 2nd molar
C. Maxillary 1st molar
D. Maxillary 2nd molar

178. The lingual surface of which incisor is the most concave?

A. Maxillary central
B. Maxillary lateral
C. Mandibular central
D. Mandibular lateral

179. In right lateral excursion, which of the following is correct?

A. The mandibular teeth move to the right.
B. The mandibular teeth move to the left.
C. The left mandibular teeth are on the working side.
D. Both A and C.
E. Both B and C.

180. Which anterior tooth has the greatest mesiodistal length when viewed from the facial?

A. Maxillary central incisor
B. Maxillary lateral incisor
C. Maxillary canine
D. Mandibular central incisor
E. Mandibular lateral incisor

181. Which premolar is typically the largest?

A. Maxillary 1st premolar
B. Maxillary 2nd premolar
C. Mandibular 1st premolar
D. Mandibular 2nd premolar

182. All of the following muscles are involved in right lateral excursive movement EXCEPT

A. right masseter.
B. right temporalis.
C. right medial pterygoid.
D. left medial pterygoid.
E. left lateral pterygoid.

183. By age $9^1/_2$, how many teeth will a young boy have?

A. 12 primary and 12 permanent teeth
B. 10 primary and 12 permanent teeth
C. 10 primary and 14 permanent teeth
D. 8 primary and 16 permanent teeth
E. 6 primary and 16 permanent teeth

184. Which of the following regions in the sagittal view of Posselt envelope of motion below represents a free opening or closing of the mandible?

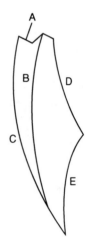

A. A
B. B
C. C
D. D
E. E

185. Failure to properly close a proximal contact when restoring a posterior tooth can lead to which of the following?

A. Mesial drifting of the tooth
B. Gingival inflammation
C. A food trap
D. All of the above
E. None of the above

Dental Anatomy and Occlusion

186. Which anterior tooth has the greatest faciolingual-to-mesiodistal length ratio when viewed from the occlusal?

    A. Maxillary central incisor
    B. Maxillary lateral incisor
    C. Mandibular central incisor
    D. Mandibular lateral incisor
    E. Mandibular canine

187. The mesial proximal contact is more cervical than the distal in which of the following?

    A. Primary maxillary canine
    B. Primary mandibular canine
    C. Permanent maxillary 1st premolar
    D. Permanent mandibular 2nd premolar
    E. None of the above

188. In an ideal occlusion, the lingual cusp of the mandibular 2nd premolar sits between which of the following?

    A. MARGINAL ridges of the maxillary 1st and 2nd premolar
    B. Marginal ridges of the maxillary 2nd premolar and 1st molar
    C. Central fossa of the maxillary 2nd premolar
    D. Lingual embrasure of the maxillary 1st and 2nd premolar
    E. Lingual embrasure of the maxillary 2nd premolar and 1st molar

189. The oblique ridge on a maxillary molar extends between what two cusps?

    A. MB and DB
    B. MB and ML
    C. MB and DL
    D. DB and DL
    E. DB and ML

190. A synovial membrane covers the articular disc, enabling smoother movement along the articular eminence. The glenoid fossa is lined with a layer of hyaline cartilage.

    A. Both statements are true.
    B. Both statements are false.
    C. The first statement is true; the second statement is false.
    D. The first statement is false; the second statement is true.

191. How many embrasures are present per contact area?

    A. 1
    B. 2
    C. 3
    D. 4
    E. 5

192. The mandibular 1st molar may have a 4th canal in which root?

    A. Mesial
    B. Distal
    C. Buccal
    D. Lingual

193. In an ideal occlusion, the distal cusp of the mandibular 2nd molar articulates with which of the following?

    A. The central fossa of the maxillary 2nd molar
    B. The marginal ridges of the maxillary 2nd and 3rd molars
    C. The buccal groove of the maxillary 2nd molar
    D. The central fossa of the maxillary 3rd molar
    E. None of the above

194. Which of the following ridges is not located on the corresponding tooth type?

    A. Cervical ridge: All molars
    B. Labial ridge: All anterior teeth
    C. Oblique ridge: Maxillary molars
    D. Marginal ridge: All teeth
    E. Buccal cusp ridge: All premolars

195. From which view is only one root visible on a mandibular 1st molar?

    A. Mesial
    B. Distal
    C. Buccal
    D. Lingual
    E. Occlusal

196. Following root canal therapy, gutta percha extending beyond the apex of which tooth is most likely to impinge on the mental foramen?

A. Mandibular canine
B. Mandibular 1st premolar
C. Mandibular 2nd premolar
D. Mandibular 1st molar
E. Mandibular 2nd molar

197. The closer a tooth is to an occlusal determinant, the _____ it will be influenced by that determinant. The _____ teeth ideally guide the mandible in lateral excursive and protrusive movements.

 A. less; anterior
 B. more; anterior
 C. less; posterior
 D. more; posterior

198. What mandibular position is represented by the point in the frontal view of Posselt envelope of motion below?

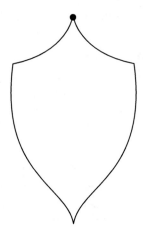

 A. Centric occlusion
 B. Retruded contact
 C. Anterior edge-to-edge position
 D. Maximum opening
 E. Maximum protrusion

199. The TMJ is what type of joint?

 A. Synovial synarthrosis
 B. Synovial amphiarthrosis
 C. Synovial diarthrosis
 D. None of the above

200. Which of the following tooth roots is most likely to be pushed into the maxillary sinus during extraction?

 A. Maxillary canine
 B. Maxillary 1st premolar
 C. Maxillary 2nd premolar
 D. Maxillary 1st molar
 E. Maxillary 2nd molar

1. **The correct answer is C.** From an occlusal view, the major feature distinguishing the mandibular lateral incisor from the mandibular central incisor is the presence of a distolingual twist found in the distal half of the lateral's incisal edge. This distolingual twist follows the natural arch shape of the mandible and, therefore, also allows one to easily distinguish right from left mandibular lateral incisors. The mandibular central incisor, on the other hand, is bilaterally symmetrical with a centered cingulum, making it very difficult to determine right from left.

Answer A is incorrect. Unlike maxillary incisor crowns, where the central is larger than the lateral, the mandibular lateral incisor crown is slightly larger in all dimensions.

Answer B is incorrect. The cingulum of the mandibular lateral incisor is slightly distal of center (similar to the maxillary central incisor and mandibular canine). Anterior teeth that have a centered cingulum on the lingual surface include the mandibular central incisor, maxillary canine, and maxillary lateral incisor.

Answer D is incorrect. Both the mandibular central and lateral incisors have incisal edges that are lingual to the root-axis line, and therefore is not a distinguishing feature.

2. **The correct answer is D.** All 5 cusp tips can be seen from the buccal. The somewhat staggered arrangement of the 3 buccal and 2 lingual cusps allow the tips of the lingual cusps to peak above the buccal and distobuccal grooves.

Answers A, B, and C are incorrect. Minimally, the 3 buccal cusps would be visible.

3. **The correct answer is C.** The lingual inclination of the crowns of mandibular posterior teeth helps define the curve of Wilson, not the curve of Spee. When viewed from the anterior, the lingual cusps of the posterior teeth in both arches are aligned at a more inferior level than the buccal cusps, thus giving rise to the curve of Wilson, or mediolateral curve.

Answers A, B, and D are incorrect. When viewed from the buccal, the cusp tips of posterior teeth follow a gradual curve that is convex in the maxillary arch and concave in the mandibular arch (relative to a flat plane of occlusion between the two arches). The curve of Spee runs anteroposteriorly, and is sometimes referred to as the anteroposterior curve.

4. **The correct answer is E.** Both maxillary and mandibular canines have characteristic labial and lingual ridges, but those on maxillary canines are more prominent. The vertical lingual ridge extends to the cingulum of the canines, creating mesial and distal fossae on either side of the lingual ridge.

Answers A, B, and C are incorrect. None of these teeth have labial or lingual ridges. Instead, these teeth have a single concave lingual fossa bounded by mesial and distal marginal ridges, and a convex cingulum on the lingual surface.

Answer D is incorrect. The question asks for the tooth with the most prominent lingual ridge. The lingual ridge on the maxillary canine is more prominent.

5. **The correct answer is A.** The palatal root is the longest of the three roots in a maxillary molar, but 3rd longest among roots of maxillary teeth, after the maxillary canine and 2nd premolar roots.

Answers B, C, and D are incorrect. See above.

6. **The correct answer is C.** The buccinator muscle assists in mastication by compressing the cheek against molar teeth, thus holding food under the teeth. It originates from the pterygomandibular raphe and maxillary and mandibular buccal alveolar processes. Its upper and lower fibers crisscross to insert into

the lower and upper lip, respectively. The buccinator receives its innervation from the facial nerve (CN VII, buccal branch).

Answers A, B, D, and E are incorrect. These are the four muscles of mastication, all innervated by CN V3.

7. **The correct answer is A.** Overjet is defined as horizontal overlap of the incisors, normally 2-3 mm.

   Answer B is incorrect. Overbite is defined as the vertical overlap of the incisors, normally 1-2 mm.

   Answer C is incorrect. There is no vertical overlap of the incisors in an openbite. Anterior openbite can result, for example, from a persistent thumb-sucking habit.

   Answer D is incorrect. Crossbite is a reversed horizontal overlap relationship of the teeth. If the lower incisors are anterior to the upper incisors in centric occlusion, the condition is called anterior crossbite or reverse overjet. Posterior crossbite exists when the maxillary posterior teeth are lingually positioned relative to the mandibular teeth in centric occlusion.

8. **The correct answer is A.** The primary mandibular 2nd molar resembles the mandibular 1st molar; however, the three buccal cusps of the primary tooth are nearly equal in size, whereas the permanent 1st molar bears a distal cusp which is typically considerably smaller.

   Answer B is incorrect. No primary tooth resembles the permanent mandibular 2nd molar.

   Answer C is incorrect. The primary maxillary 2nd molar resembles the permanent maxillary 1st molar. They are similar in most respects (albeit the primary 2nd molar is smaller), with an oblique ridge and fossae (and sometimes even a cusp of Carabelli) corresponding to those of the permanent maxillary 1st molar.

   Answer D is incorrect. No primary tooth resembles the permanent maxillary 2nd molar.

9. **The correct answer is C.** Central incisors (A) erupt around 6 months of age, lateral incisors (B) at 9 months, primary 1st molars (D) at 12 months, primary canines (C) at 18 months, and primary 2nd molars (E) at 24 months. Mandibular primary teeth typically erupt before the maxillary primary teeth with the exception of the primary lateral incisors. Remember: ABDCE at 6,9,12,18,24.

   Answers A, B, and D are incorrect. See above.

10. **The correct answer is C.** When viewed from the mesial or distal aspects, all anterior teeth (centrals, laterals, and canines) have a triangular or wedge-shaped outline.

    Answer A is incorrect. When viewed from the proximal aspect, all mandibular posterior teeth (premolars and molars) have a rhomboidal shape because the crowns tilt lingually from the cervix.

    Answer B is incorrect. All maxillary posterior have a trapezoidal crown outline when viewed from the mesial or distal, with longest uneven side at the base of the crown. Unlike mandibular posterior crowns which tilt lingually from the cervix, maxillary crowns are aligned directly over the roots from the proximal view.

    Answer D is incorrect. The outline form of this tooth from the proximal aspect is rhomboidal, as it is with all mandibular posterior teeth.

11. **The correct answer is D.** Both gemination and fusion can be described as conditions in which "double teeth" occur. They occur most often in the maxillary and anterior regions and are differentiated by counting the number of teeth in the dentition. In gemination (or twinning), one tooth bud splits to form what appears to be two teeth (1 root, 2 teeth). The single root is not split and has a common pulp canal. Both twinned and fused crowns typically appear double in width compared to a single tooth but notched since the division is incomplete.

Answer A is incorrect. Concrescence occurs when the roots of two or more unique teeth are united by cementum.

Answer B is incorrect. Hypercementosis is the nonneoplastic deposition of excessive cementum. Blunting of the roots is frequently seen upon radiographic examination.

Answer C is incorrect. In fusion, two adjacent tooth germs fuse during development (2 roots, 2 teeth). Unlike gemination, radiographs usually reveal two separate but fused roots with separate pulp chambers.

Answer E is incorrect. Fibrous dysplasia is a developmental condition in which bone is progressively replaced by fibrous tissue. The key radiographic appearance of fibrous dysplasia is described as "ground glass." There is no association between any of the above conditions and fibrous dysplasia.

12. **The correct answer is C.** Angle classification is primarily based on molar relationships. For example, a class I molar relationship is one in which the MB cusp of the maxillary 1st molar opposes the buccal groove of the mandibular 1st molar. If the maxillary 1st molar is mesial to this position, a class II molar relationship exists. If it is distal, a class III molar relationship exists.

    Answer A is incorrect. This has no bearing on Angle classification of occlusion.

    Answer B is incorrect. Although the canine relationship can be classified as class I (ie, maxillary canine tip falls between the mandibular canine and 1st premolar), class II, or III, it is the molar relationship that *primarily* defines Angle classification of occlusion.

    Answer D is incorrect. This has no bearing on Angle classification; however, excessive overjet may be seen as a sequela of class II, division I occlusion.

13. **The correct answer is C.** Primary teeth are more constricted at the cervical 3rd than permanent teeth. Pulp chambers are comparatively larger in primary teeth, especially in the mesial horns. Therefore, great care must be

taken when preparing class I and class II cavity preps, especially on the mesial half.

Answers A, B, and D are incorrect. See above.

14. **The correct answer is E.** On 2-cusped premolars, the triangular ridges of the buccal and lingual cusps converge at the central groove and join together to form a transverse ridge. However, the three triangular ridges of the 3-cusped mandibular 2nd premolar (one large buccal and two smaller lingual cusps resulting in a Y-shaped occlusal groove pattern) do not meet, and thus no transverse ridge is formed.

    Answers A, B, C, and D are incorrect. A transverse ridge crosses the occlusal surface of these premolars, running between the buccal and lingual cusps. Specifically, the triangular ridges of the buccal and lingual cusps unite to form the transverse ridge.

15. **The correct answer is B.** During left working movement, the right (nonworking) condyle rotates and translates anteriorly, downward along the articular eminence, and medially to the left. The left (working) condyle rotates forward and typically translates slightly laterally to the left (a Bennett shift).

    Answers A, C, D, and E are incorrect. See above.

16. **The correct answer is C.** Both the mesial contact and marginal ridge is more cervical than the distal, which is a feature that is unique to the mandibular 1st premolar.

    Answers A, B, and D are incorrect. These premolars have mesial marginal ridges located more occlusally than the distal marginal ridge. Recall that mesial marginal ridge grooves are almost always present on maxillary 1st premolars. Furthermore, the mesial marginal ridge of the mandibular 2nd premolar is more horizontal than the cervically sloping mesial marginal ridge of the mandibular 1st premolar.

17. **The correct answer is B.** The lingual cusps of the maxillary premolars tilt mesially and,

therefore, will articulate with the distal triangular fossae of their mandibular premolar counterparts. Recall that mandibular teeth are situated mesially and lingually to their counterparts in the maxilla. Therefore, as a general rule, a maxillary tooth will articulate with its mandibular counterpart and the tooth distal to it; likewise, a mandibular tooth will articulate with its maxillary counterpart and the tooth mesial to it. Accordingly, the maxillary 1st premolar will occlude with the mandibular 1st premolar (counterpart) and the mandibular 2nd premolar (the tooth distal to the counterpart).

Answers A, C, D, and E are incorrect. Nothing rests in these fossae in ideal intercuspation.

18. **The correct answer is C.** The 1st premolars in both arches have the longest and sharpest buccal cusps relative to the 2nd premolars. Remember that all premolars except the mandibular 1st premolar have a longer buccal cusp than lingual cusp.

    Answers A, B, and D are incorrect. See above.

19. **The correct answer is E.** Primary molars have a shallow occlusal anatomy relative to their permanent counterparts. Cusps are short, ridges are not as pronounced, and the fossae are not as deep.

    Answer A is incorrect. The roots of primary molars are very divergent, which allows for the eruption of the permanent premolars. They are also much less curved, and there is little to no root trunk.

    Answer B is incorrect. The mesial cervical ridge of primary molars is very prominent, and the cervical lines course more apically on the mesial half due to this prominence. Recall that all primary anterior teeth also have prominent cervical ridges.

    Answer C is incorrect. Enamel is approximately 1 mm thick and of relatively uniform thickness in primary molars as opposed to that of permanent molars, which is 2.5 mm thick on the occlusal surface.

Answer D is incorrect. Primary molars have much shorter root trunks than their permanent counterparts. This allows their roots to diverge at a more coronal level, accommodating the size of the underlying permanent tooth.

20. **The correct answer is A.** There are no premolars in the deciduous (primary) dentition. Premolars are only found in the adult permanent dentition, and succeed the primary molars.

    Answer B is incorrect. In the permanent (not the primary) dentition, there are 2 premolars per quadrant, 4 premolars per arch, for a total of 8 premolars in both arches (maxilla and mandible).

    Answers C, D, and E are incorrect. See above.

21. **The correct answer is C.** Remember that supporting cusps are the maxillary lingual and mandibular buccal cusps. These cusps (also called working cusps) function by grinding against the opposing teeth. Supporting cusps tend to be rounder and located than nonsupporting cusps. The tips of the supporting cusps rest in the opposing marginal ridge areas with the exception of the ML cusp of maxillary molars and DB cusps of mandibular molars which rest in the opposing central fossa.

    Answers A, B, and D are incorrect. All mandibular lingual and maxillary buccal cusps are nonsupporting cusps. These cusps tend to be taller and sharper than supporting cusps, and their function is to help disarticulate the teeth during excursive jaw movements. Note that nonsupporting cusps do not occlude in any fossae or marginal ridge areas, but they do oppose grooves and embrasure areas.

22. **The correct answer is B.** Anodontia refers to the total lack of tooth development. These individuals do form any teeth. Someone with partial anodontia is congenitally missing one or more teeth. Remember that an edentulous patient does not necessarily suffer from anodontia.

Answer A is incorrect. Hyperdontia is the development of an increased number of teeth, which may be associated with conditions such as cleidocranial dysplasia, Down syndrome, Gardner syndrome, and Sturge-Weber angiomatosis.

Answers C, D, and E are incorrect. See above.

23. **The correct answer is A.** The auriculotemporal nerve conducts the primary innervation to the TMJ. It transmits pain within the capsule, and also provides parasympathetics to the parotid gland. The auriculotemporal nerve is a branch of CN V3. Two other nerves also supply sensory fibers to the TMJ: the nerve to the masseter and the posterior deep temporal nerve, both of which are innervated by CN V3. Remember that the TMJ only receives sensory innervation, not motor.

Answers B, C, D, and E are incorrect. See above.

24. **The correct answer is B.** The maxillary 2nd premolar, with its oval occlusal outline, is typically much more symmetrical than the 1st premolar, which has a decidedly more asymmetric, hexagonal occlusal outline. In fact, the only part of the occlusal outline of the maxillary 1st premolar that appears symmetrical is the buccal surface, with its rounded, inverted V-shape due to the prominent buccal ridge. The remaining lingual three-fourths of the 1st premolar, on the other hand, appears bent to the mesial.

Answer A is incorrect. An asymmetric occlusal outline is a distinguishing feature of the maxillary 1st premolar that is not present on the 2nd premolars. The mesial outline appears straight or concave, and is bisected by a mesial marginal ridge groove not present on the distal. Moreover, the mesial marginal ridge is shorter buccolingually than the more convex distal marginal ridge such as the lingual three-fourths of the crown appear bent to the mesial. Lastly, the lingual cusp tip is positioned more to the mesial and the buccal cusp tip more to the distal, versus 2nd premolars which are more symmetrical overall.

Answer C is incorrect. With its prominent mesiolingual cusp and oblique ridge connecting to the distobuccal cusp, it's quite evident that the occlusal outline is asymmetric.

Answer D is incorrect. The mesiolingual groove that separates the mesial marginal ridge from the lingual cusp renders this tooth relatively asymmetric when viewed from the occlusal. There is more bulk on the distal half, and the mesial side of the crown appears pushed in on the mesiolingual corner.

Answer E is incorrect. The presence of a minor fifth cusp (distal cusp) on the buccal creates an asymmetric occlusal outline. Overall, there are 3 buccal cusps (MB, DB, distal) and 2 lingual cusps (ML, DL).

25. **The correct answer is C.** Only the DB cusps of mandibular molars and ML cusps of maxillary molars reside in their counterpart's central fossa in ideal intercuspation. The remaining supporting cusps reside in the mesial marginal ridge areas of their counterparts.

Answer A is incorrect. The buccal cusp of the 2nd premolar resides in the mesial triangular fossa of the maxillary 2nd premolar.

Answer B is incorrect. The MB cusp contacts the mesial marginal ridge of the maxillary 1st molar and the distal marginal ridge of the 2nd premolar.

Answer D is incorrect. The DB cusp of the mandibular 1st molar resides in the central fossa of the maxillary 1st molar; the distal cusp of the mandibular 1st molar opposes the distal fossa of the maxillary 1st molar.

Answer E is incorrect. The DB cusp contacts the central fossa of the maxillary 2nd (not the 1st) molar.

26. **The correct answer is D.** Both maxillary incisors and maxillary canines have a functional lingual surface. The maxillary canines are unique as the only cusped teeth with a functional lingual surface. The lingual surfaces, in part, help guide the mandible in excursive and protrusive movements.

Answers A, B, C, and E are incorrect. The incisofacial aspect of mandibular incisors and canines function against the lingual surfaces of maxillary incisors and canines, respectively. They aid in disarticulating the posterior teeth during protrusive and excursive movements (anterior guidance versus canine guidance).

27. **The correct answer is D.** Remember that a point angle is formed by the junction of 3 surfaces. All teeth have 4 point angles. In the example in question, tooth No. 11 is the maxillary left 1st premolar, which has mesio-facial-occlusal, disto-facial-occlusal, mesio-lingual-occlusal, and disto-lingual-occlusal point angles.

Answers A, B, C, and E are incorrect. See above.

28. **The correct answer is A.** The MB cusp tip of the mandibular 1st molar contacts the interproximal marginal ridges of the maxillary 1st molar and 2nd premolar.

Answers B, C, and D are incorrect. Remember: the DB cusps of mandibular molars and ML cusps of maxillary molars occlude in the central fossae of their opposing counterparts in ideal intercuspation.

29. **The correct answer is B.** The Universal Number System numbers the permanent dentition 1 through 32 starting with the maxillary right 3rd molar as No. 1 and the mandibular right 3rd molar as No. 32.

Answer A is incorrect. If the question had asked you to use the Federation Dentaire Internationale (FDI) system, then this answer choice would be correct. In the FDI numbering system, the 1st digit represents the quadrant and arch in which the tooth is found, as well as whether or not the tooth is primary or permanent; the 2nd number denotes the tooth position relative to the midline, from closest to farthest away.

Answer C is incorrect. The primary, not the permanent, canines are identified with the Universal Numbering System in this answer.

Recall that the primary teeth are identified by letter rather than number in this system, starting with the primary maxillary right 2nd molar as A, lettering across the maxillary arch to J (primary maxillary left 2nd molar), dropping down to K (primary mandibular left 2nd molar), and ending at T (mandibular right 2nd molar).

Answer D is incorrect. Tooth No. 12 identifies the permanent maxillary left 1st premolar using the Universal Numbering System; however, tooth No. 12 in the FDI system identifies the permanent maxillary right lateral incisor.

Answer E is incorrect. This choice identifies the primary canines according to the FDI System. In the primary dentition, the upper right (UR) quadrant is designated "5", the UL is "6", LL is "7", and LR is "8", and the canine is the 3rd ("3") tooth from the midline, numbering distally.

30. **The correct answer is A.** Mandibular lateral incisors, which are single rooted, frequently have two canals (up to 40%).

Answer B is incorrect. The mandibular canine is typically single rooted with one canal. Although a two-rooted (buccal and lingual), two-canal variant exists (4%-20%), the question asks for the tooth that has 2 canals within a single root.

Answer C is incorrect. The mandibular 2nd premolar will have a single canal within a single root 97.5% of the time.

Answer D is incorrect. Invariably, the maxillary central incisor has 1 root and 1 canal.

Answer E is incorrect. Like the maxillary central incisor, expect a single root with 1 canal in the maxillary canine.

31. **The correct answer is C.** The articular eminence is located just anterior and inferior to the articular (glenoid) fossa. The functional portion is on the posterior inferior aspect of articular eminence where the mandibular condyle (and intervening articular disc) rubs against during mandibular movement.

Answer A is incorrect. This portion of mandibular fossa does not articulate with any part of the condyle or disc.

Answer B is incorrect. Only when the condyle and disc slip past the articular eminence, can the anterior aspect of the articular eminence be engaged. However, this is a pathologic, painful condition resulting in an open-locked jaw.

Answer D is incorrect. The anterior three-fourths of the mandibular fossa, also called the articular (glenoid) fossa, is considered nonfunctioning because, when the teeth are in tight centric occlusion, there is no contact among the condylar head, disc, and this part of the temporal bone.

32. **The correct answer is D.** In general, the crowns of primary anterior teeth are wider mesiodistally compared to their incisocervical height. Hence, primary teeth appear "short and squat" relative to their permanent counterparts.

    Answers A, B, and C are incorrect. See above.

33. **The correct answer is B.** The large palatal root spans the entire width of the lingual surface, tapering from the CEJ to a blunted or rounded apex. No furcation can be detected on this surface. Remember: palatal roots are wider in the mesiodistal than in the buccopalatal direction.

    Answer A is incorrect. The buccal furcation entrance may be detected between the MB and DB roots an average of 4.2 mm from the CEJ.

    Answer C is incorrect. The mesial furcation entrance may be detected between the MB and palatal roots an average of 3.6 mm from the CEJ. This furcation is most easily accessed from the palatal given the relatively large breadth of the MB root buccolingually.

    Answer D is incorrect. The distal furcation entrance may be detected between the DB and palatal roots an average of 4.8 mm from the CEJ. Since the DB root is not as wide as

the MB root buccolingually, this furcation is centered buccolingually.

34. **The correct answer is E.** The proximal surfaces are the sides of a tooth generally next to an adjacent tooth. The mesial surface is closer to the midline, whereas the distal surface is farther from the midline.

    Answer A is incorrect. The facial surface rests against the lip or cheek.

    Answer B is incorrect. The lingual surface is nearest the tongue.

    Answer C is incorrect. The incisal surface is the cutting edge of an anterior tooth.

    Answer D is incorrect. The buccal surface is the same as the facial surface, but more commonly used for posterior teeth.

35. **The correct answer is A.** Just like an ideal 1st molar relationship, the MB cusp of the maxillary 2nd molar opposes the buccal groove of its counterpart, the mandibular 2nd molar.

    Answer B is incorrect. The DB cusp of the maxillary 2nd molar opposes this groove in ideal intercuspation.

    Answer C is incorrect. An MB groove does not exist on the mandibular 2nd molar which has only 2 buccal cusps and a single buccal groove (opposed by the MB cusp of the maxillary 2nd molar).

    Answer D is incorrect. This relationship could exist in a class II malocclusion in which the buccal groove of the mandibular 1st permanent molar is distal to the MB cusp of the maxillary 1st permanent molar. However, the question asks for the molar relationship in the ideal intercuspal position.

36. **The correct answer is D.** Longitudinal root depressions exist on both sides of the mandibular canine root, and when deep enough, clearly bifurcate the root labiolingually.

    Answers A, B, and C are incorrect. Maxillary central incisors, laterals incisors, and canines almost always have one canal and are invariably single rooted.

Answer E is incorrect. Careful! This tooth is not normally single rooted; rather, it typically has two roots and a bifurcation.

37. **The correct answer is C.** Typically the maxillary 2nd premolar has only one root, and the shallow mesial developmental groove that exists on the root does not extend onto the crown, as it does on the maxillary 1st premolar. The root depression on the distal is often deeper than on the mesial.

    Answer A is incorrect. The cross-section of the root at the cervix of the maxillary central incisor is somewhat triangular in shape and there are no prominent root depressions. The distal root surface is convex; and at the very most, the mesial surface may be flattened or have a very slight longitudinal depression.

    Answer B is incorrect. A shallow longitudinal root depression is often found in the middle of the mesial root surface on a maxillary lateral, but not on the distal.

    Answer D is incorrect. Longitudinal depressions are not common on the mesial root surface, but are frequent on the distal surface. In contrast, the mandibular 1st premolar has root depressions present on both sides, deeper on the distal. Sometimes these depressions may be quite deep and end in a buccolingual apical bifurcation.

38. **The correct answer is C.** A class III lever is comparable to "tweezers" in which the effort is between the fulcrum and the load. In the case of the mandible, the fulcrum is the TMJ. The effort is supplied by the masseter, medial pterygoid, and temporalis muscles which attach at locations anteroinferiorly to the TMJ (ie, coronoid process, inferior border of mandible, lateral and medial aspects of the ramus, etc), and the load is imparted upon incising food.

    Answer A is incorrect. A class I lever is a "see-saw" in which the fulcrum is between the effort and the load.

    Answer B is incorrect. A class II lever is a "wheelbarrel" in which the load is between the fulcrum and effort.

Answer D is incorrect. This is not a simple lever classification type.

39. **The correct answer is C.** Follow the eruption sequence of permanent teeth until you get to 12 permanent teeth: 4 first molars + 4 central incisors + 4 lateral incisors = 12 permanent teeth. Eight primary incisors were replaced by the 8 permanent incisors (20 − 8 = 12 primary teeth remaining). The child described above is at the end of the early mixed dentition phase and is most likely $8^1/_2$ years old.

    Answer A is incorrect. At most, only 8 permanent teeth (4 first molars and 4 [upper and lower] central incisors) would be expected at this age. All primary teeth except the lower and upper central incisors would remain (20 − 4 = 16 primary teeth).

    Answer B is incorrect. It is likely that the permanent maxillary lateral incisors would not have erupted by this age (usually around age 8-9).

    Answer D is incorrect. At the very least, one would expect the mandibular canine and/or the maxillary 1st premolar to have erupted at this age, yielding 14-16 permanent teeth and 8-10 primary teeth.

    Answer E is incorrect. By this age, no primary teeth should remain. The permanent 2nd molars likely would have erupted (at about age 11-13).

40. **The correct answer is B.** The FOA has the potential to make contact with the inner incline of guiding cusps.

    Answers A, C, D, and E are incorrect. The lingual inclines of the maxillary anterior teeth are guiding inclines.

41. **The correct answer is C.** All posterior teeth, when viewed from the occlusal, have proximal contacts that are slightly buccal to the middle 3rd.

    Answer A is incorrect. No tooth in an ideal dentition has a proximal contact that is lingual to the middle 3rd when viewed from the occlusal.

Answer B is incorrect. If the question asked you to evaluate the proximal contact from the buccal or lingual views, then this answer would have been correct.

Answer D is incorrect. The occlusocervical position of a proximal contact cannot be evaluated when viewing a tooth from the occlusal. Rather, one would have to look from the buccal or lingual views. Nonetheless, when viewed from the buccal or lingual, the contact described in the question above would be in the middle 3rd (as it is for all posterior teeth).

42. **The correct answer is D.** All anterior teeth (incisors and canines) in both the permanent and primary dentitions have a cingulum, or bulge, on the cervical 3rd of the lingual surface. 4 central incisors + 4 lateral incisors + 4 canines = 12 teeth.

    Answers A, B, C and E are incorrect. See above.

43. **The correct answer is D.** In posterior cross-bite situations, the supporting and guiding cusps are reversed. That is, the maxillary buccal and mandibular lingual cusps would be supporting, while the maxillary lingual and mandibular buccal cusps would function as guiding (nonsupporting) cusps.

    Answers A, B, and C are incorrect. In both working and nonworking movements of an ideal intercuspal relationship, the supporting cusps are the maxillary lingual cusps and the mandibular buccal cusps.

44. **The correct answer is D.** Mamelons are small enamel tubercles on the incisal edges of anterior teeth formed from the three facial developmental lobes. They normally wear away when the tooth comes into functional contact with its opposing tooth. In an anterior open bite situation, there is no contact between the maxillary and mandibular anterior teeth. The age of the patient suggests that if the teeth were in contact, the mamelons would have been worn away.

Answer A is incorrect. In a posterior cross-bite, the anterior teeth would most likely remain in function during excursive movements, and the mamelons would have worn away.

Answer B is incorrect. In an anterior cross-bite, the anterior teeth would most likely remain in function during excursive movements, and the mamelons would have worn away.

Answer C is incorrect. The presence of mamelons is considered normal only when they are present on newly erupted teeth that haven't yet contacted their antagonists.

Answer E in incorrect. Grinding of the teeth at night would lead to attrition, flattening the incisal edges or cusp tips, thus wearing mamelons away.

45. **The correct answer is C.** The superior fibers of the lateral pterygoid originate at the roof of the infratemporal fossa, and insert in the articular capsule and disc. Its inferior fibers originate on the lateral side of the lateral pterygoid plate, and insert on the anterior condylar neck. Functions of the lateral pterygoid muscle include mandibular protrusion, depression, and contralateral excursion.

    Answer A is incorrect. The superior fibers of the lateral pterygoid originate at the roof of the infratemporal fossa, and insert in the articular capsule and disc. Its inferior fibers originate on the lateral side of the lateral pterygoid plate, and insert on the anterior condylar neck. Functions of the lateral pterygoid muscle include mandibular protrusion, depression, and contralateral excursion.

    Answer B is incorrect. The medial pterygoid originates at the medial side of the lateral pterygoid plate, and inserts on the medial side of the mandibular angle. Functions of the medial pterygoid muscle include mandibular elevation, protrusion, and contralateral excursion.

    Answer D is incorrect. The temporalis originates at the lower temporal line, temporal fossa, and temporal fascia, and inserts on the medial coronoid process and anterior ramus. Functions of the temporalis muscle include mandibular elevation, retrusion, and ipsilateral excursion.

46. **The correct answer is C.** In general, mesial contact areas of anterior teeth are located in the incisal 3rd, and distal contact areas are positioned more cervically. The only exception is the mandibular central incisors. Due to the highly symmetric nature of the mandibular centrals about their root-axis line, both mesial and distal contacts exist at the same level (the incisal 3rd).

Answer A is incorrect. Although the mesial contact is in the incisal 3rd, the distal contact is located at the junction of the incisal and middle 3rds.

Answer B is incorrect. Both maxillary lateral incisor and maxillary canine have mesial contact areas at the junction of the incisal and middle 3rds, and distal contacts located in the middle 3rd.

Answer D is incorrect. Although both mesial and distal contacts are located in the incisal 3rd of the mandibular lateral incisor, the distal contact is located slightly more cervically than the mesial (ie, they are not at the same height occlusocervically).

Answer E is incorrect. With a mesial contact in the incisal 3rd and a distal contact area in the middle 3rd, the mandibular canine has the greatest difference in height between its proximal contacts than any other tooth.

47. **The correct answer is C.** All posterior teeth (premolars and molars) have a lingual HOC in the middle 3rd, and a buccal HOC in the cervical 3rd, when viewed from the proximal.

Answer A is incorrect. No tooth has a buccal or lingual HOC in the occlusal 3rd of its crown. Remember, though, that the *proximal* HOC is located in the occlusal 3rd in most anterior teeth.

Answer B is incorrect. The buccal HOC of posterior teeth is in the cervical 3rd.

Answer D is incorrect. All anterior teeth (incisors and canines) have a lingual HOC in the cervical 3rd (at the cingulum).

48. **The correct answer is C.** The maxillary 1st premolar has an oval-shaped pulp chamber, flattened mesiodistally (like an hourglass). Remember that it generally has two roots. Mandibular incisors also have pronounced hourglass-shaped pulp chambers. The mesiodistal constriction of the oval is less pronounced in the canines and other premolars.

Answer A is incorrect. Although no tooth has a perfectly round pulp chamber (at the level of the CEJ), the maxillary central incisor has the roundest.

Answer B is incorrect. The maxillary lateral incisor has an egg-shaped pulp chamber.

Answer D is incorrect. No teeth have an oval-shaped pulp chamber that is flattened buccolingually.

Answer E is incorrect. The mandibular 1st molar has a rectangular-shaped pulp chamber.

49. **The correct answer is D.** The buccal cusps of the mandibular posterior teeth are supporting cusps, which mean that they contact the opposing dentition in areas called centric stops. Not only do these buccal cusps contact their maxillary antagonists in the intercuspal position, they also can contact their maxillary antagonist during working and nonworking lateral movements. The lingual cusps of the mandibular molar, on the other hand, are nonsupporting, and do not rest in a central fossa or marginal ridge area of a maxillary antagonist. However, the buccal incline of the lingual cusps can serve as a guiding incline for the maxillary lingual supporting cusps during mandibular movement.

Answer A is incorrect. On the working side during lateral excursion, the outer aspect of the mandibular buccal (supporting) cusp can glide along the inner or lingual incline of the maxillary buccal guiding (nonsupporting) cusp.

Answer B is incorrect. On the nonworking side, the lingual supporting cusps of the maxillary teeth can be guided along the inner aspect of the buccal cusps.

Answer C is incorrect. The lingual aspect (nearest the cusp tip) of the lingual maxillary supporting cusps can be guided along the inner incline of the lingual mandibular cusps during excursive movements (working side).

50. **The correct answer is C.** Tooth J is the primary left maxillary 2nd molar, which is replaced by the maxillary left 2nd premolar, No. 13.

    Answer A is incorrect. The maxillary right permanent 3rd molar is not a succedaneous tooth.

    Answer B is incorrect. Tooth No. 10, the maxillary left lateral incisor, replaces the primary left lateral incisor, G.

    Answer D is incorrect. Tooth No. 20, the mandibular left 2nd premolar, replaces the primary left mandibular 2nd molar, K.

    Answer E is incorrect. Tooth No. 21, the mandibular left 1st premolar, replaces the primary left mandibular 1st molar, L.

51. **The correct answer is A.** Generally, teeth have a greater proximal cervical line curvature mesially than distally. The curvature is greatest on the incisors and decreases toward the last molar, in which there may be no curvature at all.

    Answer B is incorrect. The mesial and distal proximal cervical line contours of the anterior teeth have more curvature than on posterior teeth.

    Answer C is incorrect. The mesial surface generally has a greater curvature than the distal.

    Answer D is incorrect. The least amount of curvature (if any) can be expected on the distal aspects of posterior teeth.

52. **The correct answer is B.** This is one of the most obvious characteristics that distinguishes 1st, 2nd, and 3rd molars from each other. In

fact, the smaller DL cusp of the maxillary 2nd molar, compared to the wider, prominent DL cusp of 1st molars, gives the appearance of more taper (narrowing) from buccal to lingual on 2nd molars.

Answers A, C, and D are incorrect. See above.

53. **The correct answer is C.** Working interferences are premature contacts of posterior teeth on the working side during lateral excursive movement. Recall that nonworking interferences occur on the nonworking side. Protrusive interferences occur between the distal aspects of maxillary posterior teeth and mesial aspects of mandibular posterior teeth.

    Answers A, B, and D are incorrect. See above.

54. **The correct answer is E.** The narrow mandibular incisor opposes a relatively wide central incisor, and therefore only contacts this tooth. Also recall that the maxillary posteriors are positioned distally to their mandibular counterparts, so the maxillary 3rd molar can contact only the mandibular 3rd molar. The mandibular 3rd molar, on the other hand, can contact the distal marginal ridge of the maxillary 2nd molar, as well as the central fossa of the maxillary 3rd molar via its MB and DB cusps, respectively.

    Answer A is incorrect. The width of the maxillary central incisor allows it to be contacted by both the mandibular central and lateral incisors.

    Answer B is incorrect. The mandibular lateral incisor and canine can articulate with the maxillary lateral incisor.

55. **The correct answer is B.** An impacted tooth is one that does not erupt within the expected time. Although 3rd molars are the most commonly impacted teeth in the adult dentition, it is not represented as a choice. Maxillary canines are the 2nd most common impacted teeth, followed by mandibular premolars. Recall that maxillary canines are the last non-molar teeth to erupt in the maxillary arch,

emerging after all the incisors and premolars have erupted. Given their long path of eruption, and the possibility of insufficient arch space, they may become impacted, typically to the palatal.

Answer A is incorrect. Although impaction of these teeth is not unheard of, the frequency is less than that of 3rd molars and maxillary canines.

Answers C, D, and E are incorrect. See above.

56. **The correct answer is E.** The cervical ridge runs mesiodistally in the cervical 3rd of the buccal surface of all primary teeth (as well as all permanent molars). The cervical ridge is prominent in primary anterior teeth, and is best seen when viewed from the proximal. The cervical ridge of primary molars is most prominent on the mesial-facial aspect.

Answers A, B, C, and D are incorrect. See above.

57. **The correct answer is A.** The large ML cusp has one triangular ridge that meets the MB triangular ridge to form a transverse ridge. Its 2nd triangular ridge extends toward the DB cusp and forms part of the oblique ridge.

Answer B is incorrect. The DL cusp has only one, inconspicuous triangular ridge that abuts with the oblique ridge at a roughly perpendicular angle.

Answer C is incorrect. The cusp of Carabelli does not have a triangular ridge.

Answer D is incorrect. The MB cusp has only one triangular ridge (forming a transverse ridge with ML cusp)

Answer E is incorrect. The DB cusp has only one triangular ridge, which joins with one from the ML cusp to form part of the oblique ridge.

58. **The correct answer is B.** In an ideal occlusion, the cusp tip of the maxillary canine sits between the mandibular canine and 1st premolar.

Answer A is incorrect. The incisal edge of the maxillary lateral incisor opposes the mandibular lateral incisor and canine.

Answer C is incorrect. The cusp tip of the maxillary 1st premolar resides between the mandibular 1st and 2nd premolars.

Answer D is incorrect. The cusp tip of the maxillary 2nd premolar lies in the facial embrasure between the mandibular 2nd premolar and 1st molar.

59. **The correct answer is C.** Maxillary 2nd molars rarely have a cusp of Carabelli. It is also noteworthy to mention that the DL cusp is absent in more than one-third of these teeth!

Answers A, B, D, and E are incorrect. See above.

60. **The correct answer is B.** During the bud stage, epithelial cells from the primary epithelial band proliferate into the underlying ectomesenchyme.

Answer A is incorrect. The primary epithelial band forms at about week 6 in utero.

Answer C in incorrect. The cap stage, in which the bud splits into a caplike structure, and where the enamel organ, dental papilla, and dental follicle begin to take shape, starts at about week 9 in utero.

Answer D is incorrect. The bell stage of tooth development, in which cells differentiate in preparation for the formation of hard tissues, starts at about week 11 in utero.

Answer E is incorrect. At approximately 18 weeks in utero, the tooth enters the crown stage in which enamel and dentin are actively synthesized.

61. **The correct answer is B.** Remember the four determinants of occlusion: the right and left TMJs, the neuromusculature, and the teeth. As a dentist, the only one that can be directly controlled is the teeth (by restorations, orthodontics, and equilibration).

Answers A, C, D, and E are incorrect. See above.

Dental Anatomy and Occlusion

62. **The correct answer is C.** Maxillary 1st molars can present with a wide, prominent DL cusp that results in a wider lingual half than buccal half. Keep in mind, though, that all molar crowns in general will taper from buccal to lingual, even maxillary 1st molars. It's only those maxillary 1st molars with large distolingual cusps that serve as an exception to this rule.

    Answer A is incorrect. With three buccal cusps and two lingual cusps, the mandibular 1st molar clearly tapers to the lingual.

    Answer B is incorrect. Although this tooth exhibits less crown taper from buccal to lingual than the mandibular 1st molar, the lingual side is still narrower.

    Answer D is incorrect. Compared to maxillary 1st molars, 2nd molars taper more from the buccal to the lingual due to their smaller distolingual cusp.

63. **The correct answer is C.** The maxillary canines contact mandibular canines (anterior segment) and mandibular 1st premolars (posterior segment). Likewise, the mandibular 1st premolar contacts the opposing maxillary canine (anterior) and 1st premolar (posterior). Thus, 2 maxillary canines + 2 mandibular 1st premolars = 4 total teeth. Remember: Maxillary teeth contact their opposing counterpart and the tooth distal to it. Mandibular teeth contact their opposing counterpart and the tooth mesial to it.

    Answers A, B, D, and E are incorrect. See above.

64. **The correct answer is A.** Maxillary 1st molar: ML > MB > DB > DL > cusp of Carabelli.

    Answers B, C, and E are incorrect. See above.

    Answer D is incorrect. No distal cusp exists on this tooth. Instead, a distal cusp is found on the mandibular 1st molar.

65. **The correct answer is B.** The MB cusp is always the largest and longest cusp, occupying nearly two-thirds of the buccal surface.

Answer A is incorrect. It has a very well-developed mesial marginal ridge.

Answer C is incorrect. The occlusal table is much larger on the distal side of the transverse ridge compared to the mesial side.

Answer D is incorrect. The occlusal table has a small mesial triangular fossa and a large distal fossa, but no central fossa due to the presence of a prominent transverse ridge extending between the MB and ML cusps.

Answer E is incorrect. The mesiodistal length is greater than the buccolingual width.

66. **The correct answer is E.** Cervical enamel projections (CEPs) are apical extensions of enamel located at furcation entrances on *molar* teeth (28% mandibular, 17% maxillary). CEP size can vary greatly from small projections at the CEJ to larger extensions into the furcation proper. They are most commonly found on buccal surfaces. In decreasing order of incidence: Mandibular 2nd molars > Maxillary 2nd molars > Mandibular 1st molars > Maxillary 1st molars. Like enamel pearls, CEPs can predispose a tooth to periodontal attachment loss since connective tissue does not attach to the enamel (where cementum would normally be located).

Answers A, B, C, and D are incorrect. See above.

67. **The correct answer is E.** This arrangement is found in an ideal class I canine occlusion.

Answer A is incorrect. In an ideal occlusion, the maxillary canine occludes with the mandibular canine and 1st premolar.

Answer B is incorrect. This arrangement may be found in a class II occlusion.

Answer C is incorrect. In an ideal occlusion, the maxillary 1st premolar occludes with the mandibular 1st and 2nd premolars.

Answer D is incorrect. In an ideal occlusion, the maxillary lateral incisor articulates with the mandibular canine and lateral incisor.

68. **The correct answer is A.** The maxillary central incisor has the roundest pulp chamber (although it is not perfectly round). It is slightly egg shaped with the widest portion buccally.

Answer B is incorrect. The maxillary lateral incisor has an egg-shaped pulp chamber with the widest portion buccally.

Answer C is incorrect. The maxillary canine has an oval-shaped pulp chamber, flattened mesiodistally (hourglass shaped).

Answer D is incorrect. The mandibular central incisor has an oval-shaped pulp chamber, flattened mesiodistally (hourglass shaped).

Answer E is incorrect. The mandibular lateral incisor has an oval-shaped pulp chamber, flattened mesiodistally (hourglass shaped).

69. **The correct answer is E.** When the mandible is at rest, the teeth generally do not contact each other. In order for the teeth to touch in centric occlusion, muscles that elevate the mandible must contract. The major elevators of the mandible are the masseter, medial pterygoid, and temporalis muscles.

Answers A, B, C, and D are incorrect. See above.

70. **The correct answer is D.** The mandibular 1st molar has 3 grooves: buccal, distobuccal, and lingual. The 2nd molar has 2 grooves: buccal and lingual.

Answers A, B, C, and E are incorrect. See above.

71. **The correct answer is E.** Primate spaces are located mesial to the primary canines in the maxilla (between the lateral incisors and canines), and distal to primary canines in the mandible (between the primary canines and primary 1st molars). The primate spaces (so named because most subhuman primates have these spaces throughout life) are normally present from the time the primary teeth erupt, and close with the eruption of the permanent 1st molars (early mesial shift).

Answer A is incorrect. Spacing is normal throughout the anterior part of the primary dentition, but is most notable in the primate spaces mentioned above.

Answer B is incorrect. Careful! Primate spaces are found only in the primary dentition (premolars are only found in the permanent dentition).

Answer C is incorrect. The primate space is mesial to the primary canines in the maxilla.

Answer D is incorrect. This answer choice most closely resembles the definition of leeway space, which is the difference between the sum of the mesiodistal widths of the primary canine, 1st and 2nd molars, and the succeeding permanent canine, 1st and 2nd premolars.

72. **The correct answer is B.** Each maxillary molar has one transverse ridge, which runs between the MB and ML cusps.

Answers A, C, D, and E are incorrect. See above.

73. **The correct answer is C.** In centric relation, lateral excursions, and mandibular protrusion, the mandibular central incisor will only articulate with the lingual or incisal aspect of the maxillary central incisor.

Answer A is incorrect. The mandibular 1st molar articulates with the maxillary 1st molar and 2nd premolar in maximum intercuspation and during lateral excursive and protrusive movements.

Answer B is incorrect. The mandibular lateral incisor can articulate with the maxillary lateral and central incisors.

Answer D is incorrect. The maxillary lateral incisor can articulate with the mandibular lateral incisor and canine.

Answer E is incorrect. Both the mandibular central and lateral incisors can contact the lingual surface of the maxillary central incisor.

74. **The correct answer is C.** Each maxillary molar has 4 fossae: mesial triangular, central

(bounded by the mesial transverse ridge and the oblique ridge), distal triangular, and distal (within the distal oblique groove, and between the oblique ridge and DL cusp). Each mandibular molar has 3 fossae: mesial, central, and distal.

Answers A, B, and D are incorrect. See above.

75. **The correct answer is B.** Maxillary 1st molars are typically rhomboidal in shape when viewed from the occlusal, and often a prominent distolingual cusp exists such as the lingual portion of the occlusal surface is in fact wider than the buccal portion. Mandibular 1st molars have a somewhat trapezoidal occlusal outline, with the shortest side (mesiodistally) on the lingual. In general, maxillary 1st molars are wider on the lingual, and mandibular molars are wider on the buccal.

    Answers A, C, and D are incorrect. See above.

76. **The correct answer is B.** The spheno-mandibular ligament is a remnant of Meckel cartilage, originally derived from the 1st branchial arch. It extends from the spine of the sphenoid bone to the mandibular lingula.

    Answers A and D are incorrect. The temporomandibular ligament (also called the lateral ligament) does not directly derive from one of the branchial arches.

    Answer C is incorrect. The stylomandibular ligament is not originally derived from one of the branchial arches. It extends from the styloid process to the mandibular angle.

77. **The correct answer is A.** A mesiodens is a small supernumerary tooth that typically forms between maxillary central incisors. It has a cone-shaped crown with a short root, and may remain unerupted.

    Answer B is incorrect. A supernumerary 4th molar is often called a distodens, or distomolar.

    Answer C is incorrect. Dens-in-dente (tooth-within-a-tooth) is a deep surface invagination

of the crown or root that is lined by enamel. In order of decreasing frequency, the permanent teeth most commonly affected are the following: Lateral incisors > Central incisors > Premolars > Canines > Molars.

Answer D is incorrect. A supernumerary tooth situated lingually or buccally to a molar tooth is termed a paramolar.

Answer E is incorrect. A talon cusp (dens evaginatus of an anterior tooth) is a well-delineated additional cusp (not an additional tooth) that is located on the surface of an anterior tooth. These cusps occur most commonly on maxillary lateral and central incisors, projecting from the lingual surface, and forming a three-pronged pattern resembling an eagle's talon.

78. **The correct answer is A.** Recall that, in an ideal occlusion, the MB cusp of the maxillary 1st molar opposes the buccal groove of the mandibular 1st molar. As the mandible moves to laterally to the working side, the MB cusp tip slides through the buccal groove.

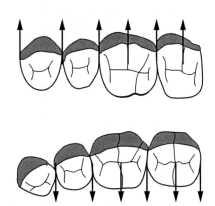

Answers B, C, D, and E are incorrect. See above.

79. **The correct answer is C.** Although they can resemble each other, there are enough differences that you will not confuse them. Even though the primary tooth has 4 cusps, the DB and DL cusps are inconspicuous, making the larger MB and ML cusps look like maxillary premolar cusps. The grooves form an "H" pattern, which is somewhat similar to a

maxillary premolar. However, a distinct notch can be seen separating the large MB cusp from the diminutive DB cusp when viewed from the buccal.

Answer A is incorrect. The primary mandibular 2nd molar most closely resembles the adult mandibular 1st molar.

Answer B is incorrect. No primary tooth resembles the permanent mandibular 2nd molar.

Answer D is incorrect. The primary maxillary 2nd molar most closely resembles the adult maxillary 1st molar.

Answer E is incorrect. No primary tooth resembles the permanent maxillary 2nd molar.

80. **The correct answer is E.** Remember that the buccal/facial HOC of all permanent teeth is located in the cervical 3rd of the crown. The lingual HOC of all anterior teeth is also located in the cervical 3rd (at the cingulum).

    Answer C is incorrect. The lingual HOC of all posterior teeth (premolars and molars) is located in the middle 3rd of the crown.

    Answers A, B, and D are incorrect. See above.

81. **The correct answer is C.** The 8 permanent teeth include 4 permanent central incisors and 4 permanent 1st molars. All of the primary teeth are present except the four primary central incisors (20 − 4 = 16), which exfoliated when the permanent central incisors erupted at approximately age 6-7.

    Answer A is incorrect. This is likely a 6-year-old child with permanent 1st molars that hasn't yet exfoliated any primary central incisors.

    Answer B is incorrect. This is an unlikely scenario in which the permanent mandibular central incisors erupted prior to the permanent 1st molars, for example.

    Answer D is incorrect. This is an older child (about 8 years old) with permanent 1st molars (4), central incisors (4), lateral incisors (4), and primary canines (4) and molars (8).

In a couple of years (ages 10-12), the child should expect the eruption of the permanent mandibular canine and permanent mandibular and maxillary premolars, followed by the permanent maxillary canine.

82. **The correct answer is A.** A class III canine relationship occurs when the maxillary canine occludes distal to the distal cusp ridge of the mandibular canine.

    Answer B is incorrect. This defines an Angle class I occlusion.

    Answer C is incorrect. This defines an Angle class II occlusion.

    Answer D is incorrect. See above.

83. **The correct answer is B.** For a mandibular 2nd molar, the order from largest to smallest cusps is ML > DL > MB > DB. The same is true for the four major cusps of the mandibular 1st molar; the minor 5th distal cusp is the smallest of all (ML > DL > MB > DB > D).

    Answers A, C, D, and E are incorrect. See above.

84. **The correct answer is B.** Remember that the articular disc (meniscus) is composed of dense fibrocartilage, providing the most protection against compression and tension.

    Answers A and C are incorrect. The disc is elliptical and biconcave, consisting of thick anterior and posterior bands. The central intermediate zone is much thinner and completely avascular.

    Answer D is incorrect. The superior insertion areas of the lateral pterygoid muscle are the anterior portion of the articular disc and capsule. Its inferior insertion site is the anterior condylar neck.

    Answer E is incorrect. Because it is biconcave, the disc has two reciprocal articular surfaces: one between its superior aspect and the glenoid fossa and articular eminence; the other between the inferior aspect and the condyle. The spaces between these structures create superior and anterior compartments.

85. **The correct answer is A.** A fourth canal may be found in the mesiobuccal (30% prevalence). The MB II canal is located about 1.8-mm lingual to the MB I canal.

   Answers B, C, and D are incorrect. See above.

86. **The correct answer is D.** Don't be troubled if you missed this question since it's unlikely that anyone would get it correct unless you like to memorize random tables. If anything, this question is an exercise in reading a question carefully and thinking about it before answering. Many may have chosen the maxillary canine, since it has the longest root in the permanent dentition. However, it also has a relatively long crown length (only the mandibular canine and maxillary central incisor are longer), making the root-to-crown ratio less than thought. The answer is a tooth with a relatively squat crown and reasonably long roots. The mandibular 1st molar fits this bill: its root-to-crown ratio is 1.87. The maxillary 1st molar is a close 2nd with a 1.78 root-to-crown ratio.

   Answer A is incorrect. Root-to-crown ratio = 1.24 (the lowest of all teeth).

   Answer B is incorrect. Root-to-crown ratio = 1.70.

   Answer C is incorrect. Root-to-crown ratio = 1.45.

87. **The correct answer is C.** The vertical dimension of rest (VDR) is the vertical dimension of the face with the mandible in the postural (rest) position. The vertical dimension of occlusion (VDO) is the vertical dimension of the face when the teeth contact in centric occlusion (CO). For a dentate patient, then, VDR > VDO. The difference between the two is the freeway space (FS), the distance the teeth are separated when the mandible is in the postural position (typically 1-3 mm). Thus, VDR = VDO + FS.

   Answers A, B, D, and E are incorrect. Another way to state it is VDO = VDR – FS.

88. **The correct answer is C.** Erosion is the loss of tooth structure from chemical means, such as acids. It typically affects smooth surfaces, including lingual and occlusal surfaces, resulting in cup-shaped defects. Erosion limited to the facial surfaces of the maxillary anterior teeth is often associated with dietary sources of acid (eg, sucking on lemons); whereas palatal erosion is often associated with regurgitation of gastric acids (eg, GERD or bulimia). The amalgam restoration extending above the remaining occlusal surface of No. 30 suggests that an erosive process is at play, rather than attrition.

   Answer A is incorrect. Abfraction is the loss of tooth structure resulting from abnormal occlusal stresses. As a tooth flexes under stress, enamel rods fracture just coronal to the CEJ, leading to V-shaped cervical-facial lesions.

   Answer B is incorrect. Attrition is wear caused by tooth-tooth contact. Large, flat, smooth, and shiny wear facets are the typical presentation.

   Answer D is incorrect. Abrasion is wear caused by abnormal mechanical means (often overzealous oral hygiene or other factitious habits). Toothbrush abrasion typically presents as a V-shaped notch in the cervical region, frequently in the canine-premolar area.

89. **The correct answer is A.** Both mandibular premolar and molar crowns tilt toward the lingual (relative to the root-axis line) when viewed from the proximal. Moreover, the cusp tips of the mandibular canines, as well as the incisal edges of the mandibular incisors, are typically positioned lingual to the root-axis line. The opposite is true of the maxillary incisors and canines, which typically have incisal edges/cusp tips that are positioned slightly labial to the root-axis line. Maxillary molar and premolar crowns do not tip noticeably in any direction, and appear aligned directly over the roots.

   Answers B, C, and D are incorrect. See above.

90. **The correct answer is B.** Just like its permanent counterpart, the primary maxillary

canine has the longest root of all deciduous teeth, averaging 13.5 mm in length.

Answer A is incorrect. The primary maxillary central incisor has one of the shorter roots, measuring about 10 mm in length. Remember that the mandibular central incisor has the shortest primary root (9 mm in length).

Answer C is incorrect. The primary maxillary 2nd molar roots average 11.7 mm in length.

Answer D is incorrect. The primary mandibular canine root averages 11.5 mm in length.

Answer E is incorrect. The primary mandibular 2nd molar roots average 11.3 mm in length.

91. **The correct answer is B.** The incisors begin to calcify around $4^{1}/_{2}$ months, the canine and 1st molar around 5 months, and the 2nd molar around 6 months in utero.

Answer A is incorrect. Although tooth development starts at about 6 weeks in utero, calcification has not yet started by 16 weeks.

Answer C is incorrect. At 6-8 months in utero, all of the primary teeth are in a stage of calcification, but none of the permanent teeth have begun to calcify.

Answer D is incorrect. The 1st permanent teeth start to calcify at birth.

Answer E is incorrect. By 16 weeks postpartum, all of the primary central and lateral incisors have completed calcification, but none have erupted.

92. **The correct answer is C.** The lateral pterygoids are the primary protractors of the mandible. It also functions in mandibular depression and contralateral excursion.

Answer A is incorrect. The masseter functions in mandibular elevation (primary function), retrusion, and ipsilateral excursion.

Answer B is incorrect. The medial pterygoid functions in mandibular elevation, protrusion, and contralateral excursion.

Answer D is incorrect. The temporalis functions in mandibular elevation, retrusion, ipsilateral excursion, and maintaining its rest position.

93. **The correct answer is D.** Centric relation (CR) is the intercuspation of the teeth when the condyles are located in the most anterior and superior position of the glenoid fossae. Because the condylar position of CR is anatomically defined, it is relatively easy for dentists to consistently position the mandible there when changing a patient's VDO.

Answers A and B are incorrect. These mandibular positions may present challenges in reproducibility because occlusal interferences or tooth-to-tooth contacts may shift the mandible slightly in another direction.

Answer C is incorrect. Any variation is muscle contractility can alter the postural position dimension.

94. **The correct answer is B.** Mandibular molars have a larger mesial root and a smaller distal root.

Answer A is incorrect. All anterior teeth, as well as mandibular premolars and maxillary 2nd premolars, are typically single rooted.

Answer C is incorrect. Maxillary molars have three roots.

Answer D is incorrect. No tooth typically has four roots.

Answer E in incorrect. Come on—are you kidding me!

95. **The correct answer is B.** The central groove of the mandibular 1st molar zigzags mesiodistally between the three buccal cusps and two lingual cusps.

Answer A is incorrect. The mandibular 2nd molar has buccal and lingual grooves that align to intersect with the central groove to form a "plus-sign" occlusal pattern.

Answers C and D are incorrect. Maxillary molars have an oblique ridge running diagonally across the occlusal surface separating the DL cusp from the other cusps, and creates a discontinuous occlusal pattern.

Answer E is incorrect. The maxillary 2nd premolar has a short central groove with multiple supplemental grooves.

96. **The correct answer is C.** Centric occlusion is typically the most superior position, but retruded contact (D) is the most posterior. In some individuals, however, RC may coincide with CO, but it is never more anterior than CO.

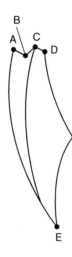

Answer A is incorrect. This is maximum protrusion.

Answer B is incorrect. This is the anterior edge-to-edge position.

Answer D is incorrect. This is retruded contact.

Answer E is incorrect. This is maximum opening.

97. **The correct answer is C.** Three facial lobes and one lingual lobe (cingulum) comprise the four developmental lobes of anterior teeth. Canines and most premolars also develop from four lobes (three of which comprise the facial aspect). The only exception is the three-cusped mandibular 2nd premolar which develops from five lobes (three facial lobes of the buccal cusp and two lobes for each of the two lingual cusps).

Answers A and B are incorrect. No tooth develops from only 2 or 3 lobes. Four lobes is the minimum.

Answer D is incorrect. As a general rule, each molar cusp forms from one lobe. Therefore, the mandibular 1st molar develops from five lobes (three buccal and two lingual).

Answer E is incorrect. A variant of the mandibular 1st molar bears six cusps (a 3rd lingual cusp called tuberculum intermedium), each of which is developed from a single lobe.

98. **The correct answer is C.** A TMJ dislocation occurs when the condyle translates anteriorly, in front of the articular eminence. To correct, you should apply firm downward pressure on the posterior mandible and ramus, with concomitant upward pressure on the chin. This motion, coupled with natural TMJ muscular guidance, will allow the condyle to move back over the articular eminence into its original position within the glenoid fossa. Reduction attempts should be made as soon as possible to prevent severe pain and/or muscle spasm.

Answers A, B, D, and E are incorrect. See above.

99. **The correct answer is A.** The most frequently congenitally missing teeth: 3rd molars > Maxillary laterals > Mandibular 2nd premolars.

Answers B, C, D, and E are incorrect. See above.

100. **The correct answer is D.** The 1st primary teeth to erupt are the mandibular central incisors at about 6 months of age; the last are the 2nd molars at about age 2. The 1st permanent teeth to erupt are the 1st molars around age 6. Therefore, the answer to this question must be between ages 2 and 6 years.

Answer A is incorrect. By age 1, all of the primary 1st molars may not have erupted.

Answer B is incorrect. By age $1\frac{1}{2}$, all of the primary canines may not have erupted.

Answer C is incorrect. By age 2, all of the primary 2nd molars may not have erupted.

Answer E is incorrect. By age $6\frac{1}{2}$, the permanent 1st molars have most likely erupted.

101. **The correct answer is C.** All mandibular incisors are quite small relative to the rest of the dentition, yet the mandibular central incisor is smaller in mesiodistal width, faciolingual width, crown height, and root length compared to the mandibular lateral incisor.

    Answers A, B, and D are incorrect. See above.

102. **The correct answer is B.** Remember that mandibular lingual cusps occlude in the embrasure between their maxillary counterpart and the tooth mesial to it. However, the DL cusps of mandibular molars articulate with the lingual grooves of their maxillary counterparts.

    Answers A and C are incorrect. The MB cusp of the mandibular 1st molar occludes with these two marginal ridges.

    Answer D is incorrect. The DB cusp of the mandibular 1st molar occludes here.

    Answer E is incorrect. The ML cusp of the mandibular 2nd molar articulates here.

103. **The correct answer is B.** A type II canal system has two separate canals leaving the pulp chamber, but later merge together just short of the apical foramen.

    Answer A is incorrect. A type I canal system has a single canal from the pulp chamber to the apical foramen.

    Answer C is incorrect. A type III canal system has two separate canals leaving the pulp chamber which exit the root at two separate apical foramina.

    Answer D is incorrect. A type IV canal system has a single canal leaving the pulp chamber, but dividing into two separate canals which exit the root at two separate apical foramina.

104. **The correct answer is E.** The primary mandibular 1st molar is unique in that it does not resemble any other primary or permanent tooth.

Answers A, B, C, and D are incorrect. See above.

105. **The correct answer is A.** As a general rule, the mesial cervical line curvature is always greater than the distal on any given tooth. Furthermore, the convexity of the curvature will diminish (or flatten more) as one moves away from the midline (posteriorly). The proximal cervical lines curve toward the incisal (convex), whereas the facial or lingual cervical lines curve apically.

    Answers B, C, D, and E are incorrect. See above.

106. **The correct answer is B.** The lingual cusps of the maxillary premolars tilt mesially and, therefore, will articulate with the distal triangular fossae of their mandibular premolar counterparts.

    Answers A, C, D, and E are incorrect. Nothing rests in these fossae in ideal intercuspation.

107. **The correct answer is A.** A fracture of the right condyle will result in the right lateral pterygoid to not function, allowing the left lateral pterygoid to act unopposed. The mandible will thus deviate to the right side as it is pulled forward and downward. Remember that the mandible deviates to the same side as the damaged condyle or articular disc.

    Answers B, C, D, and E are incorrect. See above.

108. **The correct answer is E.** The mandibular teeth are housed within the confines of the maxillary teeth, so it's not surprising that the incisal edges of the anterior teeth reside lingual to the root-axis line.

    Answer A is incorrect. The incisal edge of maxillary incisors is located slightly labial to the labiolingual center of the root.

    Answer C is incorrect. The incisal edge of the maxillary canine is located slightly labial to the labiolingual center of the root.

Dental Anatomy and Occlusion

109. **The correct answer is C.** Teeth that have a centered cingulum include the maxillary lateral incisor, maxillary canine, and mandibular central incisor. The cingula of the maxillary central incisor, mandibular lateral incisor, and mandibular canine are slightly distal of center.

   Answers A, B, D, and E are incorrect. See above.

110. **The correct answer is C.** Humans have a heterodont, diphyodont dentition. A heterodont dentition is one in which the teeth have a different morphologies; whereas a homodont dentition has the same morphology throughout. Diphyodonts have two sets of teeth throughout their lifetime (eg, in humans, deciduous and permanent dentitions). As their names suggest, monophyodonts have only one set of teeth, and polyphyodonts have multiple sets of teeth.

   Answers A, B, D, and E are incorrect. See above.

111. **The correct answer is B.** Permanent incisors typically erupt *lingual* to their primary counterparts. This is why the facial part of the remaining primary root will usually be longest and most securely attached to the gingiva.

   Answers A, C, and D are incorrect. See above.

112. **The correct answer is B.** The maxillary oblique ridge directly opposes the DB developmental groove of the mandibular molar counterpart.

   Answers A, C, D, and E are incorrect. See above.

113. **The correct answer is D.** Mandibular canines have a mesial crown contour that appears continuous with the root surface when viewed from the labial. This feature allows one to easily identify right from left mandibular canines, as well as maxillary from mandibular canines since the mesial aspect of maxillary canines bulges beyond the root outline.

Answers A, B, C, and E are incorrect. See above.

114. **The correct answer is E.** The primary mandibular 2nd molar has five cusps: MB, ML, D, DB, and DL. Unlike the permanent mandibular 1st molar, the distal cusp is typically just as large as the MB and DB cusps.

   Answer A is incorrect. All incisors and canines (both primary and permanent) have only one cusp.

   Answer B is incorrect. No primary tooth has two cusps.

   Answer C is incorrect. No primary tooth has three cusps.

   Answer D is incorrect. Both primary maxillary 1st and 2nd (although this may have a five-cusp variant) molars, and the mandibular 1st molar have four cusps.

115. **The correct answer is B.** The temporomandibular ligament (also called the lateral ligament) prevents the inferior and posterior displacement of the condyle. Its fibers run downward and posteriorly from the lateral aspect of the articular eminence to the posterior aspect of the condylar neck.

   Answer A is incorrect. The sphenomandibular ligament is an accessory ligament, which runs from the spine of the sphenoid bone to mandibular lingula.

   Answer C is incorrect. The stylomandibular ligament is an accessory ligament, which runs from the styloid process to the angle of the mandible.

   Answer D is incorrect. This ligament does not exist.

116. **The correct answer is E.** Posterior bite collapse occurs when posterior teeth are lost, leading to tipping and migration of adjacent teeth. This results in overclosure and bite deepening, which causes the mandibular anterior teeth to impinge on the palatal surfaces of the maxillary anterior teeth. Over time, these teeth often flare anteriorly, collapsing the face, and resulting in a decreased VDO.

Answer A is incorrect. As VDO decreases, the freeway space will increase.

Answer B is incorrect. The postural position will likely remain the same.

Answer C is incorrect. Because the rest position will be similar, so will the VDR.

Answer D is incorrect. The maximum opening length will likely remain the same.

117. **The correct answer is B.** The mandibular 2nd premolar has three occlusal schemes: (1) Y-shaped pattern (most common) has three cusps with a unique lingual groove and central fossa; (2) H-shaped pattern has a mesial fossa, central groove, and distal fossa; and (3) U-shaped pattern has a curved central groove.

    Answer A is incorrect. The mandibular 1st premolar has a prominent transverse ridge without a central groove, separating the mesial and distal fossae. It typically has a distinct mesiolingual developmental groove.

    Answer C is incorrect. The mandibular 1st molar has two transverse ridges, three fossae with pits, two buccal grooves, and a short lingual groove. The central groove zigzags, resembling a "+<" pattern.

    Answer D is incorrect. The mandibular 2nd molar has two transverse ridges, three fossae with pits, three secondary grooves, one buccal groove with a pit, and a short lingual groove. The central groove is relatively straight with a "+" pattern.

118. **The correct answer is C.** The maxillary canine has the longest root in the permanent dentition (averaging 17 mm).

    Answers A, B, and D are incorrect. See above.

    Answer E is incorrect. The mandibular canine has the longest mandibular root (averaging 16 mm).

119. **The correct answer is A.** Nonworking interferences occur between maxillary lingual cusps and mandibular buccal cusps (both are supporting cusps). This is the only time that these areas contact each other outside the intercuspal position.

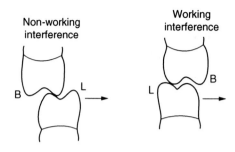

Answers B, C, and D are incorrect. See above.

120. **The correct answer is D.** The lingual canal is most frequently missed during root canal therapy when the access preparation does not extend far enough lingually. Remember that mandibular lateral incisors will frequently (up to 40%) have a second canal.

    Answers A, B, C, and E are incorrect. See above.

121. **The correct answer is A.** Ankylosis is the fusion of the tooth to the alveolar bone. Because of this, it is difficult to discern a PDL space (as there isn't one) on a radiograph. Teeth that are ankylosed need to be surgically removed.

    Answer B is incorrect. A taurodont is a molar with an elongated root trunk, which typically has an enlarged pulp chamber. Although not always the case, taurodontism generally occurs in patients with amelogenesis imperfecta, Down syndrome, or Klinefelter syndrome. These teeth would not pose a problem during routine extraction.

    Answer C is incorrect. A dilaceration is a bend in the root of a tooth. Depending on its location and severity, the dilacerations in the root tip may increase the difficulty of an extraction. If you are not careful, the root may fracture within the alveolar bone.

    Answer D is incorrect. Hypercementosis is the excess deposition of cementum along a root. Care must be taken during extraction to widen the alveolar bone enough to successfully deliver the tooth. If severe enough, these teeth may need to be surgically removed.

Dental Anatomy and Occlusion

Answer E is incorrect. Cervical enamel projections are apical extensions of enamel located at furcation entrances on molar teeth. Although they do not pose a problem during routine extraction, they may put a molar at a higher risk for periodontal attachment loss (connective tissue will not attach to enamel).

122. **The correct answer is D.** The apices of primary teeth are complete 1-2 years after eruption. Since the last tooth erupts by age 2, complete root formation will occur between ages 3 and 4.

   Answer A is incorrect. By age 1-1$\frac{1}{2}$, only the primary central incisors are close to being complete.

   Answer B is incorrect. By age 1$\frac{1}{2}$-2, all of the primary incisors have completed root formation.

   Answer C is incorrect. By age 2-3, the apices of the primary 1st molars are complete.

   Answer E is incorrect. The primary root apices will have been well-completed by this time.

123. **The correct answer is C.** The postural position is the physiologic rest position of the mandible, creating the vertical dimension of rest (VDR). It is a purely muscle-guided position since no teeth contact in this position. The resulting 1-3 mm space is called the freeway space (FS).

   Answer A is incorrect. Centric occlusion (CO) is a purely tooth-guided position, in which the maxillary and mandibular teeth contact each other in maximum intercuspation. This position creates the vertical dimension of occlusion (VDO).

   Answer B is incorrect. Centric relation (CR) is a purely ligament-guided position, in which the condyles are in the most anterior and superior position of the glenoid fossa.

   Answer D is incorrect. See above.

124. **The correct answer is E.** All other answer choices are features characteristic of the maxillary canine.

Answer A is incorrect. The cusp angle of the maxillary canine is sharper than the more blunt cusp of the mandibular canine.

Answer B is incorrect. The vertical labial ridge is less pronounced on the mandibular than maxillary canine.

Answer C is incorrect. Mandibular canines have more incisally positioned proximal contacts in comparison to their maxillary counterparts. Most notably, the mesial contact of the mandibular canine is in the incisal 3rd due to its nearly horizontal mesial cusp ridge. The distal contact area, as expected, is more cervical than the mesial, at the junction of the middle and incisal 3rds.

Answer D is incorrect. The cingulum on a mandibular canine is often slightly offset to the distal, whereas the maxillary canine has a centered, more prominent, cingulum.

125. **The correct answer is A.** Just like their permanent counterparts, primary maxillary molars have 3 roots, and primary mandibular molars have 2 roots.

   Answers B, C, and D are incorrect. See above.

126. **The correct answer is D.** Anterior guidance enables all of the posterior teeth to disarticulate during protrusive and excursive movements. The maximum disarticulation occurs when the anterior teeth are edge-to-edge. Cusp height is highly influenced by the overbite-overjet relationship of the incisors and canines. A deep overbite with minimal overjet is associated with long cusps. Conversely, a long overjet with minimal overbite is associated with short cusps.

   Answers A, B, and C are incorrect. See above.

127. **The correct answer is A.** Similar to premolars, mandibular incisors, and maxillary molars (but in contrast to maxillary central incisors and mandibular molars), canine crowns are wider faciolingually than mesiodistally. Another general class trait of

canines is that the mesial cusp ridge is shorter than the distal cusp ridge due to a more incisally located mesial proximal contact area.

Answers B, C, and D are incorrect. See above.

128. **The correct answer is D.** On mandibular canines, the distal cusp ridge bends distolingually, following the curvature of the lower arch.

    Answer A is incorrect. Mandibular centrals are highly symmetrical, and their incisal edges have no twist, running at right angles to a line bisecting the facial and lingual heights-of-contour when viewed from the incisal.

    Answer B is incorrect. Maxillary lateral incisor ridges run mesiodistally with no twist.

    Answer C is incorrect. Incisal ridges on maxillary canines are straighter mesiodistally than on mandibular canines when viewed from the incisal.

129. **The correct answer is A.** The condyles are in the terminal hinge position during centric relation (CR). This is the most superior and anterior position along the articular eminence of the glenoid fossa, with the articular disc located in between. Only condylar rotation can occur in this position.

    Answers B, C, D, and E are incorrect. See above.

130. **The correct answer is C.** Calcification of the 1st permanent tooth to erupt, the mandibular 1st molar, typically starts at birth. By age 3, all of the permanent 1st molars have completed calcification. The last permanent tooth to erupt, the 3rd molar, usually finishes calcification by age 16.

    Answer A is incorrect. Calcification of the 1st primary teeth begins at about 18 weeks in utero. The primary central and lateral incisors have completed calcification by 12 weeks postpartum. The last primary tooth to erupt, the 2nd molar, usually finishes calcification by age 1.

Answer B is incorrect. At 6-8 months in utero, all of the primary teeth are in a stage of calcification, but none of the permanent teeth have begun to calcify.

Answer D is incorrect. By 8-weeks postpartum, only the primary central incisors are close to completion.

Answer E is incorrect. By 16-weeks postpartum, all of the primary central and lateral incisors have completed calcification, but none have erupted.

131. **The correct answer is C.** You will typically find proclined maxillary laterals with concomitant retroclined maxillary centrals, creating a deeper overbite. Remember that any class II malocclusion is defined as one in which the MB cusp of the maxillary 1st molar articulates mesial to the MB groove of the mandibular 1st molar; and the maxillary canine occludes mesially to the distal surface of the mandibular canine.

    Answer A is incorrect. Class I occlusions are the most prevalent. A class I occlusion is defined as one in which the MB cusp of the maxillary 1st molar articulates with the MB groove of the mandibular 1st molar; and the maxillary canine occludes between the mandibular canine and 1st premolar.

    Answer B is incorrect. In a class II, division I malocclusion, all of the maxillary anterior teeth are flared, creating a large overjet. Molar and canine relationships are the same as for any other class II malocclusion.

    Answers D and E are incorrect. There are no separating divisions of class III malocclusions. It is defined as one in which the MB cusp of the maxillary 1st molar articulates distal to the MB groove of the mandibular 1st molar; and the maxillary canine occludes distally to the distal surface of the mandibular canine.

132. **The correct answer is B.** Maxillary lateral incisors have the most morphological variability of all incisors. They are often narrow, conical, and peg shaped. They are also the

most common tooth to exhibit both dens invaginatus (dens-in-dente) and dens evaginatus (talon cusp). Maxillary laterals have a 1%-2% incidence of being congenitally absent.

Answers A, C, and D are incorrect. See above.

133. **The correct answer is B.** The canines are the only teeth with a distinct vertical labial ridge. Shallow developmental depressions lie mesial and distal to the labial ridge, which runs incisocervically near the center of the crown in the middle and incisal 3rds. The labial ridge can be quite prominent on the maxillary canine.

Answer A is incorrect. Two shallow vertical developmental depressions separate the facial surface of incisors into three lobes (mesial, middle, and distal), but no labial ridge exists.

Answer C is incorrect. Although premolars have a similar looking ridge on the labial surface, it is called a buccal ridge, not a labial ridge.

Answer D is incorrect. No molar has a labial ridge.

134. **The correct answer is D.** The root trunks of primary teeth are generally shorter than those of permanent teeth.

Answer A is incorrect. Primary teeth are whiter than permanent teeth.

Answers B and C are incorrect. Primary crowns appear much more bulbous, largely because their CEJs are more constricted compared to permanent teeth.

Answer E is incorrect. Primary teeth have larger pulp chambers than permanent teeth.

135. **The correct answer is B.** On average the permanent maxillary arch is only about 2 mm longer than the mandibular arch (128 mm vs 126 mm). Primary dental arches are much rounder than the permanent arches.

Answers A, C, and D are incorrect. See above.

136. **The correct answer is E.** The lingual HOC of all anterior teeth (incisors and canines) is the cingulum, located in the cervical 3rd of the crown.

Answer C is incorrect. Remember that the lingual HOC of all posterior teeth (premolars and molars) is located in the middle 3rd of the crown.

Answers A, B, and D are incorrect. See above.

137. **The correct answer is B.** A Bennett shift occurs during lateral excursive movements in which the working-side condyle bodily moves laterally, toward the working side. The mean length of the movement ranges from 0.5 to 1 mm. An immediate or early Bennett shift occurs in about 86% of lateral excursive movements.

Answers A, C, D, and E are incorrect. See above.

138. **The correct answer is A.** The maxillary 1st premolar will typically have 2 canals. Remember that this tooth often has a bifurcated root.

Answer B is incorrect. The mandibular 1st premolar most commonly has one pulp canal.

Answer C is incorrect. The maxillary 2nd premolar most commonly has one pulp canal.

Answer D is incorrect. The mandibular 2nd premolar most commonly has one pulp canal.

139. **The correct answer is D.** The mandibular 2nd premolar has a shorter and blunter buccal cusp than lingual cusp.

Answer A, B, C, and E are incorrect. All other premolars have a longer buccal cusp than lingual cusp. On some occasions, though, the two cusps of the maxillary 2nd premolar may be the same length (but the lingual is never larger than the buccal).

140. **The correct answer is B.** Chronic thumb sucking generally causes openbite, protrusion

and proclination of maxillary incisors (and sometimes mandibular incisors), and often a high palatal vault. On occasion, posterior crossbite may occur due to lowered tongue posturing.

Answer A is incorrect. Chronic mouth breathing is associated with a narrow upper arch (but not a high palatal vault), anterior open bite (due to supereruption of posterior teeth), and posterior crossbite (due to low tongue posturing).

Answer C is incorrect. Chronic tongue thrusting typically results in anterior open bite with or without pronounced overjet.

Answer D is incorrect. Nocturnal bruxism is more likely to occur in adults, resulting in tooth attrition, wear facets, widened PDL spaces, and other dentoalveolar lesions associated with occlusal trauma.

141. **The correct answer is D.** The mandibular central incisor is the 1st succedaneous tooth to erupt. Remember that succedaneous teeth are permanent teeth that replace the position of primary teeth. Only permanent incisors, canines, and premolars are succedaneous teeth (molars are not).

Answers A, B, C, and E are incorrect. See above.

142. **The correct answer is D.** The occlusal table of the mandibular 2nd premolar is the most square shaped.

Answers A and B are incorrect. Both maxillary premolars have a relatively rectangular occlusal table shape.

Answer C is incorrect. The occlusal table of the mandibular 1st premolar is more oval shaped than the 1st premolar.

143. **The correct answer is C.** A microdont is a tooth that is smaller than normal. Remember that maxillary lateral incisors exhibit great variability, one form of which is narrow and peg shaped, smaller than the normal size.

Answer A is incorrect. A geminated incisor will look slightly larger than a normal incisor.

Answer B is incorrect. The cusp of Carabelli is a small part of a normally sized tooth.

Answer D is incorrect. A dens evaginatus (talon cusp) is a small part of a normally sized tooth.

Answer E is incorrect. A mulberry molar is larger than a normal molar.

144. **The correct answer is E.** Both maxillary and mandibular primary canines have defined cingula, and pentagonal-shaped crowns when viewed from the facial. Remember that the mesial cusp ridge is longer in the maxillary canine so that it will enable proper intercuspation with the mandibular canine, which has a longer distal cusp ridge. Their roots are the longest in each arch, with the maxillary canine having the longest root of all primary teeth. The cusp of the primary maxillary canine is longer and sharper than that of the permanent maxillary canine.

Answers A, B, C, and D are incorrect. See above.

145. **The correct answer is A.** On posterior teeth, the FOA of the supporting cusps will contact the inner inclines of the guiding cusps close to the central fossa line. For anterior teeth, the FOA of the mandibular incisors will contact the guiding inclines of the maxillary anterior teeth.

Answers B, C, and D are incorrect. See above.

146. **The correct answer is E.** The genioglossus is the main muscle that protrudes the tongue anteriorly. Its origin is on the genial tubercles. The inferior portion inserts on the hyoid bone; the superior portion inserts in the tongue. The genioglossus, like the hyoglossus and styloglossus, is innervated by the hypoglossal nerve (CN XII).

Answers A, B, C, and D are incorrect. See above.

147. **The correct answer is A.** The maxillary molar root trunk averages about 32% of the total root surface area. Thus, when periodontal

attachment loss occurs to the furcation entrances on this tooth, it has already lost about one-third of its support.

Answer B is incorrect. MB root surface area averages 25% of the total root surface area.

Answer C is incorrect. DB root surface area averages 19% of the total root surface area.

Answer D is incorrect. Palatal root surface area averages 24% of the total root surface area.

148. **The correct answer is D.** The cusp tip of the permanent mandibular canine lies lingual to the root-axis line, as it does on all lower anterior teeth. The cusp tip on the maxillary canine, on the other hand, may lie on or labial to this line.

Answer A is incorrect. A shorter mesial cusp ridge is common (characteristic) to all canines.

Answer B is incorrect. Since the mesial contact area on the mandibular canines resides in the incisal 3rd just below the mesioincisal angle, the mesial cusp ridge appears almost horizontal.

Answer C is incorrect. One of the most recognizable features of a mandibular canine is that its mesial crown outline is almost flat and nearly in line with the mesial side of the root (a feature not seen on maxillary canines). The distal side of the mandibular canine is convex in the incisal two-thirds, and concave in the cervical 3rd (when viewed from the labial), yielding noticeably more crown distal to the root-axis line than mesial to it.

149. **The correct answer is C.** The anterior edge-to-edge position is anterior to the CR and CO, but posterior to maximum protrusion. It is usually located near the center of the tracing mediolaterally.

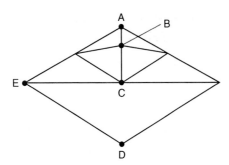

Answer A is incorrect. This is retruded contact.

Answer B is incorrect. This is centric occlusion.

Answer D is incorrect. This is maximum protrusion.

Answer E is incorrect. This is the maximum right lateral contact position.

150. **The correct answer is A.** The maxillary 1st premolar has a longer mesial buccal cusp ridge than distal cusp ridge.

Answers B, C, and D are incorrect. All other premolars have a longer buccal distal cusp ridge than mesial cusp ridge.

151. **The correct answer is D.** Teeth generally erupt into the oral cavity when their roots are $^1/_2$-$^2/_3$ developed.

Answers A, B, C, and E are incorrect. See above.

152. **The correct answer is B.** The glenoid (articular) fossa is a part of the temporal bone. Its anterior border is the articular eminence, while its posterior border is the tympanic portion of the temporal bone.

Answer A, C, D, and E are incorrect. See above.

153. **The correct answer is A.** The primary maxillary 1st molar is the smallest primary molar.

Answers B, C, and D are incorrect. See above.

154. **The correct answer is A.** An enamel pearl is a focal mass of enamel located near the furcations of molar teeth. They have about a 3% prevalence rate, and are most common on maxillary 2nd and 3rd molars. Their presence will predispose those tooth surfaces to periodontal attachment loss.

Answer B is incorrect. CEPs are much smaller and less protrusive than enamel pearls. Furthermore, they are more commonly found in buccal furcations and will not likely be seen on a radiograph.

Answer C is incorrect. A taurodont is a molar with an elongated root trunk, which typically has an enlarged pulp chamber.

Answer D is incorrect. A distodens is a super-numerary 4th molar, often found distal to the 3rd molar.

Answer E is incorrect. Hypercementosis is an excessive deposition of cementum on the root of a tooth.

155. **The correct answer is E.** Remember that unworn cusps and grooves are curved, not straight and flat. Thus, the occlusal contacts between opposing teeth will be on many points, or very small contact areas. It is only in pathologic occlusions (such as bruxism) that one will find area-to-area contacts.

   Answers A, B, C, and D are incorrect. See above.

156. **The correct answer is E.** Maxillary central and lateral incisors, canines, and 2nd premolars commonly only have one canal. Mandibular central incisors, canines, and 1st and 2nd premolars will typically have one canal.

   Answers A, B, C, and D are incorrect. See above.

157. **The correct answer is C.** Because maxillary molars have three roots, they will have three furcations. Keep in mind, however, that maxillary 2nd and especially 3rd molars may have fused roots, preventing them from having true trifurcations, only deep depressions.

   Answer A is incorrect. The maxillary 1st premolar often has a bifurcation as it typically has two roots.

   Answer B is incorrect. The mandibular 1st premolar generally has a single root, and thus has no furcation. It does, though, have developmental depressions along the length of the proximal surfaces of the root.

Answer D is incorrect. The maxillary 1st molar has two roots, and thus has a bifurcation.

158. **The correct answer is C.** Tooth No. 18 is the mandibular left 2nd molar. All mandibular posterior crowns have a rhomboidal shape when viewed from the proximal. Recall that their crowns are tilted lingually from the cervix.

   Answer A is incorrect. No tooth is square shaped when viewed from the proximal.

   Answer B is incorrect. No tooth is rectangular shaped when viewed from the proximal.

   Answer D is incorrect. All maxillary posterior crowns have a rhomboidal shape when viewed from the proximal. Unlike mandibular posterior crowns, which tilt lingually from the cervix, maxillary crowns are aligned directly over the roots from the proximal view.

   Answer E is incorrect. No tooth is oval shaped when viewed from the proximal.

159. **The correct answer is C.** Both the masseter and the medial pterygoid muscles form a sling around the mandible. The superficial fibers of the masseter insert onto the lateral angle of the mandible; the medial pterygoid inserts onto the medial angle of the mandible. Both function in elevation of the mandible.

   Answers A, B, D, and E are incorrect. See above.

160. **The correct answer is D.** During working-side movements, the FOAs of the supporting cusps slide slightly mesially or distally (depending on the arch) over the inner aspects of opposing guiding cusps, such that cusp tips pass between opposing cusp tips.

   Answers A, B, C, and E are incorrect. See above.

161. **The correct answer is D.** The maxillary canine has its mesial contact in the junction of the incisal and middle 3rds, and the distal contact in the middle 3rd.

Answer B is incorrect. The mandibular canine has its mesial contact in the incisal 3rd, and the distal contact in the middle 3rd.

Answers A, C, and E are incorrect: See above.

162. **The correct answer is A.** In general, girls' teeth erupt prior to boys' teeth.

Answers B, C, D, and E are incorrect. See above.

163. **The correct answer is B.** The maxillary 1st molar has a rectangular occlusal surface, with the shortest sides being the mesial and distal marginal ridges. Recall that the mandibular 2nd molar also has a rectangular occlusal surface.

Answer A is incorrect. No primary tooth has a square-shaped occlusal surface.

Answer C is incorrect. No primary tooth has a trapezoidal-shaped occlusal surface.

Answer D is incorrect. The maxillary 2nd molar and the mandibular 1st molar have a rhomboidal occlusal surface.

164. **The correct answer is B.** Hypodontia is a type of partial anodontia in which there is a congenital absence of one or a few teeth. Patients with congenitally missing maxillary lateral incisors also have hypodontia. It is generally not associated with systemic disease or developmental disturbances.

Answer A is incorrect. Anodontia is the complete congenital absence of teeth. This is generally caused by developmental abnormalities such as ectodermal dysplasia. Do not confuse anodontia with edentulism. All patients with anodontia are edentulous, but not all edentulous patients have anodontia (they may have lost their teeth to periodontitis, caries, trauma, etc).

Answer C is incorrect. Oligodontia is a type of partial anodontia in which there is a congenital absence of most, but not all teeth. This is typically caused by developmental abnormalities such as ectodermal dysplasia.

Answer D is incorrect. Hyperdontia is the presence of one or more supernumerary teeth in addition to a complete dentition.

Answer E is incorrect. Metadontia is not a dental term.

165. **The correct answer is D.** In nonworking movement, mandibular supporting cusps move mesiolingually to their opposing maxillary supporting cusps. Contrarily, maxillary supporting cusps move distobuccally to their opposing mandibular supporting cusps. Remember that the potential for nonworking contacts (interferences) occur on maxillary distal inner inclines and mandibular mesial inner inclines of supporting cusps.

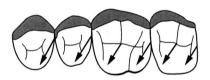

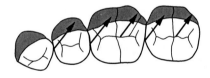

Answers A, B, and C are incorrect. See above.

166. **The correct answer is C.** Tooth No. 29 is the mandibular right 2nd premolar. Both of its mesial and distal contact areas are in the middle 3rd of the crown. In fact the mesial and distal contact points of all maxillary and mandibular posterior teeth (premolars and molars) are located in the middle 3rd.

Answers A, B, D, and E are incorrect. See above.

167. **The correct answer is A.** The vertical muscle fibers run inferior superiorly. When contracted, they will broaden and flatten the tongue.

Answer B is incorrect. The muscle fibers that run mediolaterally comprise the transverse muscle. See answer D below.

Answer C is incorrect. The longitudinal muscle fibers run anteroposteriorly. They will shorten the length of the tongue, curling it upward or downward (depending on which fibers contract).

Answer D is incorrect. The transverse fibers arise from the median fibrous septum and run laterally. When contracted, they will narrow and elongate the tongue.

168. **The correct answer is B.** Anterior teeth have 6 line angles: mesiofacial, distofacial, mesiolingual, distolingual, incisofacial, and incisolingual. Posterior teeth have 8 line angles: mesiobuccal, distobuccal, mesiolingual, distolingual, occlusobuccal, occlusolingual, mesioocclusal, and distoocclusal.

    Answers A, C, and D are incorrect. See above.

169. **The correct answer is A.** A centric slide is more common than not, with some studies showing a prevalence of up to 78%-90%. If present, it is usually about 1 mm long.

    Answers B, C, and D are incorrect. See above.

170. **The correct answer is A.** The maxillary central incisor has the greatest horizontal axial inclination when viewed in the sagittal plane. However, when viewed in the facial plane, it is almost vertical within the alveolar bone.

    Answers B, C, D, and E are incorrect. See above.

171. **The correct answer is C.** Between the two lingual cusps found on this tooth, the ML cusp is by far the largest, obscuring the view of the smaller DL cusp when viewed from the mesial.

    Answers A, B, and D are incorrect. See above.

172. **The correct answer is A.** The maxillary canine is typically the last primary tooth to exfoliate, usually around age 12. It is replaced by the permanent maxillary canine. The mixed dentition ends with the exfoliation of the last primary tooth. Remember that mandibular teeth generally erupt prior to maxillary teeth.

    Answers B, C, D, and E are incorrect. See above.

173. **The correct answer is A.** Remember that the size of a pulp horn is directly proportional to the size of its cusp. Since the MB cusp is the largest cusp in a mandibular 1st molar, it also has the largest pulp horn. Contrarily, the distal cusp has the smallest pulp horn.

    Answers B, C, D, and E are incorrect. See above.

174. **The correct answer is C.** In the anterior edge-to-edge position, the incisal edges of the anterior teeth occlude, providing the greatest VDO while teeth are still in contact.

    Answers A and B are incorrect. Although there may be an increase in VDO during centric relation and maximum protrusion positions, the change is not as large as it is in the anterior edge-to-edge position.

    Answers D and E are incorrect. Be careful! Clearly, the maximum opening position will create the greatest vertical dimension of the face, but it (and the rest position) does not involve any tooth-to-tooth contacts. Thus, these positions do not contribute to VDO.

175. **The correct answer is D.** Remember that abrasion is the loss of tooth structure due to abnormal mechanical means. Long-time pipe smokers often have a notch in one or two of their incisors, where they typically hold the pipe stem.

    Answer A is incorrect. GERD is associated with dental erosion.

    Answer B is incorrect. Nocturnal bruxism is associated with dental attrition.

    Answer C is incorrect. Occlusal trauma is associated with dental attrition.

    Answer E is incorrect. Cigarette smoking is not associated with dental wear.

176. **The correct answer is A.** When you swallow, the normal position of the teeth is in centric occlusion, and the tongue moves superiorly to touch the palate.

    Answers B, C, D, and E are incorrect. Remember that during a tongue-thrust habit, the tongue is positioned anteriorly between the incisors.

177. **The correct answer is D.** Recall that the primary maxillary 2nd molar most closely resembles the permanent maxillary 1st molar, which will appear next to each other in the arch until the primary molar exfoliates to make room for the 2nd premolar.

    Answers A, B, and C are incorrect. See above.

178. **The correct answer is B.** The most concave lingual surface is on the maxillary lateral incisor. Compared to mandibular incisors, the maxillary lateral has a more prominent cingulum, which creates more of a lingual depression.

    Answers A, C, and D are incorrect. See above.

179. **The correct answer is A.** The *working side* is defined as the side to which the mandible moves in an excursive movement. In an excursive movement of the mandible to the patient's right side, both the maxillary and mandibular right side are the "working side," while the left side is considered the "nonworking side."

    Answers B, C, D, and E are incorrect. If the mandible moves to the right, then the right mandibular (and maxillary) teeth are on the working side. The left mandibular (and maxillary) teeth are on the nonworking side.

180. **The correct answer is A.** The maxillary central has the widest crown of all anterior teeth. In order of decreasing size, the widths of maxillary anterior teeth: central incisor > canine > lateral incisor. For mandibular anterior teeth: canine > lateral incisor > central incisor.

Answers B, C, D, and E are incorrect. See above.

181. **The correct answer is A.** The maxillary 1st premolar is usually the largest permanent premolar.

    Answer C is incorrect. The smallest permanent premolar is typically the mandibular 1st premolar.

    Answers B and D are incorrect. See above.

182. **The correct answer is C.** During right-side excursive movement, the left medial pterygoid contracts, not the right. Remember that both of the pterygoid muscles function in contralateral excursive movement, while the masseter and temporalis provide ipsilateral excursive movements.

    Answers A, B, D, and E are incorrect. All of these muscles contribute to right-side mandibular excursive movement.

183. **The correct answer is C.** By age $9\frac{1}{2}$, this child will likely have 24 teeth (10 primary and 14 permanent): 4 primary 1st molars, 4 primary 2nd molars, 2 primary canines (maxillary), 4 permanent centrals, 4 permanent laterals, and 2 permanent canines (mandibular). Remember that the permanent mandibular canines erupt around age 9-10, while the permanent maxillary canines erupt at age 11-12.

    Answer A is incorrect. This configuration would likely be found in an $8\frac{1}{2}$-9 year old.

    Answer B is incorrect. This configuration of 22 teeth would not likely exist. Remember that the mixed dentition has 24 teeth by age 7 (when all of the permanent 1st molars have erupted).

    Answer D is incorrect. This configuration might be found in a 10 years old, but would not last for a long time as more primary teeth would quickly be replaced by their permanent counterparts.

    Answer E is incorrect. This configuration might be found in a 10-11 years old, but would not last for a long time as more primary teeth would quickly be replaced by their permanent counterparts.

184. **The correct answer is B.** Remember that this tracing represents the extreme borders of mandibular movement in the sagittal plane. Normal chewing and mastication generally occurs somewhere in between all of the borders.

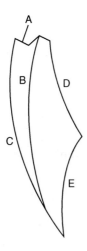

Answer A is incorrect. This represents protrusive movement from the anterior edge-to-edge position to maximum protrusion.

Answer C is incorrect. This represents the most anterior position of the mandible as the jaw opens from maximum protrusion to maximum opening.

Answer D is incorrect. This represents the rotation of the condyles in their most posterior position as the jaw opens.

Answer E is incorrect. This represents the translational movement of the condyles in their most posterior position as the mandible reaches maximum opening.

185. **The correct answer is D.** The contact point between adjacent teeth has three important functions: (1) it stabilizes the position of teeth within the dental arches (preventing drift), (2) it prevents food impaction, which can contribute to decay and periodontal disease, and (3) it protects the interdental papillae by shunting food toward the buccal and lingual "spillways."

Answers A, B, C, and E are incorrect. See above.

186. **The correct answer is C.** When looking down on a mandibular central incisor from the occlusal, its faciolingual length is greater than its mesiodistal length. It has a 1.2 faciolingual-to-mesiodistal length ratio. Recall that this is the smallest tooth in all dimensions.

Answers A and B are incorrect. The maxillary central and lateral incisors are the only anterior teeth with a larger mesiodistal length than faciolingual length (when viewed from the occlusal). The maxillary central faciolingual-to-mesiodistal length ratio is 0.82. The maxillary lateral faciolingual-to-mesiodistal length ratio is 0.92.

Answer D is incorrect. Faciolingual-to-mesiodistal length ratio is 1.18.

Answer E is incorrect. Faciolingual-to-mesiodistal length ratio is 1.07.

187. **The correct answer is A.** Both the primary maxillary canine and permanent mandibular 1st premolar are unique in that the mesial contact is more cervical than the distal.

Answers B, C, D, and E are incorrect. All other teeth, primary or permanent, have the distal contact area located more cervically than on the mesial.

188. **The correct answer is D.** Mandibular lingual cusps are guiding cusps, so they will not articulate with central fossae or marginal ridges. Instead, they always oppose lingual embrasure spaces. The only exception to this rule is the DL cusp of mandibular molars, which occlude with their maxillary counterpart's lingual groove.

Answers A, B, C, and E are incorrect. See above.

189. **The correct answer is E.** The oblique ridge is present on all maxillary molars and connects

the DB and ML cusps. It separates the MB and DL cusps.

Answers A, B, C, and D are incorrect. See above.

190. **The correct answer is B.** Although the synovial membrane secretes synovial fluid which lubricates the TMJ, it lines the internal surface of the articular capsule, not the articular disc (meniscus). Unlike most synovial joints, the articular surfaces of the glenoid fossa and mandibular condyle are lined by a layer of dense fibrous tissue (there is still debate as to whether this is true fibrocartilage). Recall that the articular disc itself is composed of avascular fibrocartilage.

Answers A, C, and D are incorrect. See above.

191. **The correct answer is D.** All teeth have four embrasures per contact area: buccal, lingual, occlusal, and cervical. In health, the gingival papilla fills the cervical embrasure. The other three embrasures aid in deflecting food away from the contact area.

Answers A, B, C, and E are incorrect. See above.

192. **The correct answer is B.** The mandibular 1st molar may have a 4th canal in the distal root (25% prevalence). In general, two canals are located in the mesial root (MB and ML), and one canal is found in the distal root.

Answer A is incorrect. See above.

Answer C is incorrect. The mandibular 1st molar does not have a buccal root.

Answer D is incorrect. The mandibular 1st molar does not have a lingual root.

193. **The correct answer is E.** Remember that a distal cusp does not usually exist on a mandibular 2nd molar. If the question had asked about the distal cusp on the mandibular 1st molar, however, it occludes with the distal triangular fossa of the maxillary 1st molar.

Answers A, B, C, and D are incorrect. See above.

194. **The correct answer is B.** The labial ridge is only found on canines. It runs incisocervically in the center of the facial crown surface, and is more prominent on the maxillary canine.

Answer A is incorrect. All molars have cervical ridges which run mesiodistally in the cervical 3rd of the buccal crown surface. Recall that all primary teeth also have prominent cervical ridges.

Answer C is incorrect. Only maxillary molars have an oblique ridge which runs from the DB cusp to the ML cusp on the occlusal surface.

Answer D is incorrect. All teeth have mesial and distal marginal ridges.

Answer E is incorrect. Only premolars have a buccal cusp ridge which runs occlusocervically in the center of the buccal crown surface. It is more prominent on 1st premolars.

195. **The correct answer is A.** The mandibular 1st molar has two roots, mesial and distal. The mesial root is very broad buccolingually, with a blunt and wide apex, hiding the distal root.

Answer B is incorrect. From the distal view, the less broad (buccolingually) and shorter distal root, as well as the larger mesial root, can be seen.

Answers C and D are incorrect. Both the mesial and distal roots can be seen from the buccal as well as the lingual. Often, the roots of the mandibular 1st molar are described as looking like "plier handles."

Answer E is incorrect. Most likely, no roots can be seen from the occlusal given the large occlusal outline of the 5-cusped mandibular 1st molar.

196. **The correct answer is C.** The root of the mandibular 2nd premolar is typically closest to the mental foramen. Remember, though, that this anatomy is variable: the mental foramen can be closer to the apices of 1st premolars and even canines at times. A periapical radiograph will help you evaluate the local anatomy.

Answers A, B, D, and E are incorrect. See above.

197. **The correct answer is B.** A tooth closer to the anterior of the mandible will be more influenced by anterior guidance, and less by the TMJs. Conversely, a posterior tooth will be less influenced by anterior guidance, and more by the TMJs. In an ideal occlusion, it is the anterior teeth that provide the guidance in lateral excursive and protrusive movements. The anterior teeth (especially the canines) will allow the posterior teeth to disarticulate preventing interferences and frictional wear.

Answers A, C, and D are incorrect. See above.

198. **The correct answer is A.** Remember that the most superior position is typically maximum intercuspation during centric occlusion (see also the sagittal view of Posselt envelope of motion).

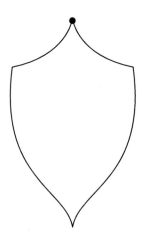

Answer B is incorrect. The retruded contact point would likely be located just below the centric occlusion point (assuming that they do not coincide).

Answer C is incorrect. The anterior edge-to-edge position would likely be located just below the centric occlusion point.

Answer D is incorrect. The maximum opening position is the most inferior point on the tracing.

Answer E is incorrect. The maximum protrusive point will not be seen from the frontal view (only the sagittal and horizontal).

199. **The correct answer is C.** The vast majority of joints are synovial, meaning that they are lined by a synovial membrane, which secretes synovial fluid (a lubricant). A diarthrosis is a fully moveable joint, such as the shoulder, hip, and TMJ.

Answer A is incorrect. A synarthrosis is an immoveable joint, such as the cranial sutures.

Answer B is incorrect. An amphiarthrosis is a slightly moveable joint, such as the symphysis pubis.

Answer D is incorrect. See above.

200. **The correct answer is D.** The roots of the maxillary 1st molar are generally closest to the maxillary sinus floor, and are most commonly pushed through if fractured during extraction. Depending on the individual's anatomy, though, any tooth in close proximity to the maxillary sinus is at risk for penetration through the floor.

Answers A, B, C, and E are incorrect. See above.

CPSIA information can be obtained
at www.ICGtesting.com
Printed in the USA
FFOW01n0010280215
11420FF